"For all his continuing sociological interest, Dreitzel's concerns are those of a practicing therapist who is interested in expanding the context and role of psychotherapy… This feature is what makes *Human Interaction and Emotional Awareness in Gestalt Therapy* a particularly valuable book for Gestalt therapists – for any psychotherapist, in fact. No matter how far ranging his social interests take him, Dreitzel brings them to bear on the character and quality of individual life, particularly in his detailed examination from the standpoint of Gestalt therapy of the ways in which we suffer physical and psychological pain and how we distinctively make use of our emotions in episodes of contact."

— **Michael Vincent Miller**, PhD,
from the foreword

"Based on his unique sociological expertise and longstanding psychotherapeutic practice, H. Peter Dreitzel presents a provocative call for simultaneous interpersonal and ecological awareness. Human individuality requires respectful co-evolution with the others and with nature, both being inseparable environments. This highly recommended book provides a close look at the complexity of our continuous 'contacts'. It encourages emotionally charged, self-reflexive and collective actions, which may maturely face, tackle and change the many man-made social and climate destructions, which are already endangering our survival as a species."

— **Professor Helmut Milz**, MD,
psychosomatic medicine; psychotherapist;
former in-house consultant, WHO; author,
The Self-Sensing Human

Human Interaction and Emotional Awareness in Gestalt Therapy

In *Human Interaction and Emotional Awareness in Gestalt Therapy* H. Peter Dreitzel explores a model of the contacting processes between human beings and their environments and presents a phenomenological exploration of the emotions guiding such contacts.

The book makes an important contribution to our understanding of the role of psychotherapy in the modern world, especially in the context of change and crisis. Dreitzel sets out a new perspective of how we interact with each other, how we frame our encounters and differentiate them from one another, how we give them meaning, and how they are related to our needs and wants. This is followed by a unique phenomenological exploration of the emotions guiding such contacts, the first time the world of human feelings has been explored in depth and systematically analysed in Gestalt thought. These innovative explorations are framed first by a discussion of the historical development of Western conventions regarding everyday behaviour, and secondly by an examination of perspectives on climate change. Dreitzel analyses the mental and emotional states of potential clients as they are affected by these global processes and the book also includes an epilogue which evaluates how to work with climate anxiety.

Dreitzel's conception of social change, with Gestalt therapy at its core, is relevant to all aspects of humanistic psychology. It elevates empathy, emotional development and the prevention of suffering at all levels of society, filling important gaps in Gestalt therapy theory and expanding it into exciting new territory. *Human Interaction and Emotional Awareness in Gestalt Therapy* also contains an insightful foreword by Michael Vincent Miller, PhD, and will be essential reading for Gestalt therapists, other professionals with an interest in Gestalt approaches and readers interested in social interaction, climate change and the role of psychotherapy in a changing world.

H. Peter Dreitzel, PhD, was born in Berlin in 1935. Between 1960 and 1970 he was Assistant Professor of Sociology, University of Göttingen, Germany, and Graduate Faculty of the New School for Social Research, New York, USA. From 1970 to 2000 he was Professor of Sociology at the Free University of Berlin, and in 1973 he co-founded the Berlin Gestalt Center (GZB). Inspired by his most significant teacher in the field, Isadore From, Dreitzel has been a Gestalt therapy practitioner since 1975 and has been a trainer and supervisor at several training institutes in Germany and other European countries. He is the author of several publications on Gestalt therapy.

Gestalt Therapy Book Series

The Istituto di Gestalt series of Gestalt therapy books emerges from the ground of a growing interest in theory, research and clinical practice in the Gestalt community. The members of the Scientific and Editorial Boards have been committed for many years to the process of supporting research and publications in our field: through this series we want to offer our colleagues internationally the richness of the current trends in Gestalt therapy theory and practice, underpinned by research. The goal of this series is to develop the original principles in hermeneutic terms: to articulate a relational perspective, namely a phenomenological, aesthetic, field-oriented approach to psychotherapy. It is also intended to help professions and to support a solid development and dialogue of Gestalt therapy with other psychotherapeutic methods.

The series includes original books specifically created for it, as well as translations of volumes originally published in other languages. We hope that our editorial effort will support the growth of the Gestalt therapy community; a dialogue with other modalities and disciplines; and new developments in research, clinics and other fields where Gestalt therapy theory can be applied (e.g., organizations, education, political and social critique and movements).

We would like to dedicate this Gestalt Therapy Book Series to all our masters and colleagues who have sown fruitful seeds in our minds and hearts.

Istituto di Gestalt
www.gestaltitaly.com HCC Italy

Series Editor **Margherita Spagnuolo Lobb**

Gestalt Therapy Book Series

Series editor: Margherita Spagnuolo Lobb

Enchantment and Gestalt Therapy
Partners in a Communal Awakening
Erving Polster

Sexuality, Masculinity and Culture in Gestalt Therapy
An Autoethnographic Approach
Adam Kincel

Human interaction and Emotional Awareness in Gestalt Therapy
Exploring the Phenomenology of Contacting and Feeling
Peter H. Dreitzel

For more information on the titles in this series, please visit:
www.routledge.com/Gestalt-Therapy/book-series/GESTHE and
www.gestaltitaly.com

Human Interaction and Emotional Awareness in Gestalt Therapy

Exploring the Phenomenology of Contacting and Feeling

H. Peter Dreitzel

Foreword by Michael Vincent Miller

Routledge
Taylor & Francis Group
LONDON AND NEW YORK

First published 2021
by Routledge
2 Park Square, Milton Park, Abingdon, Oxon OX14 4RN

and by Routledge
605 Third Avenue, New York, NY 10158

Routledge is an imprint of the Taylor & Francis Group, an informa business

Translated by Michaela von Britzke

Hans Peter Dreitzel, Reflexive Sinnlichkeit I. - Emotionales Gewahrsein - Die Mensch-Umweltbeziehung aus gestalttherapeutischer Sicht © EHP-Verlag Andreas Kohlhage, Bergisch Gladbach 2007

British Library Cataloguing in Publication Data
A catalogue record for this book is available from the British Library

Library of Congress Cataloging-in-Publication Data
A catalog record has been requested for this book

ISBN: 978-0-367-64456-7 (hbk)
ISBN: 978-0-367-64454-3 (pbk)
ISBN: 978-1-003-12458-0 (ebk)

Typeset in Times New Roman
by Taylor & Francis Books

Dedicated
to Isadore From, † 27. Juni 1994
whose critique would have excited me,
and to Jonathan Franzen who forestalled me.

Contents

Acknowledgements

I am much obliged to my translator *Michaela von Britzke* for her generous offer to translate this book without any financial compensation but purely out of interest and in recognition of our long-standing friendship. Also, I am extremely grateful for the help and collaboration of *Judy Newton-Davies* for taking a close look at the language and style of the translation and offering many useful suggestions. I am greatly indebted to these two in ways which words cannot express: without their interested and engaged work this book would not be able to reach the worldwide community of English reading Gestalt- and other psychotherapists – as I hope it will.

I also thank Claudia Thelen-Ellison for helping with the proof reading!

I am grateful for Margherita Spagnuolo Lobb's courageous decision to publish this book in her *Gestalt Therapy Book Series* which was the precondition for reaching the English reading world.

My special thanks go to Jeff Allison and his editorial help with the final version of this book!

My wife Brigitte Stelzer-Dreitzel was my intellectual and dialogical companion during all stages of the development of this book in addition to giving me constant emotional support when I was close to giving up this endeavour! Without her this book would never have reached its final stage; nothing can express my gratitude.

Translator's note

Michaela von Britzke

Ever since I received "Reflexive Sinnlichkeit" in 1992, when the original was hot off the press, I wanted to share it with my English therapists' community and friends because it achieves something very rare: an integration of all aspects of human being-in-the-world, including the place of therapy in an endangered natural world.

There were some particular difficulties arising from the adaptations which the original text underwent in the course of its re-publication in 2007 and the current updating for this translation for the English-speaking Gestalt community. Emotion theory, presented by Peter at its cutting edge in 1992, has since made more general progress, forcing very specific attention to the differential translation of "Gefuehl" - whether to choose "feeling" or "emotion". In the text there are occasional rubs when everyday language would require "feeling" as in guilt feeling, while academic usage demands "emotion". The reader will have to use his/her own language sense here. Occasionally there are sentences which I would have liked to translate into common parlance, such as "I want to get in touch with my feelings", but for the sake of the central concept of the "contacting process", I chose the word "contact" as in the original text. Also in some cases I have added the German word in brackets, especially when I had to deal with typically German philosophical notions. More technical issues concerned translations of citations: except for core texts like Perls, Hefferline, and Goodman, *Gestalt Therapy* (Perls et al., 1951), Perls, *Ego, Hunger and Aggression* (Perls, 1992) and publications by Manfred Clynes, most quotations are translated into English with their official English/American sources provided when available, and translations from German sources cited when there was no English equivalent. This procedure was endorsed as commonly used by English academic publishers.

I could not have achieved this translation without the security of knowing that the text would be critically reviewed by Judy Newton-Davies, a native English speaker and language friend, who made many suggestions to facilitate the transition from "German academic writing" into a text which for her efforts reads far more smoothly than I could have achieved on my own. The task was to retain the academic clarity and complexity of Peter's text, saving the English language reader from too many German academic nested period constructions while retaining Peter's immediacy, his ability to converse directly with the reader, which makes this book so special.

Even though there is always something lost in translation, the text is now available for a wider circle of readers and practitioners. For me this was a work of bridging the languages which help me word my worlds – a great joy and privilege and a path of integration in another way.

Foreword

Michael Vincent Miller

More than forty years ago, when I was still a graduate student, I came across an anthology on the sociology of marriage and the family edited by Hans Peter Dreitzel. I don't recall very much all these years later about the content of the book's multitude of articles by a multitude of authors. What I do remember are the themes that Dreitzel set forth in his introduction to the volume. His introduction was an early statement concerned with how a series of liberation movements – the women's liberation movement (as it was called in those days); the gay rights movements shortly after the 1969 Stonewall Riots in Greenwich Village; and a cultural broadening of sexual freedom in general – were changing the nature of sex roles as well as the battle of the sexes in marriage and other intimate social structures. He also lamented the degree to which sociology at the time was lagging well behind cultural change in understanding how these movements were altering conventional family values. The point of his anthology, in my recollection at least, was to bring together articles that moved the social sciences forward through analysing these important changes that were taking places in western societies.

During that culturally volatile period, Peter Dreitzel was a Professor of Sociology at the University of Berlin. His anthology was one of the more interesting books on the changing dynamics in intimate relations and family life that I had read up to that point. It had a lasting effect on me, even many years later, when I was trying to think through how romantic love brought a couple together and then often turned longing for romance into a conflict-making and anxiety-producing pressure because the roles of husband and wife at the time left them too depleted and alienated to continue to be lovers. Dreitzel's anthology thus took its place as part of the supportive background for my writing, some twenty-three years later, my own first book on unhappy couples *Intimate Terrorism*, a book about the relations among love, anxiety, and power in marriages and other long-term intimate relationships.

When I first became familiar with this book of Dreitzel's from the early 1970s, I was already well on my way to becoming a Gestalt therapist. I was working on my PhD, had been in workshops with Frederick Perls, collaborated with Paul Goodman on writing for the socialist journal *Dissent*, trained with the Polsters before they left Cleveland, and before long, co-founded the Boston Gestalt Institute, with Laura Perls as a visiting faculty member. Imagine my intrigued surprise, then, when I began to see Peter Dreitzel's name appearing as a participant in the growing world of international Gestalt therapy. In the interim between the 1970s and the early 1990s, he had become a Gestalt therapist and a writer about Gestalt therapy. But he had never given up his concern with exploring how we inhabit the social and cultural environments. His interests, however, had now become differently focused; he began to examine the ways in which those environments impact the meaning and practice of psychotherapy.

In this respect Dreitzel reminds me somewhat of Paul Goodman, who also combined social thought and cultural criticism with Gestalt therapy and made such significant contributions to all three fields. Dreitzel is aware of his resemblance in interests, at least, to Goodman; he announces in his own introductory section that he is "taking up the political and sociological impetus of Paul Goodman" because he is "convinced that beyond our clients' individual family backgrounds we urgently need to consider in what kind of society our lives and therapies are embedded." Goodman, however, practiced psychotherapy only briefly and wrote about it at length only in his collaboration with Frederick Perls, resulting in the classic work, *Gestalt Therapy: Excitement and Growth in the Human Personality* by Perls, Hefferline and Goodman (PHG). Goodman's attention after that always went toward interpreting and hoping to influence the possibilities for radical social and political change, although many ideas from Gestalt therapy still made appearances, mostly indirectly or in cameo roles, in his outlook. That is where Dreitzel differs most with Goodman. For all his continuing sociological interest, Dreitzel's concerns are those of a practicing therapist who is interested in expanding the context and role of psychotherapy.

This feature is what makes *Human Interaction and Emotional Awareness* a particularly valuable book for Gestalt therapists — for any psychotherapist, in fact. No matter how far ranging his social interests take him, Dreitzel brings them to bear on the character and quality of individual life, particularly in his detailed examination from the standpoint of Gestalt therapy of the ways in which we suffer physical and psychological pain and how we distinctively make use of our emotions in episodes of contact. Dreitzel's work is especially fresh and original in his handling of these two themes. Neither in PHG nor in subsequent theorizing in Gestalt therapy have these issues been explored with such detail and specificity; if anything, they have largely been absent from much of the writing about the theory of Gestalt therapy. Yet they are surely an essential part of what any worthwhile psychotherapy is about.

Perhaps the most original expansion beyond well-travelled territory in the book is the author's phenomenological treatment of suffering and pain. This is a theme that PHG does not take up, nor have subsequent writers to the degree that Dreitzel does, as though the subject is beyond general theory. And in a way that may be true — a real understanding of pain and suffering seems to call for poetry, tragic theater, or opera. Dreitzel does manage to come close: He addresses the mystery and inevitability of pain by refusing to reduce its nearly inexplicable presence to cause and effect. Instead he shows us how its giving way to a shout or scream as well as its ultimate falling silent all lead us to understandings beyond words. From there he suggests that the very nature of intense pain is exactly where the self paradoxically is most unified in the sense of being a body, not of having one. That is an intriguing extension of Aristotle's famous remark that when you have a sore thumb, the self is in the thumb.

The other equally valuable section of the book comprises Dreitzel's extensively detailed exploration of emotions as aspects of contact-making. And it is where we get the clearest sense of his perspective as a working therapist. He points out that there has been relatively little study of the role of specific emotions and how they function in contact, which is true from the standpoint of theory, although some Gestalt therapists, of course, do look in depth at specific emotions in their clinical studies and case histories. But there are only intimations of how our emotional life functions in general in PHG; as Dreitzel himself puts it, "Perls & Goodman's text does little more than hint at the role of emotions."

From the standpoint of making contact, the best way to think of the emotions is that they yield a particular kind of information about how it is in one's world, and they mobilize one to act. They have an "evaluative, relational character regarding the environment," as Dreitzel points out, and they "have a powerful action orientation" as well. He makes a useful distinction between moods and emotions. Moods, he says, "are lacking emotions' cognitive function" in that "moods disregard the specifics of a particular contacting situation, don't take account of the special new quality of phenomena."

That seems to me exactly right as a view of the emotions in terms of their important role in orienting and mobilizing one through the process of making contact. You can see this basic function of emotions clearly in anger or sadness, for example. Anger informs you that there is a frustrating or threatening obstacle in your path, and at the same time mobilizes you to remove it. Sadness tells you that something important to you in your world is missing. If the sadness is about the recent past, it moves you to grieve the loss, which is a necessary healing process. If it is about the future, something you are hoping or longing for, then sadness may motivate you to seek it.

Dreitzel feels strongly, as I do, that the fullest understanding of matters such as suffering and emotion inevitably takes us, even as therapists, beyond clinical diagnostic categories. He writes, "More useful than any system of personality diagnostics is the grand world of literature with its rich and nuanced descriptions of human character. We can learn more from Balzac's novels, his *Comedie Humaine*, or Tolstoy's *War and Peace* than from psychological teachings about character." The late Isadore From, a superb therapist and very important teacher of Gestalt therapists, who was my supervisor for many years and a mentor of Dreitzel's as well, once told me that he learned more about how to do therapy from Henry James and Proust than he did from Freud.

At the same time, no serious psychotherapy would underestimate the damage that our emotional life has suffered in the process of growing up. The tendency ever since Freud entered the picture has been to put the blame on the family. Dreitzel takes this into account, but he sees the causes as well as the kinds of damage across a broader spectrum. Speaking as an experienced psychotherapist, he points how common it is for people to enter therapy because they can't feel much of anything. The way clients-to-be announce this as their major symptom when they first come to the office is to tell the therapist that they hope psychotherapy will get them in touch with their feelings. But Dreitzel feels that this way of experiencing their dilemma already indicates the heart of the problem. It shows how fragmented we have become, as though our senses of ourselves and our feelings are two different realms of existence that are disconnected from each other. It points to the degree to which not just our families but our very culture has led us into a non-existent, delusional conception of ourselves as divided, dualistic beings.

Since looking at a client's family background does not go far enough for Dreitzel, he argues that psychotherapists need to take a reading on a client's cultural background, because the behaviour and values of peer groups and the impact of the media has at least equalled, if not surpassed, the influence of the family in shaping our subjectivity. Of course, when you dig down even a little, you see varieties of repetition and compulsion in choice of partners and erotic behaviour that still reflect the powerful influence of mom and dad, both in how they were with the client as a child and how with each other. Those effects won't disappear unless or until we give up the nuclear family. But it certainly appears to be the case, in what I have been observing, that nowadays the peer group and social media, as well as TV, have a shaping influence that is equal to that of the family for models of love, sex, and intimacy.

Given the way that Dreitzel looks at its functioning, one could say that culture is his notion of field, though he doesn't use that term for it. From his viewpoint, culture is what we as individuals are embedded in, often without awareness, and it shapes our subjectivity, our feelings, and our contact with others. And over time and across our groupings according to social class, religious belief, ethnic or racial background, and countercultural behaviour, we gradually reshape culture. In other words, we are in culture, and it is in us. That begins to be a field-like understanding, although it lacks the immediacy of emergence from contact that characterizes field theory. Dreitzel feels strongly that in both our working and loving, contemporary culture tends to deaden our senses and emotions, replacing them with inflation of the self and calculated, strategic behaviour in place of authentic spontaneity and emotional expressiveness. One result is that we cannot give our full attention or ourselves fully to another person. A second outcome is that in place of creative aggression, primitive emotions, such as hate and violence, come to the surface in explosive ways. Nowadays even our impulses have been taken over and socialized by the state so that they can be put to use in undermining democratic institutions and creating and sustaining totalitarian structures. In addition, technology and digital media have greatly accelerated and broadened the ability of authorities to socialize people, which would mean, in the language of Gestalt therapy, that society and government can use these instruments to deliver and enforce the introjections it wants us to live by.

Dreitzel does not simply make these points; he goes on to spell them out, finding them everywhere in contemporary culture, ranging from technology to sports, from the state having taken over the job of socializing citizens to the related rise of a right-wing populism, from the benefits of sexual freedom to the spread of pornography, which he feels promotes the opposite of liberation because it distances sex from the body and therefore promotes the opposite of liberation. These are the forces, according to Dreitzel, that give the individual personality its current style and dictate its modes of feeling and behaviour, ones that he feels are wounding to our humanity along a variety of dimensions. What can be done? Dreitzel envisions Gestalt therapy as a kind of therapy of the collective, a culture-changing therapy that has the potential to initiate a healing process in a sick culture and society.

Despite being a German thinker, he is once again here reminiscent of Paul Goodman, who was a cultural radical in an American tradition that began with Emerson and Thoreau. The cultural radicals of the 19th and 20th centuries in the United States did not see much hope for social change within the political process or in politics at all; they felt government was too remote from the actualities of human life. So they evolved ideas about how to alter the consciousness of the populace through the channels of culture – art, literature, philosophy, social and cultural criticism. With Dreitzel, we have to add psychotherapy to that list of consciousness-changers. (The appearance of this tradition in Dreitzel's work may not be so surprising. He tells us he was strongly influenced by George Herbert Mead, who developed a sociology and social philosophy in the spirit of John Dewey, as did Paul Goodman.)

* * *

Dreitzel, however, is not primarily a field theorist, nor a relational one according to current understandings of these two positions. These two theoretical frameworks have pretty thoroughly overtaken modernist and postmodern Gestalt thinking. His point of departure is the theory of contact as it was put forward in PHG, which was that book's most far-reaching innovative contribution to psychology and the practice of psychotherapy. He goes on to expand this outlook in a number of fruitful ways. The view of contact in PHG is still basically an individual psychology, although it lends itself to relational and field viewpoints, as a number of contemporary writers have shown. But in itself it differs significantly from recent attempts to go beyond one-person psychologies, such as one finds in the writings of Jean-Marie Robine and Gianni Francesetti.

Insofar as Dreitzel turns toward the notion of a field specific to Gestalt therapy, he sticks to the organism/environment field put forward in PHG, a concept which mixes together in a single phrase the influence of German holistic philosophy and psychology on Perls and the influence of the American pragmatist, interactional philosophy of John Dewey on Paul Goodman. And although some Gestalt therapists treat this notion as phenomenology, it certainly is not that in any straightforward sense. The organism/environment field is more a biological than phenomenological idea; it resides more fully within the natural attitude than it does in the phenomenological standpoint. This is typical of PHG, a book that throughout is an eclectic mixture of influences: holistic and organic thinking, 19th and early 20th century American pragmatism, psychoanalytic ego psychology, a Reichian interpretation of the body as carrier of health or pathology, some ideas about the relationship of art to experience, derived mainly from Otto Rank and John Dewey, European existentialism, and phenomenological ideas that seem mostly created from scratch. That is a lot to absorb and integrate!

I am not suggesting that this mixture detracts from the ingenuity and inventiveness that characterizes PHG. In this book all these diverse ideas converge to create a radically new and promising direction for psychotherapy. But its eclecticism also gave rise to forking paths in Gestalt therapy, such that the future is still being worked out. PHG is Dreitzel's own point of departure throughout most of his book. He gives a great deal of space to elaborating fundamental ideas in PHG, as well as taking them into new territory.

And that very approach is one of the things that makes Dreitzel's text especially useful. The theoretical breakthrough that PHG brought to psychology and to psychotherapy practice nearly seventy years ago is in danger of getting buried by the variety of field theories and other approaches that have dominated recent theoretical thinking about Gestalt therapy. It is an exciting and important body of thought that is still unsettled and a little confusing. Nearly everyone who is writing about the field seems to have his or her own idea about what the field is or is not: There is the interactive field of Kurt Lewin, which derives from the action-at-a distance models of electromagnetic waves and quantum mechanics; there is the field of consciousness from some schools of phenomenology; there is the shift among certain Gestalt therapy-oriented thinkers from psychopathology as the internal life of individuals to a notion of psychopathological fields. By taking us back to the writing of Perls and Goodman and bringing it forward in a new, refreshing way, Dreitzel's book helps reground Gestalt therapy in its own actual origins. No matter how far away from its origins into new possibilities Gestalt therapy theory goes, it can no more dismiss Perls and Goodman than self psychology and intersubjective psychoanalysis can dismiss Freud.

Dreitzel also makes it clear at the outset that his book is not a discussion of clinical work per se. It doesn't tell one how to do Gestalt therapy. It has no case histories. Although he does give a summary of the Gestalt therapy approach to clients, he announces that his main intention is to present his "analysis of the contacting process," but not so much toward clinical aims as toward a "focus on the pathogenic elements in our civilization." Contemporary civilization, he argues, due to the political and economic misuses of its advances in technology, and driven by fear, greed and a craving for power, has led us down a primrose path into personal and collective darkness.

In Dreitzel's view, nearly everything that we imagine has liberated us, ranging from freedom to explore, experiment with, and choose our sexual predilections all the way to our very political institutions and governments espousing democratic freedoms, from modes of transportation and technology that provide us with the run of the globe to digital developments that open up communication from nearly anywhere to anywhere so that we don't have to leave our screen – all these developments are shot through with power and manipulation of who we think we are. And most of this goes by unrecognized by us. In this line of thinking, he is a successor to Wilhelm Reich and Herbert Marcuse, a radical Freudian and a radical post-Freudian, one a psychoanalyst, the other a philosopher, both of whom he cites. He cites them, because like him, they saw much of what claims to emancipate us as a subtle manipulation to keep us under control.

Part of what is happening here is that these new freedoms are going into strengthening the individualistic self, which leads people to imagine that they are free spirits when in actuality they are becoming more alienated. There is nothing wrong with the freedoms in themselves; the problem is that they are being deployed by the state to get us to imagine that our freedom lies in being separated from each other. Therefore, in Dreitzel's view, we need a therapy, both at the personal and the collective levels, that makes contact at least as important as the sense of self. He recognizes that even those who rebelled against psychoanalysis, including Perls, still placed too much importance on the self: "Wilhelm Reich, Alfred Adler, Fredrick Perls, the rebels of the psychoanalytic movement, shifted emphasis to the subject. And all other emancipatory movements position themselves in a similar way. Yet this is one-sided, unbalanced." Individualism gives rise to an ideal of self that is too rigid, narrow, fixed in place. The need now is not to concentrate on strengthening the individualistic self, as most western psychology and psychotherapy has emphasized, but to enable us to become so absorbed in the experience of contact with others and the world that self is no longer our primary concern. A more fluid sense of self would be required, a sense of self able to flow into the ever-new and changing circumstances that Dreitzel calls the "contacting process."

The very forces that are promoting rationalization of social processes, of work and technology, of rational thought and planning, according to Dreitzel, along with more and more centralization of these forces in the state are succeeding in alienating us from our emotions and spontaneity. But without access to our feelings and spontaneity, how can we practice creative adjustment to new and changing circumstances?

To treat this widespread social sickness, Gestalt therapy as a psychotherapy can help on the personal, individual level. But like Paul Goodman, Dreitzel's final target exists on another level: He wants to bring Gestalt therapy to bear on a civilization gone wrong, such that it is headed for something approaching its own collapse. We have intimations what this might be like with the world shut down due to Covid-19, and economies everywhere sinking into massive losses. But the real approaching disaster, which Dreitzel takes on toward the end of his book, is the climax of climate change.

In an epilogue, Dreitzel proposes an important gain based on making an unusually large leap. The psychotherapist is typically concerned with the symptoms that threaten individual well-being. Dreitzel brings what Gestalt therapy has learned from that emphasis to bear on the most dire global threat of our times: climate change. The connections he makes between looming climate catastrophe and Gestalt therapy principles are one of the most intriguing and significant parts of his book. Every psychotherapeutic modality, taken seriously, implies its own particular set of ethical values. Drawing on principles that underlie Gestalt therapy practice, Dreitzel develops an ethical vision and its implications for action that he feels could be a healing force toward successfully battling climate change.

He suggests that our consciousness of the environment is more a matter of emotional responsiveness than cognitive perception. From this perspective he argues that treating climate change as an anxious-making future emergency rather than terrifyingly present emergency is a dangerous mistake that leads us to numb our sensitivities to the world around us. Anxiety, here as emergency postponed, leads readily to denial and defenses against it, whereas fear, which leads to contact with an actual present threat, propels us to action, whether fight or flight.

What kinds of action? One kind, which is neither merely fight nor flight, is renunciation: Dreitzel describes this as "Readiness to stop throwing things away while living in a throw-away society; to reduce driving in an automobile society; to use less water and cleaning materials in a society which suffers from delusional addiction to cleanliness…" He also understands how difficult renunciation is when it means a certain reduction in freedom and pleasures we have become used to. To help deal with this difficulty, he points to the need to heighten awareness, a basic move in Gestalt therapy, that would bring us into more intimate relationships with our surroundings. He notes that people who eat with awareness taste more and thus eat less, and people who explore trees with close attention learn to love them and suffer when they are burned down or turned into lumber.

He goes a step further by suggesting that thinking of ourselves as subjects and nature as an object to be lorded over, such that the markets decide what we strip from it for our needs, may have it the wrong way around. Perhaps we ought to start thinking of "society as nature's environmental problem," he writes. Dreitzel here takes a cue from Gestalt therapy's approach to a dialogical point of view inherited from Martin Buber, in which one's give-and-take with others and with nature needs to be less subject to object and more in terms of subject to subject.

There is a good deal more of serious interest in Dreitzel's epilogue, but I will leave that for the reader to discover for herself or himself.

The task he sets for Gestalt therapy is to create both a map and a method of transformation that could begin to heal the social and cultural wounds that are heading civilization even now toward the ultimate catastrophe of climate change. His conception of social change, you could say, is therapy writ large. I suspect that this numbers among the reasons he looks so closely at the nature of pain and suffering, as well as toward the guidance that comes from attending fully to the wisdom of emotional life. Emotional awareness brings us a very different kind of understanding of the human condition than that which relies on the cognitive power of reason. Staying within the confines of intellect and rationality has brought us extremely powerful instruments for making discoveries about nature from the atomic to the cosmic level. It has also enabled us to develop instruments for harnessing nature for the purposes of technological progress. Some results of this emphasis are hugely beneficial, but some are equally effective in creating destruction, including the possibility of our own. The human species at this juncture needs a different, more far-reaching kind of wisdom than that which has underwritten the forward march of civilization till now.

As I write, the entire world, immersed in the terror of Covid-19, has shut down its economies, its customary social life, and confined families to something akin to house arrest. The breathtaking scope of this event – and I intend the double meaning – feels almost biblical in its intensity. Perhaps we are only being given at most a foretaste of what appears to be inevitable at this point, of what will happen to us, as the broadening and deepening of climate change, already well underway, gathers momentum until it finally attains apocalyptic proportions. It's as if we have been led by a virus into a preview of what things might be like when climate change turns our world upside down.

Applying Dreitzel's perspective would suggest that if the cultures of country after country and their governments could become more capable of empathy, more attuned to human suffering and human emotional life in general, we might do a better job of being prepared for what is to come. It seems awfully late. We could not be further away from this possibility at the present political moment in the United States and perhaps in a number of other countries where there has been a rise in anti-immigrant right-wing populism. We have a President and an administration that is so far removed from empathy for human suffering that it must leave thoughtful people in something resembling a state of chronic shock, especially if they grew up with the teaching, as I did, that the United States was a democracy open to equality and a welcoming message for all, no matter what race, ethnic background, or religious belief. The current situation may make Dreitzel's message seem unattainably utopian. Nevertheless, it is a message that cannot be dismissed as merely utopian, because it seems that nothing less than a fundamental change of consciousness across nation states and the type of personalities they cultivate will support our future survival.

Chapter 1

Introduction

When the manuscript of this book was finished the COVID-19 virus pandemic had not yet devastated the world as we knew it. But did we know it really? And will the virus change everything as some observers claim? I doubt it. Politicians in all industrialized countries have as soon as seemed reasonable, and often against medical advice even earlier, started to get the economy going at whatever cost. It seems that beyond the corona-crisis the capitalist machinery will continue to suck up our natural resources, as it does even now in the middle of the crisis.

That means that climate change will continue, too. Therefore the last two chapters of this book will, unfortunately, continue to be as pertinent as when I wrote them.

When I started to think about this book almost 40 years ago, I had just finished my training in Gestalt therapy, a form of psychotherapy which immediately fascinated me and which I still practice with great enthusiasm. But from the beginning I was dissatisfied with the state of the literature on Gestalt therapy. To be sure, even then there was a growing literature relating to the practice of Gestalt therapy. This time was marked by the contemporary wave of therapies derived from the Human Potential Movement, spreading the news about the innovative craft skills and techniques of this new form of psychotherapy. But there were significant lacunae in Gestalt theory. The theoretical part of *Gestalt Therapy* – the ground-breaking text written by Frederick Perls and Paul Goodman in 1951 – was almost its only theoretical basis.

Especially lacking were:

1 A consistent theory of the contacting process – a mere sketch in chapters 12 and 13 in PHG;
2 A phenomenological exploration of the role of emotions in the contacting process and in Gestalt therapy;
3 The problematical issue of clinical diagnosis in Gestalt therapy, i.e. the problem of a process-oriented diagnosis;
4 A theory of growth and development consistent with Gestalt therapy;

5 An exploration of the anthropological philosophy underlying Gestalt therapy with a special focus on the question: how we can achieve a meaningful and satisfying good life in a world of catastrophic developments?

I was not surprised to realize whilst working on these issues, that the scope of the task exceeded a single book. Since then, the situation has changed, and many important contributions to Gestalt therapy theory have been published, especially by Erving Polster, Gary Yontef, and the participants in a discussion forum on theory in several issues of the *American Journal of Gestalt Therapy* during the 1990s. Meanwhile a new wave of theoretical thinking is underway focused on "relations" and a new emphasis on the "field" and the "self". Yet little of this literature has really addressed the theoretical issues I had in mind to fulfil the promise opened by Perls, Hefferline and Goodman's book (hereafter cited as "Perls & Goodman").

So I decided to start with the first two of the topics listed above. This book presents the results of this work. The third topic in the list eventually became the subject of my book on diagnostic perspectives in Gestalt therapy, published in 2010 under the title *Gestalt and Process – Clinical Diagnosis in Gestalt Therapy – A Field Guide* (Dreitzel, 2004 / 2010). A final book on issues 4 and 5 above was published in 2018 under the title *The Art of Living and the Joy of Life – Development and Maturity in a Changing World* (Dreitzel, 2018).

So the two main parts of the present book are dedicated first to an exploration of the theory of the contacting process and secondly to a theory of emotions and their relevance for Gestalt therapy. Both parts explore their topics by applying the phenomenological method of studying our consciousness and its ways to construct what we experience as our reality. This methodological approach – the basis of the Gestalt therapeutic practice – presents itself naturally as the method at hand to dive into the depths of the way human beings make contact with each other and attempt to lead a satisfying and fulfilling life. In a highly interesting recent contribution Michael Vincent Miller (Miller, 2019:97–98) has remarked that after Fritz Perls broke during his time at Easalen with Paul Goodman he also left behind any serious attempt to further incorporate phenomenology as the major method of working therapeutically in Gestalt therapy. Miller even came to the astonishing conclusion that Gestalt therapy has little to do with awareness. This is the result of Miller's analysis of the distinction between awareness, being an undirected, unintentional activity, and attention, being always an intentional act of consciousness: "My own viewpoint is that awareness is not sufficient for a Gestalt therapy theory of contact as put forth in PGH. Contact is a meeting that is emergent, creative, potential nourishing and fulfilling, and reshapes the two parties to it" (Op. cit.:101). (I will not follow up Miller's distinction which unfortunately came too late to my attention for this book.)

What I mean here (and in the subtitle of this book) by phenomenological method is not identical with what Edmund Husserl, the inventor of phenomenology as a philosophy, was after: to establish a new philosophy beyond empiricism and rationalism with its many turns including a return to metaphysics. I will not address its complicated history. Instead here I mean a methodological perspective which is focused on the "how?" rather than on the "what?". This sticks to the phenomenological method of "bracketing" all evaluations, prejudices, emotional reactions and the like as biases. It also keeps in mind the phenomenological notion of the intentionality of all acts of consciousness (which is one reason why I see the contacting process as a horizontal time line rather than a circle).

In this new revised English edition I introduce the second main part with a study of *Physical pain and the nature of suffering* and I conclude my reflections by considering *Aliveness and the joy of life* as a general goal of Gestalt therapy. Taking up the political and sociological impetus of Paul Goodman, these two central parts of this book are framed by essays reflecting on the *historical and the cultural context* of psychotherapy today, because I am convinced that beyond our clients' individual family backgrounds we urgently need to consider in what kind of society our lives and therapies are embedded. I have focused here on the Western world because it is in these countries or at least in their Western spirit that Gestalt therapy is practised internationally, even though this entailed disregarding many national differences. This partly reflects problems of space and the danger of overloading the book but this limitation may be justified considering our common fate of being subject to both hopeful and truly fearsome technological and political developments globally. As the spirit of Gestalt therapy demands that we take responsibility not only for our individual lives but also for the future of our societies, we need to think about how we can mobilize our energy and focus our motivation – and that of our clients – to actually get involved in changing the dangerous path our civilization has chosen. That is why I have added an Epilogue with some reflections on the question how Gestalt therapy could react responsibly to environmental destruction in our age of climate change. I hope they will be encouraging.

In this way a book emerged which does not just address the narrower circle of Gestalt therapists but is written for all psychotherapists, as well as for readers interested in sociological, political and philosophical analyses of our time.

I gratefully acknowledge that the theory of the contacting process was first outlined in the seminal text *Gestalt Therapy* (Perls & Goodman, 1952) – the starting point of my own contributions to the theory of Gestalt therapy. I am delighted that both volumes of *Gestalt Therapy* have been re-published (1994) with the addition of an inspiring new foreword by Michael Vincent Miller in the spirit of his friend and teacher Isadore From. Somehow it represents a kind of last will and testament of Isadore's since it was posthumously written and published shortly after his death, and presented as originally planned: theory, followed by practice as Isadore had wanted.

At the time, the particular perspective of Perls & Goodman was meant to overcome some of the deficiencies of psychoanalysis of their time. Today – when the politics of mental health seem to be governed more and more by the diagnostic imperialism of the DSM (Diagnostic and Statistical Manual) and the doubtful promises of the pharmaceutical industry – it is even more pertinent: it emphasizes

- process instead of structure;
- creativity instead of passive adjustment; and
- the autonomy of the patient instead of the disturbances of their character.

The theoretical part of *Gestalt Therapy* (Volume One) contains in its chapters XII and XIII the theory of the *contacting process,* which in my opinion represents – together with the *theory of the self* and the focus on the *contact boundary* – the heart of Gestalt therapeutic theory.

It is the intention of this book to convey to readers interested in psychology, education and other social sciences the contribution a Gestalt perspective could offer to an understanding of the interaction between man and his environment. As far as I know there is no psychotherapeutic theory which has given as much attention to the exchange processes between human beings and the environment, and the interaction (contact) between people. This makes Gestalt therapy particularly significant considering the environmental disasters which surround us today. Perls and Goodman could not have guessed at this catastrophe at the end of the 1940s. But their theoretical insights are, in my judgment, still of great importance today for learning how to deal with these developments. This assertion will be examined in the Epilogue to this book. I am convinced that the recently much-discussed notion of the "field" will *empirically* become more and more aligned with our decaying biological environment, which in turn will become the vague but anxious-making background of all our contacting processes.

Here I present the theory of the contacting process in detail. Compared to its first formulation in Perls & Goodman, I have expanded the model without too much regard for the original text: I was not concerned with exegesis, nor did I want to enter into any dispute with Perls & Goodman's assumptions. These I do not always share though I always find them stimulating. But since the first publication of *Gestalt Therapy*, almost seventy years have passed; we now have a broad range of clinical experience and insights pointing beyond the original work.[1] There have been theoretical discussions and contributions, too, especially during the 1990s, which left their traces in my reflections, and later with the advent of "relational" Gestalt therapy, which in my view is superfluous and so it remains undiscussed here. (Is not all Gestalt therapy guided by a personal relationship between the therapist and their own therapist? That is certainly as I have learned it.)

Instead an update of the original descriptions in Perls & Goodman seems pertinent today, as I hope to demonstrate in this book. While my considerations are deeply rooted in the work of Perls & Goodman, I take sole responsibility for what follows, especially since I have not always made an effort to refer in detail to where I deviate from Perls & Goodman. But to avoid misunderstandings one important difference should be mentioned right here: in Perls & Goodman the fourth phase of the contacting process denotes action *outside* the contacting process proper, whereas I use the concept of post-contact to indicate that the process still continues with slowly fading intensity *within* the contacting situation proper. This is particularly important for the therapeutic process, because it often happens that, though progressing well, a therapy fails to catch hold because the therapist does not pay sufficient attention to the post-contact process *within* the session. This, too, is why I call the third phase *"full contact"* (also known as *"integration"*) whereas Perls & Goodman called it "final contact".

Opening Chapter IV, the essay *On physical pain and the nature of suffering* has been added to turn the focus from interaction between human beings in general terms to our subjective experience. For even though the Gestalt perspective always considers the *contacting process at the contact boundary* between the person and their environment as the real battle-field where most of our construction and experience of reality happens, it is still true that at least the experience of *physical* pain is a lonely one. This is because our bodies are separated and it is very difficult to express in words the specific quality of a pain which puts it beyond any real possibility of empathic understanding. Pain and suffering are *a priori* to the emotions to which the book turns next because the incarnated nature of our bodily existence with its frailty and its transience is the undeniable condition and basis for *all* our emotional experiences.

Following this, the *phenomenology of the emotions* provides an important completion of the analysis of human interaction. For how could we conceive of contacting processes without our feelings? Our attempt to comprehend the nature of emotions in Chapter IV and V concludes with an essay on the experience of *Aliveness and the joy of life*, the other side of pain and suffering – and an essential and encompassing aim of Gestalt therapy. We all desire to enjoy our lives more deeply and with greater intensity; Gestalt therapy and meditational practice may help us to reach this goal by reviving and cultivating our senses.

Perls & Goodman's text does little more than hint at the role of emotions. This is quite astonishing since Gestalt therapy is often quite accurately described as a mode of therapy which attributes significant importance to feelings. It is the second aim of this book to close that gap. Of course, a Gestalt therapeutic understanding of emotions must be rooted in their function within the contacting process; for this reason, in Chapter III of this book I start with elaborating the theory of the contacting process and only then subsequently proceed to develop a phenomenology of emotions consonant with this model in Chapter IV and V. I could not have done this without discovering Manfred Clynes' book *Sentics – The Touch of Emotion* (Clynes, 1976). I came across it while browsing in a tiny bookshop at a bus stop in the northern woods of New York State. I learned more about emotions from this book on my way back to town than from all the academic investigations of the whole of the Psychology of the Emotions put together as they existed at the time. Clynes taught me to understand emotions from an aesthetic point of view akin to Gestalt therapy. I was so impressed that I immediately began to write the first draft of this book. Around the end of the 20th century the Social Sciences saw what has been called an "Emotional Turn": Suddenly a new interest in our emotions was blossoming, resulting in a boom in research and popular literature. Yet seen from today the harvest of this new interest in the nature of our emotions seems meagre.

Through my therapeutic and supervision work, and through my own self-experience processes including my own Gestalt therapies and forty years of meditational practice, I have learned how – when our senses and feelings come more alive – both our motivation for and sensitivity towards a more attentive kind of relationship with our social and natural environment begins to unfold. That experience has motivated me throughout the writing of this book. It is not wrong and – in my eyes – not paradoxical to say that my theoretical insights rest partly on my own self-experience. During the years when this book gradually grew in me, I worked on it with the conceptual tools I was equipped with through my training as a social scientist, especially in the theory of symbolic interaction founded by the American philosopher George Herbert Mead. Equally I am grounded in my early training in the methodology of phenomenology by my teacher, the philosopher Helmuth Plessner, at the University of Goettingen in Germany. Thus, I checked and tested everything with reference to my sensory and emotional experiences as they came alive in my own body through my training as a Gestalt therapist and in my practice of body meditations. In this way I am more personally implicated than is usually the case in this kind of text. My reflections are of course based on the findings and insights of other and greater people, but I have developed and checked them through observation and self-experiment not least in the encounter with others. But my main method of gaining knowledge and insight was the *phenomenological* method of *epoché,* of bracketing all evaluations and distancing myself from any prejudice, staying strictly with the Here-and-Now of the givenness of emotions.

Thus, I am responsible for each thesis in this book as its author and investigator – but I am grateful throughout to all my teachers, my colleagues, my students and clients who helped through cooperation and discussion and through allowing me to teach and work with them. Many of them had a lively and patient interest in the theory of Gestalt therapy without which this book would not have been written. It is dedicated to Isadore From, who died before the first draft of the English translation could reach him and so, sadly, I am left without his critical appraisal.

If the phenomenological perspective is the best approach to studying the essence of interaction processes within our natural human environments, a different perspective is needed for understanding the social and political culture in which inevitably all psychotherapeutic work is embedded. Often the therapist's view is limited by their interest in the three main influences: family of origin, family of procreation, and work situation. But there is much more to context or environment which we need to take into account. Currently, the socio-political situation of the Western world is not just in disarray: it is in deep crisis, threatening our civilization and even our survival. It is not surprising that deep anxieties and anger increasingly break through the surface of our seemingly civilized and peaceful standards of behaviour, emerging as a relevant background to our therapeutic endeavour. Therefore, the two main parts of this book are framed by chapters exploring the historical background as well as the cultural context which co-determine all psychotherapeutic work today. In working on this English edition, I revised and largely rewrote these chapters in order to take these newer political, social and environmental developments into account. Even if the present focus of attention unavoidably focuses on the sudden growth of populist movements, my own concern has long been dedicated to issues of climate change and environmental disaster, since in the long run they will completely change if not our own lives surely that of our children and our children's children.

I would like to ask the reader to bear with me if he/she feels that I have not done justice to the particulars of the actual situation in their own country. I focused on what can typically be observed in *all* Western countries, but I am well aware of deep differences, especially in regard to the United States compared with Europe or in regard to the differences between Western and Eastern Europe.

No doubt readers of this English edition will find various reasons for criticism and may object to some of my theoretical claims. And that is as it should be, since the theory of Gestalt therapy is never completed, and with such criticism the theory can continue to grow. Of course, much of what I claim for Gestalt therapy is true for other forms of therapy, too – but Gestalt therapy is my passion.

The following text does not describe the *art of doing* Gestalt therapy, how one could or should do it. The special issues of the therapeutic setting, of clinical diagnosis and therapeutic techniques are beyond my concern in this book and can – aside from easily comprehensible professional mistakes – indeed only be learned in a living encounter between teacher and pupil. But for the sake of readers not familiar with Gestalt therapy I will give a brief summary of its essence here and explain how it differs from other forms of therapy. For clarity's sake, I will mainly describe its differences delineated from psychoanalysis out of which it first grew:

1 Gestalt therapy builds on the client's *own experience* and the shared interpretation of this experience, instead of the therapist interpreting subconscious material.
2 Gestalt therapy mainly works with *experiments for self-experience* instead of free association, as in psychoanalysis; it also does not use training exercises as offered in cognitive learning therapies. The focus for such self-experiments is the way the client interrupts contact or diminishes it without being aware of it.
3 Gestalt therapy concentrates on the experience of the client in the *here-and-now* rather than their discussion of the *there-and-then*, since all experience, including that of remembering, happens only in the present as does all learning.
4 Gestalt therapy trusts in the healing power of *awareness*, where insight and experiencing create a Gestalt, not in the power of cognitive insight alone.
5 Gestalt therapy has a *paradoxical relationship with the change desired by the client*. If we accept ourselves in loving awareness just as we are right now, the river of growth and decline flows by itself; if, however, at all cost we want to be different to what we are, we simply stand in our own way.
6 Gestalt therapy starts with the assumption that the therapeutic situation can be a safe space for the client to do self-experiments; that therapist and client have an *authentic relationship*, which enables the therapist to see the client as a whole person, a subject of creative adjustment processes and not just a symptom carrier. It is also a relationship where the client can experience the therapist as a *person* and not only as a professional concerned with the diagnostics of deficits. These are real enough and Gestalt therapists, too, struggle daily to patiently reduce these deficits a little, aiming to be alongside their clients, helping to carry these burdens. But if the therapy is focused on the contacting process between the patient and the therapist one begins to develop another perspective on the social norms according to which we usually define a specific behaviour as "disturbed".

Most books written by psychotherapists are either dealing with psychotherapeutic techniques and procedures or with specific problems of psychopathology: neurosis and psychosis; early developmental problems; addictions; character neurosis and psychosomatic illnesses. They are concerned with the phenomenology of the abnormal, the pathological.

This book takes a different stand. In my reflections regarding the cultural, historical and social contexts of psychotherapeutic work in the first and the last parts of this book, I focus on the *pathogenic elements in our civilization.* In the two main parts, I deal with the theory of the contacting process and the role of emotions in it and draw on a picture of a *"normal", undisturbed person* seeking happiness and satisfaction. Perls & Goodman take the view that there is an observable objective criterion for mental health: the capacity to be involved in "good" contacting processes containing the potential of leading to satisfying experiences. The "factual difference of continuing creativity, is the crucial criterion of vitality and neurosis. It is an independent criterion, generally observable and also introspectable. It does not require norms of health for comparison" (Perls & Goodman, p. 246). This is a valid notion and I don't doubt its truth. It is certainly helpful in a pragmatic sense in therapeutic practice. In my analysis of the phenomenology of the contacting process and the nature of emotions the focus of my perspective is on this observation of mature, alive responsiveness. I do not claim that this represents normality in any statistical sense. On the contrary I believe that we are all damaged by our history and culture; we all need (Gestalt-) therapy and should seek it to rediscover our potential for change. But for that we need a model to lead us to a more humane future.

In the last few years – and in response to many people recognizing the destructive power of technical, economical and political processes – we are seeing an upswing in the search for standards of ecologically correct behaviour. But there is a danger that even where that ecologically desirable behaviour is discussed, such ethical norms are always in danger of becoming life-inhibiting introjects – or worse, instruments of power. Gestalt therapy, though, is concerned with the never-ending process of refining awareness of our processes of exchange with nature and society. Obviously, this includes a subtle sense of the other's vulnerability – in nature and in society.

Since the beginning of my work on this book the ecological catastrophe – not too alarmist a word anymore! – has reached a dimension which brought me to think about the possible potential of Gestalt therapy to help with what must be done to prevent the destruction of our planet. These considerations resulted in the suggestions collected in the Epilogue of this book. They, too, are concerned with sensual awareness, or embodied mindfulness ("Reflexive Sinnlichkeit") as I call this mental attitude of awareness where all our physical, psychological and cognitive senses are fully alive. In the final analysis this means a meditative attitude to life. Gestalt therapeutic practice, too, teaches that we can be fully emotionally involved *and* at the same time distanced in aware recognition. Even more of its power is rooted particularly in the fact that each contacting process entails the potential of "full contact", as a moment of being together in which – in Martin Buber's words – the "I" becomes a "Thou" such that momentarily awareness and experience become one and leave no room for any distance. This is a moment when our existentially given subject-object duality is suspended. The miracle is that all uninterrupted everyday contacting processes contain the potential of such a moment, depending on the degree of our awareness. The more we experience such moments of self-lessness in full awareness, the more the spiritual dimension of our lives deepens.

The reader of this book should be warned that it may be difficult to absorb it in one reading as a whole, although only reading it completely will bring the different parts and arguments together. Thus it might well be advisable to read it in parts pausing a little after each chapter to digest it. This kind of step-by-step reading of the book may considerably facilitate a comprehensive and stimulating approach to its ideas. There is also no problem in picking individual chapters regardless of their sequence in the book if curiosity has been aroused by seeing their titles – with one important exception though: the chapter on the nature of the contacting process (III "*The satisfying experience*") must be read *before* tackling the chapter on the nature of our emotions (IV "*Emotional orientation*"), because the latter is based on the theory of the former and cannot be understood without a previous reading of the first!

Peter Dreitzel, August 2020
(www.dreitzel-gestalttherapie.org)

Note

1 See the monumental collection edited by G. Francesetti et al., *Gestalt Therapy in Clinical Practice: From Psychopathology to the Aesthetics of Contact*, (2013).

Chapter II

Historical context

The fate of the body and the senses in the civilizing process

The core method of Gestalt therapy is to concentrate on what is at any given moment. First, I perceive what is offered through my senses; then I experience it through my emotions; finally I structure it cognitively in thought. Normally, the affective sensuous qualities of perceptions, sensations and emotions attain priority when we organize our experience. However, in my psychotherapeutic work I meet many people in whose life this order of priority is turned upside down: they have many categories of order, orientation and judgment at their disposal, but they do not use their senses well and feel very little. It is not surprising therefore, that they often say their motivation for therapy is wanting to get in contact with their feelings. This wish is frequently heard from clients at the beginning of therapy – a formulation which immediately shows their misery. For how could one "get in contact" with one's feelings instead of simply feeling? Such clients (there are others, of course) do not comprise a small group of "emotionally disturbed" patients, who in contrast to more "normal" people need psychotherapeutic treatment. In fact, these represent the tip of an iceberg the true size of which psychotherapists never encounter. At least these clients have noticed that there is something missing. And they have come, because they have made up their minds to discover what there is to find. But even if this means that they have already taken the first step in their healing process, psychotherapists need to know more about their clients' cultural background. Indeed, such knowledge is probably more significant today than their family background – the more traditional focus of psychotherapeutic exploration. Apart from the usual chaos of modern family life, the influence of peer groups and parental subcultures as well as that of the media have become increasingly significant. Gestalt therapy has always emphasized the importance of taking the field into account for understanding disturbances in the contacting processes between individuals – its main focus. That is why it is useful and urgent to start with the history and present state of our culture since it constitutes the general field of daily experience which thoroughly affects the life and the troubles of our clients and patients.

In the last 50 years there has been significant growth in the number of publications on the history of culture, covering aspects of the history of our senses and our sensibilities. Two very different authors have published classics in this field in the last century: Michel Foucault and Norbert Elias. Although Foucault's *History of Sexuality* (English edition 1978) made an important contribution to my observations in the opening considerations of this book, I will focus specifically on the theory of the "Civilizing Process" developed by Norbert Elias.

One good reason for this choice is that Elias' sociological theory is based on the insight that this process of cultural development is taking place behind the backs of participants, who are largely unaware of its flow and direction and do not consciously influence it. We must understand that our culture is a field or a system with its own rules and laws determining our subjective experiences at least as much as our conscious actions. Jim Tull gives a good definition in a beautiful paragraph in his *Essays on Global Transition.*

> A system is an assortment of parts making a whole by working together to achieve a unified purpose. Conscious attention typically associated with 'purpose' is not a requirement. Like all cultures, ours is a collection of parts struggling to work together to achieve a purpose as if all this had a will and mind of its own. Yet, though there is no conscious intention or intelligent design and execution, the cultural system is a unifying force pushing and shaping what we think and do. To forgive and love human individuals, I have found it very helpful to view culture in this way – always to see and understand humans in their cultural context.
>
> (Tull, 2016, p. 212)

This is exactly the same methodological position Norbert Elias has taken in his sociological theory of the civilizing process.

Another good reason for choosing Elias' theory as a starting point for our analysis of the cultural field active in the background of our patients' felt miseries is that Elias' research is mainly concerned with the changing *manners* of our everyday interactions with our fellow humans and with the changes in our *emotional* lives. For in contrast to other schools of psychotherapy, Gestalt therapy emphasizes the importance of our senses and our emotions for understanding neurotic processes, because they are the primordial way of being in the world and for making contact with our fellow beings. Along with this insight arose the socio-cultural context in which Gestalt therapy has developed simultaneously with many other cultural (or rather counter-cultural) attempts at re-vitalizing our senses and emotions. All this influenced Gestalt therapy.

Elias' eminent work had already been published in 1939 in Switzerland, but was neglected for a long time because war broke out in the year of its publication, and Elias immigrated to England, having been persecuted by the Nazis for his Jewish descent. In 1969 a new edition appeared in Germany and simultaneously an English translation became available (Elias,

1969; Gleichmann et al., 1979). In England, the importance of Elias' work was soon discovered and became the focus of much debate among social scientists from different disciplines. Norbert Elias' theory of the civilizing process certainly needs to be revised in some of its more general claims – after all it was written 75 years ago – yet in my judgment his book continues to present a challenging outline of what he called the civilizing process from late medieval society to the French Revolution. In the depth of its psychological and sociological insights, this work also provides the best departure point for an examination of what has constituted the civilizing process in Western societies during the last 150 years, which Elias did not directly take into account.[1]

Let us start with some general observations. What is prized in the world of work and in public life is hyper-meticulousness without emotion; detachment without involvement; strategic planning and calculation, and repression of spontaneity. All these behaviours are rewarded in public life. Conversely, in the world of personal relationships, a narcissistic partner choice is apparently the rule rather than the exception – i.e. a relationship where the other is "swallowed whole" in the neurotic desire for bolstering one's own Ego.

In the realm of work, our culture discourages the curious and experiential use of our senses – with the exception of the eye, as long as it is seduced by the media. It disregards spontaneous expression of emotions which motivate action. Post-modern capitalist culture rewards detached analysis, compartmentalized rules, and the passive reception of prefabricated content. At the same time, leisure culture offers a rich array of opportunities for physical and psychological, aesthetic and esoteric experiences aimed at extending physical and emotional capacities. In this way the civilization of rich Western societies in its worldwide cultural hegemony presents a conflicting, even Janus-faced picture: on the one hand, manners have become much more relaxed and less formal; on the other, the unrestrained expression of feelings has largely been confined to our private lives and to media productions. We are trained to behave in a "cool" way, in a business-like matter-of-fact manner; and yet intensive emotional attachments between individuals are the rule right from childhood. Strictly hygienic body control and exacting levels of athletic capacity – as defined by youthfulness and health – are regarded as significant cultural values, whilst more and more people search for new ways of experiencing their bodies and their emotions as a whole – a longing that is far removed from a desire merely to maximize physical achievement, in which another part of our culture excels. We accept through our very life-style deep and significant intrusions into nature's self-regulation; but "nature" and "naturalness" have never been such important values as they are in our present culture.

This picture has become even more complex since the rise of populist movements on the right wing of the political spectrum in almost all Western societies. In such an environment the civilized standards of behaviour seem to have declined to a shocking extent: vulgarity, unrestrained racism, sadistic hate, uncontrolled rage and physical violence are breaking through the strict barriers of the state's monopoly of legitimate use of force and even violence. This monopoly is still considered to be essential for living together in a civilized and democratic society, but it is challenged by the New Media and increasingly it is expressed in the street. And this is even more true for the violation of other norms and values of civilized behaviour. Insults, denunciations of morality and trolling are common, as is unreasoned denial of facts; foul language is publicly used and tactful behaviour is lacking, while contempt is shown even for diplomatic behaviour. We observe a constant attack supported by the populist movements against behavioural standards taken for granted until now at least in the upper strata of society.

This seems to be a picture conveyed mostly by New Media. We should be aware, however, that these developments are also a product of even the traditionally serious media. David Bornstein and Tina Rosenberg reported in the New York Times (14.11.16) that even in their own newspaper a tendency prevails to prefer bad news to good news in their reports and commentaries. This applies even more to the populist press, not to mention social media! It seems that the human brain, this author's included, tends to be impressed by and hence to memorize bad news much more effectively than good news. This might have been an evolutionary advantage – until the development of our global culture of news at everybody's fingertips.[2] This phenomenon does not support a friendly view of our society but rather aggressive feelings and ranting.

This then is the complex socio-cultural background which all psychotherapeutic effort must reckon with today. In order to understand what is going on here we have to take a closer look at the work of Norbert Elias. As he understands it, the "civilizing process" is at its heart the gradual internalization of more and more external controls regarding the expression of physical and emotional needs. This he calls the development of a psychic mechanism of systematic self-restraint regarding the expression of feelings and needs. The function of this mechanism, which operates outside awareness, is to facilitate the replacement of spontaneous behaviour with strategically planned behaviours.

Two stages in this process are distinguished, which may however overlap. To begin with, all behaviours are subjected to increasingly strict and formalized standards of control. We observe for instance at the courts of the *ancien régime* in Europe of the 18th century formal types of behaviour being prescribed for more and more everyday situations, so that the question of what kind of behaviour is expected of the courtiers in this or that situation became increasingly important. This led to a new kind of literature of guide books on etiquette for courtiers.

The second phase in the civilizing process begins with the development of new, more moralizing practices of socialization in the middle classes. As a result, the more formal standards become internalized. Instead of the honour of the aristocrat, now it is the virtue of the gentleman which is the guide to acceptable behaviour. Gradually the control of the body and of the emotions becomes quasi-automatic. External sanctions of deviant behaviour like losing certain privileges or even being excluded from the court are gradually replaced by psychic reactions like embarrassment, shame and guilt feelings. The modern super-ego develops as a new locus of control and soon begins to be accompanied with and supported by endless commentary given by the new psychological sciences, at a later point quite specifically by psychiatry and psychoanalysis. (Interestingly, Michel Foucault has suggested that this *"discoursization* of sexuality" as he called this development, started with the elaboration of codices for the practice of confession in the Catholic Church.) The second stage of the civilizing process results in the emergence of what David Riesman called "the inner-directed" person, the person who owns a moral compass (Riesman, 1960).

* * *

Elias emphasizes that the civilizing process always takes place amidst multiple cultural orientations and social movements and often asserts itself in spite of them – just as if it was independent of, and indifferent to, the goals and aims of the individuals acting in their historical time. We are dealing here with two forces which assert themselves unbeknown to the acting individuals but which nevertheless explain the civilizing process.

The **first** force is what today we call globalization. This is actually a much older historical force, apparent in European history at least since the beginning of the Renaissance and Europe's conquest of other cultures since the 1400s. What Elias has in mind are the ever-expanding economic exchange processes covering ever-greater distances, forming chains of relationships and increasingly requiring the ability to "look ahead", to use "foresight" ("Langsicht") as Elias calls it. He also draws attention to the development of what sociologists call the "pattern of deferred gratification". On the psychological plane this means that people need to show a capacity to *plan*, using other modes of *rational behaviour*; they need to exhibit that "tolerance of frustration" which can bear longer periods of delayed gratification. This is just that process of "disenchantment" with modern life through rationalization and bureaucratization, which Max Weber described in great detail – and which results in "affective neutrality", as his American student, Talcott Parsons, called it. This becomes the measure of rational behaviour.

The **second** force fuelling the civilizing process is the gradual monopolization of legitimate force by the state during this period. Indeed, compared to the daily experience of violence typical of peoples' lives in medieval and early modern times, we are now living in an era of over-arching physical and emotional security. Steven Pinker (2011) in his huge study of the decline of violence in the civilizing process – incidentally also starting with Elias' work – makes the same point. Of course, violent crime still exists, and we do have our share of disturbances, terrorist attacks and uprisings. But in fact, the murder rate (numbers of murders compared to size of population) has declined to an astonishing degree! This is especially true of Europe. Pinker has some difficulty explaining the "special case" of the US and he says very little about the situation in Asia, Africa and South America. But in the Western world today our anxieties seem to be focused mainly on the increased danger of accidents which come along with the use of technical machinery, instead of fearing dangers originating in fellow human beings. Day and night we travel through land, air and sea in the industrialized world without fear of bands of robbers or pirates affecting our plans. The critical factor here is not the continued existence of violence within Western countries, but that the risk of its occurrence has diminished to the point that we no longer have to take it into account in planning activity.

Though it is true that there are old and new "no-go-areas" in the world outside the Western sphere of control, globally speaking the number of relatively peaceful areas is growing everywhere. Even the recent massive terrorist attacks in New York, London, Madrid and Paris or the increasing presence of pirates in south-east Asia and around the shores of Africa have not significantly changed the global trade and travel routines – numbers of airline passengers, for instance, continue to rise worldwide. Eventually, tourists return to places once devastated by terror attacks. The fact that even in the rich countries referenced here there are still some unsafe enclaves – for example slums and city parks at night – tends to emphasize that they are the exception to the rule of general pacification.

And the same might be said of risks threatening specific groups of potential victims in our society: women have to be aware of the dangers of sexual harassment; old people are exposed to a greater risk of being mugged; racial violence is not at all extinct; minorities such as homosexuals run a greater risk of being maltreated. However – with the exception of the special case of the USA (see Pinker, 2011) – crime rates in the Western world generally tend to decline.

Also, let us acknowledge that we no longer need to fear pestilence and cholera; that in everyday life, birth and death are largely hidden from view; that sick people are quickly isolated in hospitals; that we are no longer confronted with the sight of hunger or defecation in the streets; that we eat meat, but scarcely any town dweller has ever seen an animal slaughtered. Let us concede that personal experience of physical violence (in sharp contrast to what we experience in the media) has virtually disappeared from view in our everyday lives. The same holds true for sickness, death, and most unhygienic practices. This state of affairs is to a large extent guaranteed by public institutions, in the last resort by the monopolization of legitimate violence by the state. For our context it is important to take note of the statistical fact that in our time the greatest potential for violence arises not in the public arena but in private life. Most murders, bodily injury, sexual abuse of children and rape are committed in the family circle, amongst acquaintances, or in youth peer groups.

In Europe, we experience the singular incidence of seven *almost* uninterrupted decades of peace – an entirely new phenomenon in its history! The greater therefore was the shock following the eruption of extreme violence during the Balkan Wars and the arrival of Islamist terrorism. Each was accurately understood as a breakdown of civilization, which – for the first time since the Second World War and the Holocaust – brought back into focus how fragile the layer of civilization actually is.

I will not at this point discuss the attempts Elias made to defend his theory in view of the horrors of the 20th century (Elias, 1969c). Were they interruptions of an on-going civilizing process caused by extraordinary historical circumstances – as Steven Pinker and Elias seem to think – or were they relapses into earlier stages of this process? Or did they mark the end of this civilizing process and prove that the claim of its universality, at least in the Western world, is unjustified? This is not easy to decide. Elias believes that the Holocaust can only be explained by the extraordinarily paranoid and enclosed kind of anti-Semitism cultivated by the Nazi elite. But this does not explain the normalization of violence against Jews and other minorities during the war and even before that by Germans and their collaborators, particularly in Eastern Europe but also in France and Italy.

It seems to me that in any case we would be well advised to see the civilizing process as fragile and always in need of protection. At present, a new war in Europe seems unlikely. But the experience of peace between nations and regions within Europe is too new to be trusted. The present lack of enthusiasm for the project of a pacified Europe is dangerously forgetful of the Yugoslav experience, not to speak of earlier chapters of European history. Under the veil of slow but continuous erosion of national sovereignty a new regionalism along the lines of prosperity, language and old traditions is growing. Perhaps worse, a new wave of anti-Semitism is spreading in Europe, even in Germany. At the same time the European Union is developing a strong bureaucracy with far-reaching decision-making powers but lacking democratic legitimization. These are dangerous developments, especially in times of economic crisis which have become almost normal in the south of Europe and feared everywhere as the next international financial crisis looms. Revolts and riots, uprisings and local wars threatening the civilizing process may well become a realistic prospect, even in a pacified Europe. And then there is the enormous present and future task of dealing with constant streams of refugees from Africa and Asia.

And, of course we must also take into account the situation that has developed in the United States, culminating in the presidency of Donald Trump. The slow but ongoing decay of democratic institutions in the USA is much older than the Trump administration and is, in my opinion, mostly due to the complete prioritization of economic over human concerns in American politics. But with Trump, the amoral nature of capitalism has surfaced as the normal standard of status and behaviour which – alongside a Trump-inspired revival of old American racism and his general contempt of women – until now could only be imagined by some television series. With the title of her new book – informed by her European background – former Secretary of State Madeleine Albright has courageously drawn our attention to the real danger facing us: *Fascism – A Warning* (Albright, 2018).

Viewed from a personal perspective, we find a different picture. Near-paranoid fears concerning personal security, especially in public places and on public transportation systems in the big cities, are feeding into policy developments advocating more and more surveillance. Advancements in artificial intelligence technology and the development of drones will soon erase whatever is left of a private sphere. Today, drones for observation are no larger than small birds or even insects and are ready for production. They attract the interest of police departments, as well as the military: the price for our growing security will be the loss of more and more of our privacy, and in the final analysis, of our freedom. Leviathan is growing again with less and less legitimacy. China is the forerunner here; Xi Jinping, its most powerful leader since Mao, is trying to transform Chinese society into a digitally controlled totalitarian state. But the poison is active in the West too, reinforced by the real dangers of Islamic terrorism and destructive digital attacks on democratic states by Russia, among other perpetrators.

* * *

Elias' theory is not quite as original as he claimed. Karl Marx and Max Weber each analysed the same developmental process in their different ways. They were followed by the multifaceted tradition of the theory of the modernizing process. What was new in Elias – following the inspiration of Sigmund Freud – was the application of this tradition to the realms of the body and the emotions. Elias believed that he had identified as the most significant factors determining the history of the subject in Western Europe the increasing functional interdependency of economic transactions and the gradual expansion of internal pacification of societies by public intervention – in short, in the history of capitalism and the modern state.

Indeed, it may pay to follow this thought a little further. Perhaps we can say that the first phase of the civilizing process in Europe coincided with the phase of "original accumulation" (Karl Marx) of capital during the time of mercantilism and the Age of Enlightenment, where we see powerful attempts being made at directing and training the unpredictable impulses of our human nature (see Michel Foucault's lifelong studies).

The second phase – the development of internalized thresholds of embarrassment, shame and guilt feelings – was strongly accelerated during the Industrial Revolution in a way hitherto unknown, corresponding with and facilitating the phase of competitive capitalism. I hasten to add that these process descriptions are not intended to signify a causal relationship, but more to suggest a complex network of functionally interconnected conditions, all of which require detailed investigation. Historians will always experience understandable discomfort when such phase models seem to suggest clear demarcations, since their vast quantity of facts and phenomena never fit into a simple developmental scheme. But the sociologist observing the present time must face the task of recognizing earlier patterns and stages in the development of the western Modern Era, if they want to understand our present society in Europe and America and its impact on the emerging globalized world order.

During the 18th century and before the Industrial Revolution had taken root, a surprising change in attitudes regarding cruelty against fellow human beings and even animals took place in Britain and Central Europe. A new humanism developed, resulting in the gradual abolition of extreme forms of torture, corporal punishments and eventually the death penalty. This was also evident in the abolition of slavery and ending the imprisonment of debtors, witch-hunting and other forms of violence against the body. This process is of course the early phase in the history of what we now call Human Rights – a history which continues to this day, having already made immense progress. One might think that it took a very long time but given the history of human violence – apparently part of the development of human culture since its origin in pre-human evolution – the speed is actually quite surprising. What by now has culminated in the abolition of the death penalty in many countries began during the French Revolution with the establishment of the guillotine as the standard instrument used by representatives of the state for putting people to death. This machine was the invention of a medical doctor whose intention was to *humanize* the procedure of execution, and was introduced little more than two hundred years ago!

From these observations various questions arise. How does the present period of socio-economic development, whether we call it late capitalism, digital capitalism, post-industrial society or post-modernity, relate to the civilizing process? Are we currently experiencing a third stage of the same process or are we dealing with the end of a development which for centuries pointed in the same direction, but which has now come to an end, creating space for something new?

* * *

Before addressing this question, I must mention another aspect of Elias' theory: the observation that the civilizing process usually starts with the economically significant classes and that new standards of behaviour only gradually percolate down through the class structure. Significantly, the first volume of his work has the sub-title: "Changes in the Behaviour of the Secular Upper Classes in the West" (Elias, 1969a). Formalization of behaviour started with the aristocrats and early modern patricians in the leading centres of Europe, initially in the city states of northern Italy and the mercantile centres of the Hanseatic League; then later at the courts of Paris, London, Madrid and Vienna, and eventually at smaller German courts too. Typically, the new standards of behaviour reached the economically significant families of the bourgeoisie in the cities prior to being adopted by the landed gentry. After this and often much later, we find the same behaviours in less elaborated forms of standardized "good behaviour" in the middle and lower strata of society. In the 18th century, the court of Versailles achieved the pinnacle of this formalization of behaviour with its strict rules and endless rituals. 150 years later, the rules of good behaviour at the dinner table or during the Sunday church service attended by entire middle-class families were no less strict, even if less formalized.

The constant flow of the civilizing process meant that people already educated in formal behaviours always had to anticipate the presence of people who had not yet fully undergone the process through which standards of civilized behaviour eventually became second nature. The Stanley Kubrick film "Barry Lyndon" gives an extraordinary artistic description of the extreme repression of anything to do with bodily expression and the life of the emotions achieved through the behavioural prescriptions guiding European aristocracy of the 18th century. Fellini's "Casanova", a film about the mechanization of sexuality during the same period, could be placed alongside it. The unusually beautiful sequences of Kubrick's film – amongst them for the first time the famous shots lit solely by candle light – made most critics overlook what this film is really about: i.e. the socialization of nature during a particular historical phase, when our bodily and emotional impulses were being socialized.

Kubrick shows a stage of the civilizing process where its forced nature becomes particularly clear, because the formalization of behaviour is not yet internalized – and therefore pushed to an extreme. People appear to wear masks; move like marionettes. As ever, wild aggression and anxieties break through the thin veneer of those ritualized ways of behaving: for example, when offended by subtle verbal attacks, somebody suddenly and unexpectedly beats up his opponent; or vomits right in the middle of a highly ritualized duel with pistols. Stanley Kubrick's film even encompasses the changes which occurred during this phase in our relationship to nature itself. The use of landscape photography references contemporary paintings and it is precisely their overwhelming beauty which shows perspective itself as a limiting achievement, hiding nature in its wild and untamed reality. Suddenly the image is allowed to move as a rider unexpectedly explodes into the picture, riding right across it.

More generally, the history of landscape painting illustrates a process of change in our attitude to our natural environment, corresponding to the formalization and later internalization of enforced behaviours. At first it shows the demythologization of raw nature, which did not become a legitimate subject *sui generis* for painting until it had been denuded of all magical properties; this followed a kind of aesthetic delimitation of the violence of nature, anticipated by the separate developments of still life painting; the idyllic landscape painting of the late Baroque and Rococo schools, and finally in the taming of nature through the romanticizing of its violent aspects, using them to elevate and enhance our sense of self. In the middle of the 18th century Johann Joachim Winckelmann, early archaeologist and originator of classicism in Germany, noted in his diaries that he had to close the curtains of his coach when he crossed the Alps, utterly awed by the violent and "abysmal" spectacle. At the end of that century, Immanuel Kant in his philosophy of aesthetics made the new distinction between the beautiful and the sublime, the latter referring to the beauty of wilderness. During the early decades of the 19th century, the Prussian painter Caspar David Friedrich famously romanticized the beauty of mountains and rocks as did J. M. W. Turner at the same time in England with the beauty of the sea. Finally a further hundred years later, the philosopher and sociologist Georg Simmel could write an essay about the aesthetics of the Alps (Simmel, 1911). In the meantime, photography had been invented and had revolutionized our perception of nature: today images of sublime nature are so pervasive in our culture that the real and the virtual are becoming indistinguishable.

* * *

Returning to the relationship between class structure and the civilizing process, Elias' presentation is rather vague at this point and leaves us in the dark regarding the role of the bourgeoisie in relation to the aristocracy. While some of his observations seem to indicate that the two stages of the civilizing process are always repeated on the level of each social class, much could be said for an alternative version: that the second stage of internalizing stricter behavioural standards was largely the work of the early bourgeoisie, a development which – starting slightly later – works in parallel to the formalization of aristocratic behaviour. Of course, both classes move through both stages of the process. But it was the courts of the ancient regime which saw the culmination of formalization, whereas the bourgeoisie adopted the Protestant ethic whose puritanical requirements gradually became the ruling standard of behaviour and action, following the bourgeois revolutions and culminating in the Victorian era.

The concept of a diverse class distribution of civilized standards of behaviour was particularly well demonstrated – apparently without any knowledge of Elias' work and in a different context – by the English sociologists Michael Young and Peter Willmott in their encompassing investigation of the development of modern family structures (Young / Willmott, 1975). They called it the *"principle of stratified diffusion"*. I offer a short quotation from this book:

> The image we are trying to suggest is that of a marching column with the people at the head of it usually being the first to wheel in a new direction.

> The last rank keeps its distance from the first, and the distance between them does not lessen. But as the column advances, the last rank does eventually reach and pass the point where the first rank had passed some time before. In other words, the egalitarian tendency works with a time lag. The people in the rear cannot, without breaking rank and rushing ahead, reach where the van is, but, since the whole column is moving forward, they can hope in due course to reach where the van was. Lagged equality – always partial, never including everybody – is the nearest approach there has yet been to equality…
>
> The source of momentum is not too obscure. Without industrialization the column would not be on the move.
>
> (Young / Willmott, 1975, p. 20)

This last remark requires some clarification. In Western societies, the train started to move with the Industrial Revolution but did not really gain speed until after the Second World War. In spite of all the economic crises and wars of the 20th century, it eventually led to an era of unprecedented higher standards of living and mass consumption in the Western world. For a while, it seemed that the middle-class models of behaviour, i.e. the second stage of the civilizing process, would become the general standard prevailing in (modern) Western society.

But even as Young and Willmott published their book in the middle of the 1970s, another economic development started, which in the 21st century gained supremacy: more than half of the cars were cut off from the main force of slowly but constantly increasing wealth for all: industrial production slowed; wages stagnated or decreased in real value; an upper class of owners and shareholders of industrial companies moved forward without the burden of the poorer ranks of society – thereby becoming super-rich. The development of financial and digital capitalism gave rise to economic crises gripping the whole Western world. To varying degrees all Western societies were split into new socio-economic classes.[3]

In other words, we cannot assume that the *principle of stratified diffusion* of economic riches is a sociological law which will always work in highly industrialized societies. It worked in the Western world approximately between 1945 and 1975. But now we are faced with an equality gap almost as big as that which existed before the beginning of the First World War. Yet it may well be that "lagged equality" will be, at least for some time, the new pattern of growth in some or most societies of the emerging economies. New data collected by Joerg Baten, economist at the University of Tuebingen, Germany, (Baten, 2016) suggests, that some developing countries, China and India among them, have recently succeeded in following the older Western *pattern of lagged equality* by connecting with the driving forces of industrial production. Taking the World Bank's new definition of poverty as an income below 1.90 dollars per day, it turns out that the proportion of people who live in extreme poverty has declined from 37% in 1990 to 10 % in 2015 (corrected for actual buying power).

Yet in the Western world, the principle of lagged equality has slowly lost its descriptive power since the 1970s while the concentration of capital keeps escalating, Capital is now concentrated in the hands of just 0.1 % of the population. This new and still growing inequality gap is influenced by socio-economic developments and political decisions operating differently in different Western countries. The gap is biggest in the US, followed by the UK and Germany among the bigger Western countries, and smallest in the Scandinavian countries with their traditional social-democratic governments (now also threatened by right wing populist movements).

This is not the place to discuss the multiple reasons for this change, but let us just consider one factor – the shift in the class structure of Western societies, which is the most important factor determining the fate of the civilizing process in times of peace. The most remarkable phenomenon is the disappearance or at least the shrinking of the traditional working class through automation, artificial intelligence, the rise of the service sector and to a lesser extent globalization. With the decline of traditional industries and the decay of whole cities like Detroit, or whole industrial areas – such as parts of northern England – the old working-class culture has virtually disappeared in many places in Europe and the US. The remnants of the old labour class, often well paid, highly skilled workers, are culturally alienated and isolated without their traditional homes and settlements, their pubs, bars, clubs and sports grounds. Together with the shrinking group of self-employed craftsmen and handymen they have become a *lower* middle class, separated from a new *upper* middle class mostly by lacking higher education. This new upper middle class is the result of an educational revolution, epitomized by the extraordinary increase in college and university students over the last decades. Numbers differ in different countries, but all in all the growth rate of graduates in higher educational institutions is quite staggering. Whilst traditional educational values and ideals of learning may have disappeared or be threatened by this development – as I believe they are – the traditional liberal value orientation or even prevailing social-democratic or "green" attitudes separate this new class culturally and importantly often politically from the lower middle classes. These, fearing downward mobility towards the ranks of the new lower classes of the jobless, the underpaid temporary workers, and the regionally underprivileged members of the so-called "precariat", are or may become the carriers of the de-civilizing processes described above. In any case a new cultural gap between the new lower and the new upper middle classes can be observed which may be due to different access to education, different use of the internet, different use of social media and a different leisure culture. Here sociological research is still inconclusive and in dispute.

This new class structure which can be observed in all Western countries is both the result and the driving power of the growing gap between the first and last groups of the "train". It is now a fact that every day in our societies the rich become richer and the poor get less of the cake. This is a dangerous development politically as well as culturally as far as the civilizing process is concerned. Much now depends on whether this dangerous trend will continue and globally destabilize industrialized societies. How dangerous it actually is, has long been demonstrated by the wide-ranging research of Richard Wilkinson and his collaborators at The Equality Trust in London (Wilkinson, 1996). Up to now, the principle of stratified diffusion as a dominant social mechanism for guaranteeing relative economic equality over longer periods of time, seems to have worked sufficiently well to contain the dissatisfaction of both the poor and the lower middle classes threatened by economic decline. If that trend had continued into the foreseeable future, it was unlikely that Western societies would have needed to anticipate violent class struggle – bordering on civil war. But today, it seems that the wagons of the lower economic ranks have indeed become disconnected from both the wagons at the front and the engine.

But to what extent is the economic situation of the divided middle classes responsible for the growing populism in the West? In order to find out if and to what degree this is the case we must take a number of different trends into account. One factor is *immigration*. In countries like the USA, but also in Britain, France and Germany, constant immigration changes the language of the lower classes in such a way that it is enriched to an astonishing degree, while at the same time drawing further away from the standards required by relevant educational institutions. An even more important factor is the growing influence of the new media: television, computer games and chat rooms as well as smart phones have already changed much of how we communicate, especially between younger people and their peer groups. But there are a number of other factors involved. Ten of them I will consider here more closely, without claiming that they are the only or the most important ones.

1 Firstly, there is the practice of *bringing up children*. Much sociological research has been carried out in the decades of the second half of the 20th century, studying regional and class differences in socialization procedures. That means we are relatively well informed about how such processes were carried out, but we know little about how the change in the class structure of our societies *presently* might influence these patterns. The older findings suggest typical differences of patterns of socialization between the middle classes and the lower classes. I think that we are dealing here with the two stages of the civilizing process, which in the last century were represented by and co-existed with each other in the two large classes of Western society at the time. In the 1970s, the British sociologist Basil Bernstein[4] proposed that working-class children were disadvantaged by their "restricted" language code, in contrast to middle class children whose "elaborate" language code was identical with the

language used in school. In the long debate which followed, at least one point became clear: the language of lower-class children is anything but "restricted". In fact, it is often semantically richer than that of middle-class children. Yet it was true that the rules which children are expected to follow in educational institutions would more often be explained and reasoned in ways familiar to children of middle-class families. This replicated the ways the children had experienced at home – thus favouring middle class children's success in schools. Does this mean that such a split is now to be found between the present-day academically educated members of the new upper middle class and the new lower middle class, whose younger generation is merging more and more with the new lower class? We don't know, but the almost hysterical application of the rules of "political correctness" in American elite universities might be an indication.

2 There are endless controversies among social scientists and intellectuals about how *digitalization* and the New Media affect our culture now and into the future, when today's young people will have grown up. I am convinced that in the long run this development will have a deep and lasting effect on our culture. It is no longer just a question of which people, and how many in our societies will be more or less educated. More likely, this development will change the forms and content of education itself. Even the kind of intelligence required seems to be changing significantly: during the 1990s my colleagues and I observed that our students in the university began to display less and less capacity to concentrate on lectures for more than fifteen minutes. This was, as I found out by questioning my students, directly related to the date of the first appearance of the television set in their families, when they were children: the earlier, the greater the effect. On the other hand, they became more competent and less inhibited in oral exchanges, discussions and debates; their powers of imagination seemed to grow, and, of course they became better equipped to handle computers and use the internet.

Whether and to what extent the civilizing process continues at least in the Western World cannot be discussed without taking into account what has been termed the *informalization process* which in growing steps entered what used to be counted as its second phase; since the end of the First World War the rules of behaviour have been liberated from many strict rules.

At first sight, the civilizing process seems to continue but in fact it had already changed its character and become what later was termed the informalization process, as a third stage of the whole process. In our society we can find few relics of very formal behaviour, and these are no longer sustained by harsh external punishments like exclusion from the in-group or by inflicting physical pain. In fact, all kinds of physical violence are abhorred to a degree which suggests deep internalization of rules against it. It may seem paradoxical then that violence is so prevalent in the media. But is it really? Former generations used to read their children the most gruesome fairy tales without a second thought. True, today there is a certain tendency in the movies to show extremely brutal scenes, but in my opinion they mainly serve to stabilize the internalized rules against acting out these impulses. There is always a certain attraction of the forbidden, making us shudder. It is an old insight of the sociology of law and criminology that not only the punishment of the criminal but of the crime itself has the symbolic function of upholding the law. From this perspective, what astonishes more than a perhaps growing presence of violence in the movies is the constant decline of the rate of violent crimes in real life. Also, we should realize that what is actually shown, especially to children, is censored and has little to compare with horrors quite common in everyday life and even some forms of public entertainment only two hundred years ago.

But in order to understand the present stage of the civilizing process, it helps to consider society from a *horizontal* as well as from a vertical perspective, because we now live in a society with mass consumption and a high standard of living. Apparently, the civilizing process does not just move from the top down but also moves laterally from the economic centres to the periphery of societies. Ethnic differences in countries with many immigrants, as well as characteristic differences in the comparative behaviour of city and country dwellers can be interpreted more satisfactorily in this way. In our context here, this observation applies importantly to some of the significant differences in styles of affective expression which can be observed in different regions and countries. For instance, the often-cited lively and boisterous temperament of Mediterranean peoples is usually attributed to ethnic characteristics or even "national character", while in fact this behaviour is typical for the first stage of the civilizing process when external constraints are not yet fully internalized – and will change when and where the civilizing process moves on.

This is not meant as an evaluative statement as one might speak of "civilized" or "uncivilized" behaviour in everyday speech, but a term describing a social process beyond the awareness of those involved, as Elias did not tire to emphasize in his books. The next example will show this more clearly.

3 Let's take *driving* a car as an example of how frequently national styles and modes of behaviour have been cited as examples supporting the notion of "national character". It seems that in the economic development of countries there is roughly a ten-year period within which the car becomes a means of *mass transportation.* This sudden increase in traffic forces people to drive in a more considered and controlled way. This is a process of self-training and increasing police controls probably contribute less to it than the growing emotional and physical risks attached to the situation. Travelling by car through Europe during the 1950s,

> West Germans were said to be the worst drivers ("typical German aggression"). In the 1960s it tended to be the Italians and the Belgians, followed by complaints and jokes about the "reckless" driving style of Greeks, Turks and drivers from Eastern Europe. When I first visited Palermo in the 1950s, traffic was chaotic and drivers were indeed reckless; coming back seventy years later, I was surprised about the orderly flow of the now much thicker traffic as well as by the considerate driving style of Sicilian drivers.

This example also shows that the civilizing process is greatly speeded up if *technical developments* are involved. It is literally life-endangering to physically give vent to one's aggression by standing on the accelerator. By comparison, the outbreak of physical violence among members of Parliament which can occasionally be observed in Italy is much less dangerous. To choose a more serious example, I dare not imagine what would happen with modern war machinery if those who are in control of an arsenal of atomic weapons or deadly drones were not practising continuous emotional self-control. The Cuban Missile Crisis of 1962 was an interesting (and fearful!) case in this respect: throughout the world, people were nervously listening to the radio, anxiously speculating whether Khrushchev and Kennedy would or would not be able to control their own aggressive impulses, anxieties over safety, and their frustrations (as well as those of their military!) to avoid an atomic disaster. Internalizing external restraints today has become a safety factor of our technical development. And that is why we have good reason to be afraid of President Trump, who seems to lack these internal constraints.

But even if an atomic global disaster, like a clash between America and North Korea, is not likely to happen imminently, we observe that every new technical invention, even if it only concerns driving a car, has at first to be controlled by the police or special security units empowered by the state. In other words, during the first phase of the introduction of a new technology the state now usually takes responsibility by working out rules and controls of behaviour until the larger public of consumers has sufficiently internalised them – just as in other areas of the civilizing process in former times! Every technology demands new rules to be worked out, such as governing the use of seat belts, or more recently, the use of smartphones while driving. This dimension of the civilizing process works internationally: the wealthier a society the more people fear the risks of new technologies and demand or tolerate state control of potential misbehaviour – even at the price of their individual freedom.

But how do we explain the range of emancipating movements which have freed us from the highly formalized Victorian behaviours of repressing physical and emotional spontaneity? After all, technological progress alone does not account for the social processes that led us towards our current standards of informality and the new emphasis on physical and emotional modes of expression.

Let us focus briefly on what actually happened, beyond the decline of violence in different fields of the civilizing process:

4 During the last hundred years, *sport* has become a mass phenomenon. Even if we disregard those aspects of sport relating to show-business or the cult of sporting heroes, we notice a surprisingly great interest in active sports. Together with the attraction of nature as expressed in the pleasure people have in camping, swimming, mountain climbing, skiing; in walking, surfing and para-gliding, the interest in sports indicates the significance we attribute to physical health which is confirmed by the spread of fitness centres. This is partly a reflection of the general medicalization of society and partly a reaction to alienating and unhealthy aspects of our increasingly urbanized life styles with the spread of industrially produced cheap and, thinking of the spread of obesity, potentially poisonous food.

There is also however, a different trend in sport: *extreme sport* attracts more and more attention. In fact one of the strangest phenomena in Western societies today is the number of extreme ways by which more and more people seek to reach and even to stretch the limits of what they can physically attain and endure. As of now, over 2000 people have climbed Mount Everest, one third of them in the last decade and in doing so, 233 of them lost their lives (as of 2018). Others run through the Sahara desert, swim across the Channel, throw themselves from bridges into canyons or out of aeroplanes. They hike and bike hundreds of kilometres. They engage in free climbing, canoeing, snowboarding, base jumping, and ever-new challenges. It is difficult to clarify their motives but the number of people involved in extreme sports is growing every year. One explanation is addiction: at a certain level of endurance, the brain produces hormones which reduce pain and cause the so-called "flow" experience (Csikszentmihalyi, 1990).

Another explanation for the "normal" forms of high-performance sports is to see in them a narcissistic search for the self-celebration of being the first, the strongest, and the best. But when these sportsmen and women are asked for their motivation, they often answer that they want to do something extraordinary, to experience life more intensely – as potentially we do when exposed to the risk of death. Are we to conclude that a life of saturation in modern society is so deathly boring that many seek the anti-depressive effects of "peak experiences" which in themselves seem meaningless? This would be a sad lack of awareness. As for instance any serious experience of meditation may show, the deeper we go in our embodied mindfulness, the richer and more exciting the present moments and situations become – without requiring the spice of extreme challenge.

5 Norbert Elias claimed that embarrassment and shame are the protectors of the civilising process. The internalized rules of behaviour punish each violation immediately by these very disagreeable emotions. With respect to physical *nakedness*, shame thresholds seem to be lower than they were 50 years ago. The most important step in this change occurred with the revolution in fashion before and after the First World War. This change was anticipated by the Art Nouveau movement with its emphasis on natural forms, and by various back-to-nature movements of the youth culture of the time. From then, we can trace the beginnings of a new re-evaluation of the "natural" beauty of the human body and our feelings towards it – a phenomenon not sufficiently explained by referring to short skirts, trousers and short hair being so much more practical for the growing number of working women from the middle and working classes. The end of the obligatory corset was the beginning of the end of the obligatory bra. Just compare photographs of women in the years before and during the First World War with ones from the early 1920s. In 1913, shortly before the war, a leading German fashion magazine even suggested a diet to counter (!) the slimness suffered by some unfortunate women. What a change in less than a decade! Men's clothes, too, had become much more informal and comfortable. Nude bathing has been accepted in nudist colonies since the 1920s and is now tolerated even in the city parks of some of our bigger towns in Europe. During one summer in the 1990s the Turkish population of a neighbourhood in Berlin complained that the virtue of their daughters was endangered by the nudity of many German park visitors. Their answer – in a letter to the press – went something like this: "When we come to visit your country as tourists, you demand that we respect your customs and, for instance, refrain from swimming in the nude. Here in Germany where you choose to live, we demand of you, too, that you respect our customs"! It seems to me remarkable that at the end of the 20th century nudity in public can be claimed as a "custom" in the middle of Europe. The same goes for the home: children nowadays have a greater chance to see their parents' naked bodies for longer than the traumatically fleeting moment permitted even 30 years ago. Also, nakedness has become standard practice for sexual intercourse. Kinsey, in his investigation 70 years ago, significantly reported characteristic class differences then still evident in this respect. These last developments, however, were only gaining prevalence when the informalization process really started – and that was not before the cultural change in the late Sixties and early Seventies.

6 Concerning *sexual behaviour* in general, I do not have the impression that the liberating tendencies of the 1960s and 70s deserve to be called a "sexual revolution", but doubtless there has been a loosening up of puritanical standards. In fact, we always see the most radical Puritanism in societies when just going through the phase of original *accumulation.*

Today we can easily demonstrate this process in countries in other respects quite different, such as China, Malaysia, and Egypt – with typical differences between the rising urban middle classes and the majority of the population. However, regarding sexuality there are three significant developments characteristic of late capitalism: firstly, of course, the change in the position of women – a pre-condition for an acceptance of pre-marital sex and of divorce as normal phenomena; secondly, the invention and spread of oral contraceptives, which to a large extent have removed the gravest risk of pre-marital and extra-marital sexual intercourse. And thirdly, there is the strange phenomenon that today a kind of general voyeurism seems to be culturally accepted and even promoted. The spread of sexually stimulating images shown in public advertising is only its strongest expression.

7 With the invention of photography, our culture has developed an astonishing *dominance of the eye* compared to all the other senses.[5] Again it seems that the technical medium is nothing but a vehicle for deeper processes: the capacity to see is exactly that sense which creates, emphasizes and uses distancing between my body and that of others. It looks as if the cultural dominance of the eye is yet again a phenomenon of that same civilizing process which in other areas (eating, for instance) is also concerned with creating *an ever-greater distance between the body and its object.* This voyeurism is nothing but what Michel Foucault called the "discoursization" of sexuality (Foucault, 1979), the endless interest in describing, cataloguing and differentiating all aspects of sexuality – which is the opposite of a natural and relaxed attitude towards it. This process continues in different forms: more and more pictures taking over from words as the medium of the message. Today we wonder about the future sex life of children who, via their smart phones, are familiar with pornography even before they reach puberty. This may turn out to be the real sexual revolution – another of those revolutions which do not lead to liberation.

8 In the realm of *table manners* we conduct ourselves much less formally than our grandparents did – even while we strictly observe all hygiene standards and adhere to the explicit rule that we must suppress all sounds associated with the process of eating, drinking, and digesting – a fact which seems remarkable only because other societies had so much pleasure from such expression of physical contentment. But talking about table manners may soon become irrelevant for the family dinner table is in danger of losing its traditional function and value. More and more eating takes place outside the home, in office cafeterias, fast food restaurants or in schools. Sitting at a table is no longer a prerequisite for eating: people eat while standing or walking in public; or in their homes, where often ready-to-eat food is available and no more is needed than opening the refrigerator and serving oneself with

readymade food. With fast food abounding, table manners do not apply any more.

9 It is harder to gauge what happened to *the way we express feelings.* Perhaps it is easiest to stick with *aggression.* And here, too, we find contradictory standards. On the one hand, the process of increasing control of spontaneous aggression is no doubt continuing: all forms of physical attack between adults are considered criminal acts; even verbal sparring is considered to be "deviant behaviour" while some forms of verbal insult are even legally punishable, and a code of honour – which might have been broken in the past – is nowhere in sight, except in some unassimilated immigrant families. In the public sphere, physical aggression is largely confined to the realms of war and terror. Even in wars when aggression is considered legitimate, Western soldiers often have to be systematically trained to kill, if they are to be used as special "task-forces" or torturers. Hence the preference to use bombing from airplanes and more recently the use of remote drones in the military: the more distant the object to be destroyed, the less inhibition about killing and destruction. The development of war machines illustrates most clearly how inescapably the fate of the civilizing process is now (and has been at least since World War I) interconnected with technological progress. The next stage will probably be the use of fighting robots.

10 In the private sphere we discover a different picture. While technological progress produces more formal rules of control to be observed, be it for security's sake or for making war, i.e. killing, in private a person's only controls are their internalized inhibitions against hurting our fellow human beings. Statistics show, however, that the modern nuclear family both harbours and hides an astonishing amount of violent behaviour. There can be no question that most murders, infant sexual abuses and even rapes today occur within the family circle and in intimate relationships. (Again, the US, due to anachronistic gun laws, is an exception here) But we are talking here not of premeditated murders but rather of the result of spontaneous violence, sudden outbreaks of hatred: and in men, often the rage of the defeated in the war of emotional expression. They may take refuge in their last resort, physical force being the only power they feel they have left.

All these examples support the proposition that from the end of World War I, with interruptions during periods of fascist rule in European countries during the last century, we deal either with *stronger, deeper internalizations* or a *third stage* of the civilizing process, a slow *process of informalization* following and supported by the second stage, the process of internalization of formal rules of behaviour. But it is useful to understand, that this third stage only became the *normal* standard of behaviour after the cultural revolution of the 1960s and the 1970s. Until that time authoritarian standards prevailed in family as well as in public life, apart from bohemian circles and similar marginal milieus. Many people will remember the vehement family conflicts over the changing style of how young people were dressing and the appearance of the new electronic music when the Beatles arrived on the scene. From today's perspective these conflicts are barely comprehensible. I vividly recall – driving through Colorado in 1968 – a huge billboard on the highway with the message "Beautify America: Have a Haircut!" Now informal manners have become standard, with marginal exceptions such as may for instance still be found in the banking sector. The burning question now is whether the restraints represented by the earlier internalization of rules of civilized behaviour guarded by shame barriers, remain strong enough to keep insulting and, more importantly, violent behaviour at bay. In this respect a new barrier may arise in our societies which runs along new lines of division between new social classes.

* * *

Altogether, we are confronted with a diffuse picture: some tendencies contradict each other; some follow general developmental directions – complementing one another in Western societies. There seems to be no question that the civilizing process has not come to an end, even though we had to learn that it is capable of regression and terrible relapses. Apparently, it had so far three developmental stages which may occur in historical sequence but more likely appear simultaneously in different strata and in different geographical regions of our society. These are:

1 The formalization of behaviour
2 The internalization of formal rules of behaviour
3 The process of informalization of behaviour.

Also, presently there is once more a danger of regression, the diagnosis of which is particularly difficult because it occurs at the same time as the informalization process continues to develop.

Let us first consider two different views – one pessimistic, the other optimistic – that have been proposed in the general debate of where our culture is going, each in its own way deeply rooted in the experiences of the 20th century.

There are those who maintain that we have arrived at a second or even third stage of the industrial revolution or at a post-modern society – meaning that our society has developed into an economically, technologically and socially self-regulating system, where in principle all basic material problems have been solved. This view – or something similar – lies behind many social and economic analyses, mostly of American origin, which tend to focus their optimism on technological and scientific progress. Some believe that even the threat of global warming will be averted in the long run through technological solutions. It only remains to convince the rest of the world how appropriate such solutions are for the global village, in which supposedly we all now live. Many global enterprises and corporate finance foundations claim to be busily engaged in this task already. As to the cultural developments, we can now finally afford to tolerate a certain degree of liberation from the previously necessary constraints (Bell, 1976). Now the body and the emotions can even become the vehicles of our search for authentic self–realization. We live in a permissive society where we freely choose our preferred lifestyles and may express emotions and sensuousness in our private lives, because we can easily switch to highly controlled cool and rational modalities of feeling, thinking and acting at any time that the situation demands it.

In contrast the pessimistic view has always maintained that capitalism cannot generate true liberation from the repression of feelings and the body. This view has been put forward mainly by the intellectual leaders of the student movement and the hippy sub-culture of the 1960s and 70s. In this context, two authors from the older generations were particularly popular, the first being the psychoanalyst Wilhelm Reich who proposed in his *Mass Psychology of Fascism* (Reich, 1933) that the traditional patriarchal authoritarian model of the family was characterized by strong sexual repression responsible for the murderous atrocities of the Nazis. His book on *The Function of Orgasm* was widely read on the campuses and provided ideological support for the attempted sexual revolution. The other popular figure was Herbert Marcuse, another German immigrant to the USA, holding academic positions in several universities and where his main works *Eros and Civilization* (1955) and *One-Dimensional Man* (1965) were published. In our context his *Critique of Pure Tolerance* (1965) is of particular interest, his argument running approximately as follows: today, the rigid formality of puritanical and Victorian standards of behaviour appears to be less evident but only because we have now sufficiently internalized these restraints. Emancipatory movements can be tolerated by the capitalist system as long as they remain superficial – only as long as they do not touch rationality and standards of achievement on which this economic system is based. Marcuse coined the expression "repressive tolerance" for this, in his view, essential characteristic of our society. What others celebrated as sexual revolution in the 1970s he described as "repressive de-sublimation". Michel Foucault and many feminists and cultural critics of lesser stature have followed Marcuse in denouncing the new sexual freedom as just another, more subtle form of domination – a view which was recently updated by the #MeToo debate. From this perspective, all lifestyles appear to be just another form of commodity in the cultural market, simultaneously the objects and instruments of the economic system. Today, the internalization of external restraints – albeit in more subtle ways – continues to violate human nature. Behind the mask of emancipation, the civilizing process is the process of social relations increasingly dominated by subtle, invisible power relationships, the controllers of which are the so-called "helping professions".

However, it appears to me that these two basic descriptions are insufficient to explain the developments which I have briefly sketched as characteristic of Western societies. We may note that both positions present typically middle-class views. But presently we observe a growing split in the middle classes in which the lower part, together with the traditional working class, are falling prey to the growing speed of automation and digitalization which destroy their jobs. It is this development – and not, as they themselves often seem to believe, the globalization process – which is the real cause of their justifiable fears, experienced as an alarming threat to those involved. This creates a certain confusion in the political realm. Just as Trump shouts "America First", in Europe, too, the leaders of populist movements are typically nationalistically or regionally oriented. Both claim that the dissatisfaction of a growing part of society is caused by globalization of the economy and especially the labour market. Indeed, Western societies are mostly as yet politically ignorant of the extent and the speed of radical transformation which the digital revolution will bring to every sphere of life. While Trump uses his smartphone to govern through his nightly posts on Twitter, every day jobs disappear through automation. It is no longer clear who the users are and who is misused by the New Media, except that digital capitalism is winning. Otherwise everybody, the rulers as well as the ruled, seems to be victims and offenders both at once.

With respect to the civilizing process, these developments appear as a backlash. For a considerable number of people, the restricted standards of behaviour seem insufficiently internalized to the extent that they break down under economic pressure or fears. This is not new; the civilizing process always was subject to regressions. What is new, though, is that presently such regression comes at a moment when the process of internalization is weakened by the prevalence of informality. Hence, we find on official as well as unofficial levels a resort to aggressive and vulgar language, culminating in hate mails and comments and the so-called shit storms using Facebook, Twitter etc. This goes hand-in-hand with a growing lack of inhibition concerning the use of vulgar language in society in general and perhaps more seriously in politics (see Bergen, 2016, and Adams, 2016).

The picture is more complex, however: there is also the emergence of *Political Correctness,* the history of which has still to be written. In our context it means the opposite of the informalization process: it is a new wave of external rules to control (mostly language) behaviour with a trajectory from the support of women and under-privileged minorities to the censure of literature and art. Meanwhile this development has led to what amounts at least in the States to a cultural war between "liberals" and "populists" along the lines of the new gulf between the two parts of the traditional middle class. What has importantly been overlooked by Elias' account of the civilizing process, however, is that all emancipatory developments in their first stages must seek the help of formalized legal regulations or established social rules to support their innovative ideas by membership quotas, punishment for harassments, guarantees of civil rights, and access to formerly forbidden social spaces. This phase sometimes takes a very long time to take root in society until these new rules become internalized and protected rather by the guardians of civilization: *shame* and *embarrassment*.

So, we must take yet a closer look at this process of informalization. As such it is not under debate. The notion was introduced by Cas Wouters, a Dutch disciple of Norbert Elias (Wouters, 2007). With Elias' backing (Elias, 1969d) Wouters claimed that this process is a new phase in the civilizing process. Everywhere and in almost all spheres of life and social groups, over the past hundred years the rules that govern our behaviour have step-by-step become more informal. Over a long period, dress codes have become more relaxed; the ways we greet each other or leave a meeting have lost their former stiffness; outside the family, we more easily address each other by our first names and even before the present excess of vulgarity, our language codes had become much less guarded, less limited by taboos than in our grandparents' homes where we usually maintain a standard of decency according to our internalized standards of politeness. Indeed, the theory of the informalization process seems a good description of many traits of the present culture of Western societies. It is not necessary however to go even further, as Wouters does, and stretch this theory as if it could be applied to the dimensions of universal history. Elias himself appears to have been more guarded when he said that the process of informalization is a new stage of the civilizing process and *would lead* to the "controlled loss of emotional control". I am not sure that this applies to some features of very irrational control in the fights over political correctness, though.

But to *understand* this new stage of the civilizing process we must look even deeper, to the core of that process, which is our changing relationship to our bodies and our emotions. For these attitudes form the basis of the varieties of identity formation and reality construction which are typical for our society. The body clearly is not a separate monad, but part of a field which encompasses the individual and their environment. Emotions are states of excitement which arise at the contact boundary between the self and its objects – dependent on the actual situation. It seems that flexibility between involvement and distancing in relation to groups and other people is typical for the modern social personality which therefore has a corresponding capacity for playing ever new roles.

Robert Jay Lifton, psychiatrist and social scientist, offers a similar analysis when he speaks of the "protean character" of the modern human (Lifton, 1993). In Greek mythology, Proteus was a man who could adopt any shape with ease. As with David Riesman's description of the "outer directed" social character, Lifton sees the modern human as one who without difficulty can adopt many identities in the course of their life, while developing vague feelings of guilt due to lack of rootedness.

Actually, what has disappeared is the classical *super-ego*, the internalization of clearly defined criteria for right and wrong. According to Lifton, Protean man needs to be free from the internalized Father in order to be flexible enough to play the different and sometimes contradictory social roles required of him. And yet, he/she suffers from vague guilt feelings and a hidden tendency towards self-condemnation, because our culture is bound up with the illusion of a constant self-identity; with the idea that a healthy personality must have a strong and stable character. But in fact, the symbolic structure of our society resembles a broken mirror: we see fragments of our multiple identities accurately reflected, without being able to see ourselves as a whole. The fate of the self (our ego-identity) can never be separated from an interest in the reality status of what is happening in this moment. But few psychologists or social scientists have seen the connection. Often, they are internally too strongly connected to the previous stage of the civilizing process, where the formation and support of stable, inner directed personality structures was a central function of therapy.

Importantly however, the theory and practice of Gestalt therapy is an exception to this observation: Perls & Goodman already claimed in the 50s that "character" is a result of neurotic repressions rather than a valuable goal of psychotherapy, and that the self is in fact an ongoing process of identifications and alienations in the contacting processes of human beings and their environment (Perls & Goodman, 1952). It was unfortunate – but given its revolutionary new theory of psychotherapy also perhaps inevitable – that Gestalt therapy early on became identified with the counter-culture of the 1960s and 1970s and remained so in the eyes of the psychotherapeutic establishment. Yet the cultural changes of these years not only inspired the development of Gestalt therapy but produced an immense change in the way psychotherapy now understands the importance of our physicality as a basis for and as part of our psyche. This has even reached psychoanalysis. Marcuse's critique of "one-dimensional man" (Marcuse, 1965) does not do justice to the seriousness with which many of us now look for new and creative ways to deal with our bodily nature and the natural environment.

* * *

My own hypothesis is that the present stage of the civilizing process can best be understood as the emergence of *a reflexive relationship with nature.* If it has become difficult to experience oneself as a whole. If the question "Who am I?" becomes pertinent, one tends to look first at one's own body, whose unity appears unbroken. Thus, what is new in our present culture is the reflexive use of the body, of feelings, of outer nature and – more generally – the way we construct reality in interaction. And I mean both a thoughtful attitude to choosing with full awareness the quality, the intensity and paradoxically even the degree of spontaneity in expressing physical and emotional needs – as well as the tendency to reflect upon such forms of expression and experience. One example is the flood of literature on the meaning and self-experience of mountain climbing. Another is the enormous popularity of high-quality documentaries of wildlife. The paradox here is that there is barely any wilderness left on our planet and that which persists does so through human protection. This is probably the reason a growing number of people look for nature undisturbed by human beings – in deserts, the highest mountains and even in the arctic worlds. Yet even in the desert, one hears the noise of airplanes and in 2013 and 2019 there have been accidents due to "traffic jams" on Mount Everest where climbers have had to wait in line for up to two hours to ascend a track which can only be climbed by one person at a time. "Wilderness" becomes a social construction; "real nature" becomes confined to the "death zones", where people may actually die, and which are only accessible for the rich (the charge climbing Mount Everest was about 80,000 dollars in 2017). Meanwhile, rangers direct the tourist traffic in Yellowstone Park (the biggest nature reserve in the States), protecting the animals from aggressive photographers and tourists from aggressive bears who have become beggars along the roads because the tourists are feeding them.

The hypothesis of a new reflective mode in our relationship with nature allows us to explain very diverse phenomena of our culture such as the de-ritualization of everyday life; changes in attitudes towards nakedness and sexuality; the ecology movements; the new political significance accruing to natural categories like region, gender and sexual orientation; the spread of psychotherapies concerned with the body and the emotions; the new interest in thanatology; the search for authentic religious experience; the experimental attitude towards esoteric experience and – more generally speaking – the range of different world views and experiences of alternative dimensions of reality through psychedelic drugs and mystical experiences in nature. The common denominator of all these phenomena is the new importance attached to a reflexive attitude towards both the nature of our physicality and of our environment.

This new attitude can be shown most easily in *art,* where it already has a tradition. More and more frequently, art consists in the self-reflection of its method of production and its ways of being consumed. An example would be Roy Liechtenstein's painting entitled "Masterpiece", depicting male and female comic strip characters where the first figure says (word balloon): "Why, Brad darling, this painting is a masterpiece! My, soon you'll have all of New York clamoring for your work!" But self-reflexivity does not always manifest itself as irony. An example of a more serious reflection on the method of production is Truffaut's film "An American Night", whose story is precisely that of producing the film.

In the theatre it is not just the relationship between play and reality which is reflected on, but frequently the relationship between actors and their audience. An example is Peter Handke's play "Offending the Audience", where the players do nothing for two hours but offend the audience. It becomes obvious that the moment we take the mantra "Art is Life!" seriously, the function of art consists in nothing but to indicate possible perspectives through which anyone can perceive the reality of their choice. There are many examples of this in contemporary art. Just two examples from recent exhibitions at the Museum of Modern Art in New York: at one point, the visitor passing from one room to the next walks between a naked man and a naked woman standing within each side of the door frame. At another, a woman sits in the middle of a large room, an empty chair in front of her, and everybody is invited to occupy this chair and stare at her in close proximity for a certain time. A third example is from the 2012 "documenta" (the most important exhibition of contemporary art in Europe, taking place every ten years in Kassel, Germany). Visitors first enter a large hall which is completely empty; after a while, one notices a soft wind blowing through the hall: this is it – a "piece of art" – an artist making a point. At times it seems somewhat contrived when today's artists – often with some pathos – show how fragile the experience of reality has become, when for the audience this has long been part of their everyday life. Still, works by René Magritte and Max Ernst are, of course, classics and copies are now sold in poster shops or are available as postcards! What I call the reflexive relationship with reality is to be found everywhere in modern society – today it is no longer significant that Art is Life but rather *vice versa*: Life is Art!

* * *

But self-reflexivity is not only a mode of cognitive perception – just the opposite. It seems to me that the really interesting phenomenon of the reflexive mode is the self-reflexivity of *sensuous perception* and *feeling*: we are in love with love, we are afraid of fear, we experience pain in anticipation of being wounded; we experience sexual pleasure while reading or when talking about sex or looking at an erotic picture, and we might want to express our frustration intentionally in order to release pent-up anger, and so on. Gestalt therapy makes use of the potentialities of this cultural development in many ways, while at the same time supporting it.

But reflexive use of sensuous perception is only possible because I can be directly aware of my senses and my feelings at the very moment they are active. Only this capacity for awareness – for an internal mindfulness regarding feelings and body control – allows them to become objects of reflective action. Examples might be when we intentionally use a particularly polite and formal way of behaving – be it in play or as a strategy; or when we get involved with particularly unconventional experiences – for example a "re-birthing" or an "Avatar training" – without making an enduring commitment to the requisite behaviours and world views. This gradually-evolving new attitude is a reaction to the cultural availability of roles and emotions, of identities and realities as sources of possible experiences of self and the world.[6] To be sure, the material condition for the emergence and enduring significance of these new orientations is that basic material needs are reasonably well safeguarded. The condition for their psychological effectiveness however is that we develop and refine embodied mindfulness and eventually reach a point beyond the sensory whirlwinds and emotional storms where pure awareness is the subject of experience.

Late capitalism can cope without the formation of a stable super-ego. In fact a strong but rigid character is increasingly becoming an obstacle to the individual's ability to function. Instead of being a necessary condition in the socio-economic system it is more and more replaced by the new demands of perennial readiness to life-long learning, and the capacity to be always flexible for new but not necessarily creative adjustments. On the positive side the new stage of the civilizing process, which we see unfolding slowly and through conflicts, is that of a mindful orientation towards sensuousness in which distance and involvement, planning and spontaneity condition and supplement each other – even if the price for this development is role division, forced upon us by technological developments and economic conditions. These forces not only split their exponents into different cultural worlds but even split the individual's contingent of social roles.

One of the results of this new stage of the civilizing process is that new tasks arise for education as well as for psychotherapy. We are now concerned less with internalizing cultural standards through parental injunctions and prohibitions, and more with the development of communicative competency and the ability to learn; we are concerned with creativity as well as with sensitivity for the exchange processes between human beings and their environment. The result would be reliable competency for participation in flexible and experimental constructions of reality. Such competency is founded on what I call embodied mindfulness. Gestalt therapy is an enterprise concerned with rediscovering, developing and caring for the pre-conditions of this competency. As a form of psychotherapy, it mainly deals with the dysfunctions produced by the new stage of the civilizing process itself through the very pressure on everyone to change their lives and keep learning. For with the enormous speed of development and the fast-growing complexity of modern societies, most people now experience that what they learned when young is already outdated by the time they reach middle age.

Today, common psychic dysfunctions are of two kinds. On the one hand we still see old-fashioned patterns of alienated character masks dominating the picture, especially in politics and corporations. These people tend towards depression. On the other hand, we see a growing number of people whose disturbance arises from anomic lack of orientation and narcissistic lack of boundaries. Their suffering is rooted in the growing virtualization of our worlds of experience – even though they tend to use this phenomenon as a point of refuge.

However, older stages of the civilizing process survive simultaneously and may cause conflicts. While paternalistic educational practices from a former stage of the civilizing process, focused on formal values of honour or religious virtues, may be completely outdated – though still surviving in evangelical enclaves in the US and in some traditional families of the new lower middle classes in Europe – they can also be imported by immigrants from pre-modern societies living in Western countries and struggling to adjust to their new cultural environment. Repressed rage only too easily crystallizes into resentments and prejudices, strengthening an attachment to the status quo of a consumer-orientated society, stifling creativity in human beings and damaging nature. If rigid self-control is culturally supported, it imparts an illusionary feeling of power and the capacity to achieve, but it is doomed to fail because it is a defeat of one's own nature. Hence, where people are socialized in such ways within the growing culture of the new reflective attitudes towards nature, they lack the feeling of being alive, a feeling for the sensuously adventurous nature of life. Even in 1952 Perls & Goodman noticed this:

> But suddenly the repressions begin to fail because of the general spread of luxuries and temptations; self-esteem is weakened by social insecurity and insignificance; character is not rewarded; and outgoing aggression in civil enterprise is hampered, so that aggression is wielded only against the self; in this present day situation self-conquest looms in the foreground as the centre of neurosis.
>
> (Perls & Goodman:145)

But then again, there is often the need to project what is experienced as limiting the self – and the limiting objects are always registered as "them", the outsiders who do not "belong".

Norbert Elias called our internalized mechanisms for self-repression a "machine of self-restraint" ("Selbstzwangsapparatur") – according to him the condition of the possibility of civilized behaviour in modern society. To be sure, widespread peace has been helpful in this process! But Elias says little about the losses connected with this development; peace has been bought at the price of violence against our inner nature and our natural environment. Today's world is threatened again by a new wave of aggressive resentment against people who "do not belong". This is a result of the schism in the old middle class: its lower part is confused by the liberal values held up and taken for granted by its upper echelons, now often called "elites", values which they have not yet internalized and which they believe are threatening their identities, aggravated by their not unjustified fear of downward mobility beyond their control. No wonder that Paul Goodman, who was no optimist, took neurosis to be an anthropologically unavoidable side-effect of the civilizing process.

Beyond these dysfunctions another more modern phenomenon now arises, affecting mostly the new academic upper-middle class in its urban and suburban habitats. This is the emergence of neurotically disturbed people who had no boundaries given to them in childhood, who were inundated with mechanical and digital toys, whose experience of nature was limited to a glance from the car window, whose bodily experience – in sexuality, too – is oriented towards competitive sports; who are alienated from the language of literature and from historical understanding but are very good and flexible in dealing with virtual worlds; human beings who play with alien identities because they are unable to develop their own. Increasingly, it is this kind of person who will need psychotherapeutic care today. Both groups show deep disturbances in the relationship between their human organism and its environment, and this is why Gestalt therapy may come closest to offering psychological solutions to these problems.

Notes

1 Such a procedure seems to me more in keeping with the value of Elias' sociology, rather than glorifying it and edifying it as a monument either requiring support or needing to be toppled. The first procedure is followed mostly by his disciples; the second was tried by the cultural anthropologist Hans Peter Duerr, who seems to have made the battle against Elias his life's work. However interesting the material gathered by Duerr (2005), I am not sure that it devalues the theoretical core of Elias' investigations. Although Duerr may have achieved some partial victories in his impressive enterprise – his collection of materials does not coalesce into a history of the subject in the European process of modernization. However accurate his rejection may be of any claim to general applicability of Elias' civilizing theory to extra-European cultures and pre-modern epochs of European history (something which Elias never claimed), I still think it is restricting to insist, as some ethnologists do – especially of the French structuralist school, apart from Duerr – on the ahistorical nature of anthropological constants, and thereby deny the value of any developmental perspective on the stream of human events, human behaviour and the history of our mental development

2 See also Pinker`s new book *Enlightenment Now* (2019). The Swedish author Hans Rosling has been pursuing the same arguments for a long time already. See his book *Factfulness: Ten Reasons We're Wrong about the World* (2018).

3 These new facts in world economy are presented in the book by French economist Thomas Piketty, *Capital in the Twenty-First Century* (2014) which has led to a worldwide debate among economists. For readers seeking a comprehensive summary of Piketty's research and the debates it triggered, see John Cassidy, *Piketty's Inequality in Six Charts*, in *The New Yorker* (26.3.14).

4 See Bernstein (1971). For critical expansion see Hager et al. (1973).

5 For new research on the interesting history and sociology of the senses compare: Robert Jütte (2004)

6 It seems to me that the reflexive attitude towards (our) nature is underpinning the observations of Andreas Reckwitz' much discussed new sociological theory of the society of singularities. See Reckwitz (2017).

Chapter III

The satisfying experience

The contacting process in the interaction between humans and their environments

The departure point and ongoing background of all Gestalt therapeutic work is a theory of the contacting process, which describes the exchange relationships between the human organism and its environment. The original version of this theory was first outlined in chapters XII and XIII of Perls & Goodman under the heading *"Creative Adjustment"*. In this chapter I intend to provide an explication and further elaboration of the original ideas of Perls and Goodman.

The theory of the contacting process could even be understood as a sociological or even anthropological theory of action explaining all or any human experience – an over-extension of the model which I will not discuss here. Its sole purpose was and is here to be a useful tool for (Gestalt) psychotherapy. Hence the only criterion for validity of this theory should be: does it prove to be helpful for the general orientation of the therapist, and their perceptions and interventions? This theory does not attempt to do more than fulfil such a pragmatic function – even if it should also turn out to be helpful for gaining psychological and sociological insights beyond its immediate aim. In fact I do believe that it could make a valuable contribution to a general theory of action or interaction in sociology, but this is not the point I wish to make in this book.

Each psychotherapy process starts either explicitly or implicitly with an idea of what is "normal" and what is "disturbed". This theory of the contacting process describes what is considered "normal" from a Gestalt therapeutic perspective. Such a model of "normality" is the assumed background from which the "disturbances" of the patient take shape ("weak gestalts") in the eyes of the therapist. The limits of the model emerging from this theory consist in setting boundaries around what can be considered a psychological "disturbance", and therefore as material for therapeutic work; and what are really not suitable subjects for therapy, like political adversity, economic hardship, physical illness. Still, it is part of the ethos of psychotherapy to assume, possibly contra-factually, that the potential and resources of the afflicted person are always more extensive than they assume at any given moment – therapists, too, can have astounding experiences.

I. Figure and ground

The process of Gestalt formation in the contacting situation

Each organism lives embedded in an environment, with which it exchanges energy, material and information. The same is true for the human organism; just like any other living being, they are an "autopoetic" system. It is an organization of parts, which perennially renews itself in "anabolic" (increasing) and "katabolic" (decreasing) processes, while over time no cell and no molecule remains the same.[1] These processes of change are responsive to their environmental source systems which in turn are embedded in higher order systems or aggregations of subsystems. Such an organism-in-context field never achieves complete homeostasis. It is ruled by its constant need to be replenished by material, energy and information from its environment. The organism is therefore "open" to its environment – and this in turn is open towards more encompassing systems – i.e. it is dependent on exchange and oriented towards new experience. Only by assimilating something new can an organism grow; growth in turn is the definition of life. The process by which the organism absorbs something new from its environment we call the *contacting process.* The contacting process encompasses the perception of new information from the environment, the differentiation between something that can be assimilated and something that cannot; it refers to moving towards that which is new and can be assimilated, as well as the incorporation of the new and its assimilation.

At this point it already becomes clear that the project of describing such processes in words encounters difficulties which will occur again and again as we proceed. The model of the contacting process corresponds to Heraclitus' famous saying: "Everything flows". However, our language quickly meets limitations when we try to describe processes. It is not orientated towards processes and functions, but designed to describe things and qualities. It is not oriented towards dynamic interactions, but towards static opposites. "Subject" and "object", "mind" and "matter", "biological" and "cultural", "inner world" and "outer world", "rational" and "emotional" – we could almost continue this list of opposites arbitrarily, which inform our patterns of thinking, and which in turn make it difficult to formulate and understand interdependencies in organism/environment relationships. Thus the concept of a "field of organism/environment relationships" suggests a flat plain clearly delineated with certain properties. Instead, in this context "field" is intended to suggest fluid interchanges of all functions of growth and change in shifting contexts of interactions between organism and environment.

The human organism and its specific environment show some particularities which need to be clarified before I can describe the contacting process in detail. I understand human beings as body-soul-spirit unities, as living systems, which have spiritual, emotional and bodily functions in perennial interplay with each other and never occurring separately. This should be remembered when I talk frequently about the human organism, rather than simply about human beings or individuals. Each thought is a bodily process too; each emotion has cognitive aspects, and the potential and limitations of our being a body have an effect on our mental and psychic condition – in just the same way that our thinking and feeling has an influence on our body.

Beyond this, an organism can only be defined in the context of their changing environments. Other than animals, which through the structure of their senses and their genetic codes are conditioned always to live in their specific environments, human beings can and must form and organize their environment themselves. Of course, some animals are also extremely adaptable with regard to some environmental conditions, but they adapt thanks to their organic endowment, something human beings do not have in the same way. We must compensate for our instinctual insecurity and the relatively limited development of our sensory endowment by the use of planning and technology. Humans are, as Johann Gottfried Herder said, "invalids of their higher powers".

The human organism is biologically programmed to improve its sense organs through inventions and to change its environment through discoveries. Telescopes and glasses are not external to human beings but are part of our anthropological potential. Changing our environment, indeed, is an anthropological necessity. In order to reproduce, human beings are forced to adapt nature; changing nature is not just a possibility but is imperative for survival. Of course, these adaptations have to take place according to the laws of nature. More than ever before we are confronted with the fact that we are not merely capable of making our environment more hospitable (for us!), but also of making it more inhospitable. Since we did eat of the fruit of the Tree of Knowledge, the problem here is created not so much by our knowledge, as by our ignorance and the complacency that always accompanies limited knowledge. The Tree of Knowledge is like the Hydra: each bit of knowledge generates new questions and expands our awareness that there is an infinity of things we do not know. But there is no return to pre-lapsarian times; we must continue to question, to search, to quest and explore. Therefore, the real problem at present is not that we have too much science, but that we have too little – and in some respects the wrong kind of science. Intellectual endowment is part of human nature, and the nature of our environment is its adaptability.

From the outset, working on nature has been a social process. Especially through the extremely long socialization period, cooperation with others – communication, that is – has always been a condition of human nature. In that way, the means and forms of production and reproduction are social from the beginning. In other words, the human organism is a social organism and the forms of social organization are expressions of the respective conditions of production. Also, being aware of their own death, human beings need to make sense of their existence. In this way, we "cultivate" our natural and social environment through interpretive patterning and symbolic rituals which change in interaction with and in response to particular historical conditions of production.[2] For human beings therefore, environment is always an already formed and perennially adaptable system of objects and symbolic elements with bodily, social and cultural functions.

The human organism does not encounter this environment *in abstracto,* but in specific *concrete contacting situations*, whose spatial and temporal horizons contain everything that is given here and now. In thought and fantasy we can transcend the limits of the situation, but as a body/soul unit we are always situated in a (specific) situation, and only in such situations can new things be encountered, new experiences be made. Only within given situations – no matter how they may be adapted – can the human organism undertake the task imposed on us: to adapt *creatively* to the given environment. It consists in discovering and inventing something new, the objects of our need satisfaction. This means that what is *given* in a situation is not the endless amount of physical, social and cultural data it contains, but whatever stirs our curiosity, attracting and binding our attention and demanding that we concentrate – compared with which everything else fades into the background as irrelevant, eventually becoming unnoticed.

Therefore, contacting situations are not only circumscribed by a space/time dimension but they are also contoured by a "structure of relevance of what is simultaneously given",[3] which gradually develops in the contacting situation. We distinguish between more or less relevant information and make this distinction according to our spontaneously emerging need or deferred needs active in this situation. The concept of contact boundary is crucial here. It is the point where organism and environment touch each other, the point where all sensorimotor attention increasingly gathers. It is foreground, the figure or Gestalt which arises as the most relevant information from the background, focussing according to changing degrees of relevance or irrelevance – until even this background fades, and all attention is focussed exclusively on this one point alone of encounter with the environment.

The contact boundary is therefore not identical with our skin, which we normally experience as the boundary between "inside" and "outside". Instead, the point of contact shifts from "inside" to "outside", even erasing this distinction for a brief moment and returning from "outside" back to "inside". Food intake can serve as an example. Frederick Perls took food intake to be the prototypical paradigm of exchange processes between organism and environment. I experience hunger – a bodily sensation in my stomach; my senses organize themselves so that my attention is directed towards food related contexts and gets aroused by this stimulus. I see the cold buffet, or I smell the smells which come from the kitchen. Next in line are certain processes of orientation – I choose objects for the satisfaction of my need, I weigh the costs (time, money, social and moral considerations) and perhaps I defer satisfaction of my need. Now the manipulation of the environment begins: I reach out, break the bread, cut the meat or boil the potatoes. This is where the positive aspect of aggression comes in – literally and metaphorically cutting into pieces, fragmenting – a de-structuring of whatever food the environment makes available to me: adapting nature. This aggressive process is continued in tearing apart, chewing and swallowing. In relishing the taste while chewing, the culmination of the contact process is achieved; the exclusive sensorimotor attention of the organism is now focused on the mouth, the momentary contact point between organism and environment. Finally, a sense of satisfaction is achieved, and the figure of food pales again as the arousal of the organism diminishes and at last disappears altogether. The organism can now integrate whatever it can assimilate and eliminate what is left.

This example can – with appropriate modifications – be transferred to other contacting processes. My attention can be just as much captivated by an intellectual problem as by an erotically attractive person – in an uninterrupted contacting process, my cognitive and affective capacities and my sensorimotor functions are focused on the contact boundary, where for this specific experience organism and environment merge. This specific unity of experience creates the relevant figure or Gestalt, which is set apart from the background of the remaining field of organism/environment.

The concept of figure or Gestalt is used to describe experience, illustrating how we experience "world" as that which we encounter at any time in the field of organism/environment. Therefore adjustments of the contact boundary, the point of connection, are identical with the fluid changes of figure/ground constellations, the process of Gestalt formation. Whatever is happening at the contact boundary – activated by need – rouses our attention, and this in turn organizes attention, will and action. They interact to shape the figure, which rises from a background of less relevant information. The curve described by the contact boundary is identical with the curve of the intensity of the organism's sensorimotor and affective excitement, which in our example culminates in tasting and chewing the food. The function of this *excitement* is to mobilize the organism's energies, to sharpen its capacity for attending and orienting, and to increase its power to create Gestalts, so that all its might is directed towards assimilating whatever is new.

Through this contacting process we experience and learn something about our world. Whatever we experience as real happens at the contact boundary and touches the whole of the human organism. Through experience we attain growth and maturity, a renewal of life and an increase in competency. Through this contacting process alone we experience *a feeling of reality.* Psychologically speaking, we experience subjectively as real only that which we experience at the contact boundary – that which subsequently proves successful through the satisfaction of our needs – or creates frustration by resisting satisfaction. Importantly from a sociological point of view, another aspect is relevant: that we need confirmation of such experiences by others, especially if we are dealing with symbolically mediated contacting processes. However real an experience at the contact boundary has been for a person, if it fails in the long run to gain social validation by others, it radically isolates the person from community. It can even trigger a psychotic episode. The very reality, therefore, which the human organism is capable of experiencing "body and soul", is inter-subjectively constituted in contacting processes.

2 The phases of the contacting process

The unfolding of the self

Goodman calls the energy process through which the human organism copes with their environment – perennially replenishing its lack by absorbing something new – the "self".[4] The "self" therefore is nothing substantial or static, but a process: with every arousal of need or interest the self unfolds, and with each satisfaction it disappears again.

> Let us call the "self" the system of contacts at any moment. As such the self is flexible and different in different situations, for it varies with the dominant organic needs and the pressing environmental stimuli. It is the system of responses, it diminishes in sleep when there is less need to respond. The self is the contact boundary at work; its activity is forming figures and grounds.
>
> (Perls & Goodman:11)

The model of the contacting process does not know a static Ego-identity. Human beings experience themselves when they are interested in something new, and experiences gained previously are elements of the psychic and social competencies which constitute part of what presently motivates action. The reality of our biographical continuity is being reconstructed anew in the contacting process: we re-write our history in the interest of what is currently given (Berger, 1969).

This means that the self is the energetic force behind the formation of Gestalts in the organism/environment field. The clearer the figure arising from the background, and the more our sensorimotor attention is focused on the figure as it arises at the contact boundary, the more fully the self unfolds. In essence the self is identical with the process of Gestalt formation, since the figure embodies all the interests of the self, and the self is nothing but its current interest. The figure now arises with the need and disappears as the need is satisfied. Since self and environment meet and inter-fuse in the figure, the full experience of the self is the ever new and passing experience of a deeper union of body and the surrounding field, the lived oneness of the organism/environment field. This description also enables us to define *meaningfully* the concept of *self-realization* which is frequently misused today: *self-realization* means to enter into spontaneous contact processes, to allow them to run their course, and to let go of them once satisfaction has been achieved. Letting go, then, the dissolution of the self, is death lived in life, the experience of satisfaction through life itself.

When we look more closely at the contacting process, we can differentiate various stages of self-realization: fore-contact; orientation and manipulation; integration; post-contact. During fore-contact the self awakens to the possibility of an experience of aliveness; during orientation and manipulation the self is fully engaged in the exploration and re-shaping of this new environment; during integration it achieves climax – and during post-contact it gradually fades again. With respect to the Gestalt formation process, one could describe these phases as follows:

Fore-contact: A need arises in the organism or is triggered by an environmental stimulus. Need and stimulus can barely be differentiated: a hungry person sees (or fantasizes about) nourishment, but also sight or smell of food generate appetite. Need and environmental stimulus then generate a figure which is set apart from the background of the body and less stimulating parts of the environment. The organism spontaneously senses that a need has arisen, and most likely senses which of several needs should first be satisfied. In such contact situations which mostly in our society don't arise spontaneously, rather following patterns of social arrangement for the (direct and indirect) satisfaction of regularly occurring needs (e. g. work meetings, social events, shared meals, erotic contacts), this phase of pre-contact is usually filled with rituals of greeting epitomized in small talk.

Orientation and Manipulation (in Perls & Goodman "contacting"): At this point the need – while remaining the engine of the sensorimotor activity of the organism – moves into the background of the experience, while the potential objects of need satisfaction move into the foreground. Such objects (in Freudian terms, libidinal objects) can be concrete (food) as well as virtual (ideas), but mainly they are concerned with other human beings as partners in a variety of interactions. Equally, the object of need satisfaction is not always identical to the aim and purpose of an action: the joy of climbing mountains is more than just reaching the top, and the pleasure of taking a bath is not limited to being clean by the end of the process. Feelings of attraction and aversion may develop in relation to possible objects in the contacting situation. These are initially spontaneous orientations of the organism in the given environment. In social situations we now leave behind rituals of greeting and meaningless small talk and begin to be interested in the task at hand – the challenging topic of conversation, the exciting presentation, the fascinating other. Sensual and cognitive orientation occurs simultaneously with turning physically and with resolute grasp. Differentiating situational givens into objects of relevance also implies *negation* – discarding, pushing aside of unattractive possibilities, which seem indigestible and uninteresting – as well as *affirmation* through turning towards that which is desired, moving towards it and reaching for it. Whatever is interesting is being identified and grasped; whatever is uninteresting is blanked out or pushed aside. The configuration of the contact situation according to criteria of relevance takes place through orientation and manipulation.[5] This manoeuvre is necessarily aggressive – grasping affirmatively; destroying or eliminating whatever is irrelevant.

Integration (in Perls & Goodman "final contact"): At this point, the Gestalt is discovered and invented, immediately appearing conspicuously in the foreground, pushing everything else aside. The organism merges with the object of its need. This peak of the contacting process constitutes a situation of healthy confluence of organism and environment: The "Thou" of my partner fills my experience completely, or I become as one with the task in hand, or – in aesthetic experience – I am "all ears and eyes". In sexual encounter the contacting process is completed with orgasm, an experience which is perhaps the most obvious example of what is meant by integration of need and object. The organism forsakes all intentional planning and action. Perception, feeling and motor activity work together spontaneously and allow boundaries between self and other to become permeable. The self is merged completely with their experience. I am, literally as well as metaphorically, gripped as I grip. The paradox of our existence – to have and to be a body – is momentarily resolved – and with this I leave my-self behind.

Post-contact (as Perls & Goodman use it, this is part of the full-contact-circle, with "final contact" as the last phase of this circle): The timeless moment of integration of course does not last. As I come back to "myself", organism and environment gradually separate out; slowly the figure pales. Yet, post-contact is an important stage of the contacting process. Only at this point, as the new experience slowly resonates in the organism, does assimilation of the new learning begin and the contacting process become a satisfying experience. Whatever has been assimilated has been digested in peace, the body now needs to relax and regenerate. Our capacity for absorption is exhausted and needs a break, before we can "change gear" for other contacting processes. In social interaction there are countless variations of ritualized post-contacts: the "social" part of work meetings, visiting the restaurant after the theatre, the shared breakfast after a night of love, many forms of saying goodbye. Everything that was important has been said and done – and still, there is a need to make extra time for silence, for thanking the other, for the return to the temporal and physical conditions of the organism/environment field. A contacting process without post-contact is worse than one which does not get beyond the pre-contact phase. In the one I remain hungry until the next time; in the other I am full, but not satisfied.

These four phases of the contacting process systematically build on each other. They are – from a phenomenological perspective – *grounded* in each other. In practice this means that none of the stages can be skipped without damage to the next. If the fore-contact is left out, the need remains diffuse or arises suddenly and overwhelmingly in the middle of the contacting process as an organismic impulse, as in bulimia. Attempting to leave out orientation and the setting up of an appropriate context leads to engagement without appropriate regard for distance, careless action and frequently regressive fantasies. They are bound to miscarry in view of the immediate actuality. If the contacting process is not completed through the integration of need and object, nothing new has been absorbed – and without appropriate ending through post-contact the organism has difficulties or may even be unable to integrate whatever was new.

In the normal course of events many contacts end after the fore-contact or fail to achieve satisfaction through full integration. This does not mean that they are pathological. The behaviour pattern of delayed gratification is part of the organism's characteristics and is possibly an aspect of the basic requirements of social interaction. Finally we need to consider that within the same social event different kinds of contact situations quickly follow on from each other. They can be superimposed on each other or interlaced like Russian dolls, and therefore social reality is almost always more complex than it appears in the model of the contacting process. And this is even truer when we consider that in social situations, the contacting processes of different participants in the interaction cross over or complement each other. The model of the contacting process in the first instance is primarily designed for one acting subject. To describe the whole of the interactional web of the organism/environment field in a social situation is another task, and rather one for sociological theory. For the purpose of psychotherapy it suffices to analyse the contacting process from the perspective of just one participant of the interaction: the patient.

If the self is defined as the activity of figure/ground formation in the contacting process, this of course does not mean that the process happens unconsciously. Quite the opposite – self-unfolding is experienced as an increasingly alert sensory-intellectual process of *attentiveness*, which grips the whole organism. This experience of the self experiencing itself, its deepest modus of experience, is perhaps captured best in the English word "awareness" which encompasses consciousness without being identical with its purely cognitive aspects. With these I can focus on a problem and think about its solution. But awareness as I use it here is an intense holistic experience of the world as presently given in the specific contact points between me and my environment here and now, which always includes emotional aspects.

3 The instincts

Needing and desiring

Gestalt therapy emerged from the debate with psychoanalysis. Both Perls and Goodman were deeply impressed with Freud, each in his own way struggling with him as a father figure. Therefore, it is not wrong that Gestalt therapy has occasionally been called a neo-analytical school; after all, Frederick Perls and his wife Laura, who had a deep influence on the development of Gestalt therapy, were both trained psychoanalysts. And so it is not surprising that Goodman occasionally borrows aspects of Freud's meta-psychology when he describes the different functions of the self. He speaks about *id functions, ego-functions* and *personality functions* of the self. Self-unfolding in the contacting process begins with developing needs and appetites – the *id functions.* Then it searches for objects related to these needs in its environment and creates a Gestalt through sensorimotor orientation and manipulation – the *ego-functions.* Finally new experiences and abilities gained in the contacting process are assimilated – the *personality functions.* (Gestalt therapy can do without the construction of a *super-ego*, since from the perspective of the model of the contacting process it consists entirely of neurotic introjects.[6])

Initially, these distinctions were meant to help a psychoanalytically trained public to understand Gestalt theory. Today they are still valuable in helping the therapist to be alert to the following two points:

- Disturbances in experiencing needs, i.e. in the id functions, are more serious and need to be treated differently from disturbances of personality functions. The earlier processes might lead to psychotic symptoms, whereas the latter relate to narcissistic processes and in the worst case to psychopathic processes without any awareness of the environment.
- From a Gestalt therapeutic perspective, disturbances of id functions and personality functions can only be worked with if the patient has a sensory experience of how he continually reproduces these malfunctions through blocking off different ego-functions in fore-contact, orientation and adaptation, in integration and during post-contact phases. In Gestalt therapeutic work we address the process of how the patient blocks, obstructs or weakens his ego-functions in the contacting process.[7]

Beyond this, orientation for therapeutic practice distinguishing these three functions is barely relevant and therefore will not be considered in the following more detailed examination of the activities of the self at the contact boundary.

At the beginning of each contacting process is a need. The organism experiences scarcity which can only be assuaged by assimilating something new from the environment. Each need is experienced as a lack of something, and only through this lack does a specific organism/environment constellation become fore-contact, the first phase of any contacting process.

The organism experiences lack – initially vaguely, then more clearly – and begins to reach out beyond its own resources; energy is required for doing so. But simultaneously, it opens out into its environment, takes in, processes and absorbs, compensates for lack, feels satisfied. The objects of the environment are not "libidinally charged" but are part of intentional actions of the thinking and acting human being. The self is not juxtaposed to the aims and objects of its desiring, but from the beginning it is in sensuous and cognitive contact with them, shapes them through this contact into the figure arising from the background – not only of the environment but also of the organism itself.

Being in need is the experience of lack. Some deficits need to be equalized immediately; others can wait. The air we breathe is so necessary that we assume its presence without a second thought. Only when it is acutely lacking are we anxiously aware of how dependent we are on this environmental condition. Lack of warmth and food can be borne a little longer, but have to be relieved sooner rather than later. Other needs, some of them physical, do not need to be satisfied as long as survival is not at stake. The body does not die from lack of sexual satisfaction, although the organism as a whole suffers. Such suffering can only become foreground when other, more urgent needs are satisfied. Vienna's bourgeoisie, from which Freud recruited his patients, were a satisfied rich bourgeoisie able to afford acceptance of Freud's obsession with sexuality. If it were useful at all to speak about different drives, self-preservation would have to be accorded the first priority. In relation to individual survival the organism has clear physical priorities: air, food and warmth are its unquestioned first requirements.

But of course, human beings need a lot more; even an individual is part of the species and has needs which serve the maintenance of the species – biologically as well as socially and culturally. Without sexuality there would be no procreation, and without information and communication, society could not reproduce itself either individually or culturally.

Obviously, there is an order of priority of needs – yet it is very difficult to establish such an order with any clarity, as soon as we go beyond the most elementary descriptions. Abraham Maslow, one of the founders of Humanistic Psychology, made a suggestion which can fruitfully be used with the model of the contacting process (Maslow, 1954a; Hondrich, 1975). Maslow differentiates five groups of needs which respectively are foregrounded in the phases of the psycho-social developmental process of human beings. To begin with there are the physiological needs for food and warmth; in the second phase we are dealing with needs for protection and security; thirdly there are the social needs for being loved, accepted, belonging; in the fourth phase needs for status, appreciation and esteem are in the foreground and finally, in the last phase, the focus is on "self-realization" (this expression is meant in a somewhat more extended, more existential way than the term "self-actualization" used by Maslow although the relationship should be clear) and personal fulfilment. In this model it is essential that the conditions for satisfying the needs of the prior phase are secured before the needs of the following phase can be fully experienced and become the paramount impetus for action. Of course, elementary needs are never permanently satisfied – we need nourishment daily, and of course the desire to be loved emerges again and again. But only once the individual has achieved sufficient social and psychological competency to get what it needs from its environment, and only if this environment is sufficiently equipped with resources, can it continue to unfold and develop new needs on other levels.

Maslow's model is open and flexible enough to withstand three challenges which can in principle be raised against any attempt to establish a catalogue of human needs. Psychology, sociology and anthropology each raise one particular concern.

There is no human need which can be satisfied forever. That is true even for so-called childish needs, which secretly remain adult longings; it is not the need for maternal care or paternal orientation that is childish, just a perennial fixation onto the same person to satisfy these needs. Our lives take place in a complex tangle of contacting processes initiated by our needs, some of which regularly repeat themselves while others arise afresh. Significantly, some of them gain greater importance in each life phase. Our energy flows into those contacting processes which are currently of greatest interest for us, those which are motivated by needs which focus our anxieties and hopes, the new needs, whose satisfaction we cannot yet achieve with our felt competency. For instance, sexual encounters are always exciting; but only in puberty, when sexual needs first fully unfold, do they obtain that irretrievable significance which often makes all other contacting processes pale into insignificance.

In that way, Maslow's model allows space for the ever changing and developing order of relevance of the daily contacting processes throughout life. It also shows that psychological disturbances can arise from the hierarchy of needs being turned upside down if, for example, under the pressure of (often internalized) societal expectations, we may look to satisfy needs of a higher order when the competency for a problem-free satisfaction of more elementary needs has not yet been achieved. Normally the organism automatically regulates the order of priority in such situations. But if the experience of an overriding basic need is sufficiently strong to distract us from currently active contacting processes, a significant delay of need satisfaction would diminish or disable the organism's ability to fully function. If in turn primary needs are satisfied, the organism flourishes on other levels too and begins to sense more subtle needs. Thus the psychoanalytical concept of sublimation makes no sense within the theory of the contacting process. Of course, in this theory too, sexuality is a core need – but not the only one. The model of the contacting process entails the inexhaustible range of human needs and interests in a perennially changing organism/environment field. Each contacting process is *sui generis* and has its specific needs and satisfactions. The book I write, the mental activity which I am engaged with, is not a compensation for absent sexuality. If there is a connection at all, it would be that lack of sexual satisfaction would deter me from my work. Sexual images would replace theoretical imagination.

The second proviso refers to the *historical and cultural* variability of human needs. Bertolt Brecht's famous contention that first there is food, then there is morality, was less an anthropological diagnosis than a political demand. Whatever is postulated as a basic need or even as a human right – some of them sometimes even realized! – depends on prevailing power distributions and on how rich a society is. Maslow takes this into account by measuring the relations between labour and capital (Maslow speaks about "cultures") against the same standards. Whatever can be experienced as a need at all depends on the level of economic and cultural development of a society (or a social grouping). Where hunger still prevails (even today) we will look in vain for a need for individual self-realization. And whoever in our society is threatened by loss of work, will prioritize security needs. But whoever has a secure place of work may suddenly have a question regarding whether they are receiving sufficient recognition and whether they are able to use their abilities in a satisfactory way.

The third proviso refers to an *anthropological* problem: we human beings are able to say "No" – even to our needs. Knowing about the unavoidability of dying, in the final analysis, we can even deny life itself. Appropriately, we recognize today that suicide often tends to be a neurotic solution to a problem which has nothing to do with wishing to die. But in view of this we must not forget that beyond all psychological reflection this possibility of a final irrevocable "No" is a basic figure of our human condition, which in many different ways co-determines our lives. In our current context this has two implications. First of all, as stated, the satisfaction of higher needs can be deferred; secondly, the satisfaction of all needs can be rejected once and for all.

The first case is of primary importance: without the behavioural pattern of deferred gratification there is neither cooperation nor culture. It seems that this requires no further explanation, and yet from a Gestalt therapeutic point of view we have to keep checking whether somebody has consciously chosen to defer their need satisfaction, or whether deferral derives from habitually internalized norms, of which the person is unaware, i.e. introjects. Of course, there are frequently good reasons for deferring need satisfaction – perhaps because another need satisfaction seems to be more achievable, even while it is less urgent; or the situation does not allow more than fore-contact and a first orientation; or consideration of other people may suggest this course. It remains important that the original need can still be sensed and that the deferral takes place with insight and as a free decision. Of course, however tedious, some things need to be accomplished; some rules need to be kept. But it is also possible to surrender to the tasks, surrender to learning and to the recognition that the rules of social intercourse are also rules which allow new room for play. In other words, doing *anything* can become the object of a fascinating contacting process.

Forever insisting on "self-realization" is frequently nothing more than the desire for narcissistic gratification, while on the other hand any skewed orientation towards focussed action and simply getting stuff done often merely expresses an introjected achievement orientation.

The sociological theory of deferred gratification can easily become an ideology, which conceals the problems of alienated labour (Dreitzel, 1973). From a Gestalt therapeutic perspective it is centrally important to determine whether the delayed need can still be experienced, is still allowed to be noticed and will motivate future contacting needs; or whether it is repressed to avoid having to experience the meaninglessness of those socially expected actions and the helplessness which arises in the face of overwhelming social pressures.[8]

The second case is more complicated. It is one of the unique potentials of human beings to be able to distance ourselves a little from our bodies, putting its needs on hold in favour of higher aims. Asceticism, though, is a position which has become alien to our society. It seems that even in the religious sphere, where there is a tradition of asceticism, renunciation is now rarely seen as a necessary condition for spiritual experience (the exception being the stubborn refusal of the Catholic Church to give up celibacy and its denial of homosexuality). Still, ascetic behaviour is a foundational figure of our human experiential potential. If a person's concern is focused on the beyond, such a search is beyond the range of therapeutic model (as for instance if they decide to die by refusing to eat) – except if the patient is being forced by institutional or introjected rules.

Whenever we meet attitudes of secular asceticism, we must always ask whether this is forced by a low standard of living due to lack of resources or simply a manifestation of exploitation. Today we no longer need our work to produce ever more food, but we do not know how to distribute food (or whatever else is produced in surplus quantities) except through institutionalized labour. In the work of the psychotherapist it remains of crucial importance to determine whether a person with full awareness and competency says "No" (for instance in case of sexual assault or if they fast voluntarily), or whether they find themself forced by social pressure to forego erotic satisfaction. If this kind of social pressure is internalized we are dealing with introjects which can be worked with therapeutically in the hope of extending the realm of decision-making freedom within the client. If such socio-economic pressures are consciously experienced, though, (e.g. in non-voluntary lack of work), psychotherapy can only work indirectly through strengthening personal competences, all of which always have a political dimension. Let us not forget that there is no true renunciation of anything, unless there has been a fully embodied experience of it – where we dealing with a "No" from a position of psychological and social autonomy.

It begins with small things: first I have to sense what I need, what is necessary, where the lack is located. Only after this come the desires. The order of priority of needs becomes real again in any contacting situation – in sensing what I need now, in thoughts about what I now desire. "An animal", the German philosopher Ernst Bloch says, "relates to the aim of its need in exactly the same way as is entailed in the need itself, whereas humans create an image of it as well" (Bloch, 1961:58). Bloch's critique of Freud's theory of instincts (Bloch, 1961) is relevant also for Gestalt therapy: in human beings the relation between need and object is mediated through abstractions. At first I sense a need and immediately recognize a class of objects which might serve to alleviate this lack. "Food" would satiate my hunger, "(wo)men" would assuage my sexual appetite, "something warming" would take care of feeling cold – and so on.

But only in situations of extreme scarcity will such generalizations suffice – then I don't care what I eat and which (wo)man satisfies my craving. "Beggars can't be choosers", the saying goes. A German proverb observes that "when desperate, the devil even eats flies". The devil here is the animal in the human being: our most elementary needs, our survival instinct. When lack is so desperate that it eats us up from within, there is no preferring any longer. Then I know nothing beyond my need. Normally, though, a specific desire emerges from the experience of need, the image of something concrete following the abstraction. It is *this* food I'd like to eat; I'd like to sleep with *this* person; a *hot bath* would be just right to warm me up. Our desires and hopes go beyond generalizations which would help to assuage the need – without going into the blue yonder. It is the desire which concretizes – at first just imaginatively – the objects of need satisfaction, making an initial choice which (as long as we are dealing with action-orientated wishing and not just with daydreaming) is connected to previous experience. Wishing contains an anticipation of satisfaction which of course could also become the basis for negation. Only at this stage can I tell myself that I am not going to fulfil my desire in just *this* way or not *now*. And through this, the other function of wishing becomes foreground, i.e. its capacity to consolidate into *wanting,* pointing beyond the current situation. The delayed gratification is now nothing but the unfulfilled need, which is going to determine what I want in subsequent similar contacting processes.[9] Each wanting has to arise from need. Wishes grow without limit or dissipate unless they remain rooted in the prior sense of lack. They must relate to what is actually available, not drawing energy away from the contacting process. Otherwise, desire achieved does not lead to real satisfaction, and a sense of lack remains. If on the other hand general hunger unfolds into a specific appetite – triggered and guided equally by the recollection of previous experience as well as through the appeal of the new – then we know what we want; fore-contact is complete and a new phase of the contacting process begins.

4 Sensorimotor functions

Perceiving and acting

At this point the contact boundary shifts from "inside" to "outside". Concurrently with something being noticed incidentally – which then serves to activate and animate the process through which wanting and wishing become more concrete – the picture of what is wished for and wanted becomes a template for perception. Now the organism reaches beyond itself, leaves mere fantasy behind and begins – through activating its senses – to enter the process of Gestalt formation which is always a process of discovery and invention at once. The objects which trigger interest gradually emerge from a background which takes shape according to different relevancies of the situation, and group themselves around the contact boundary like a halo becoming darker at the edges. Part of this background is the body. The image of desire already became slightly distant from it in separating itself from the mere sense of need. Only while in physical pain or when experiencing the social pain of acute embarrassment does the body – often vehemently – become foreground and physicality become figure. Normally at this point the "inner" perceptions lose interest and weight compared to what demands attention from the "outside".

The image of a halo must not seduce us to exclusively think about the eye (seeing). All our senses are involved in the contacting process at the same time; they work together syn-aesthetically, even while first this, then that sense is in the lead. This explains why, if one of the senses is disabled, the others can to some extent compensate for this failing by working together. Seeing and touching especially co-operate in such a way that by "touching" things with our eyes and "seeing" them with our hands we seem to grasp their form and significance at once. The baby learns to comprehend the world first by grasping with its hands. Today it is well understood that there is an intimate connection between the development of the senses in the child and the growth of its cognitive abilities. This means that neither the senses nor the cognitive functions can be understood in separation from the motor functions of the human body. As the philosopher Helmuth Plessner in his phenomenological research on the functioning of the human senses noted:

> Sensorimotor function is the operative word. The senses, considered on their own, do not yield the secret of their diversity. Only embedded in the complete organism whom they simultaneously serve and rule – as is always the case with serving – can we begin to understand them in their encompassing unity.
>
> (Plessner, 1970a, p. 244)

In order to fully fathom and appreciate the connection between the openness of our relationship with the environment and the experience of our physicality, we need a philosophical anthropology of the senses developed in the phenomenological tradition as worked out by Helmuth Plessner (1964), Erwin Strauss (1980) and Maurice Merleau-Ponty (Merleau-Ponty 1962). It defines the function of the senses in the contacting process by starting with our specifically human patterns of behaviour. "Looked at from the outside we are determined by our upright walk, from the inside through our instrumental relationship with our own bodies. This in turn refers back to our ability to objectify" (Plessner, op. cit.:244). Walking upright permits the hand-eye field to be freely available and thus we gain the capacity for variable space perception. In particular, our instrumental relationship with the body allows human beings to advance beyond the stimulus-response pattern. When physically we turn with all our senses to the environment, we use ourselves as instruments and thereby open ourselves to the world.

We have the ability to perceive movement in the environment along with the experience of being able to move arbitrarily; and therefore human beings can – as it were – spur ourselves on as well as reining ourselves in. Our precarious situation – to have a body and yet to be a body, to be within and outside ourselves at once – forces us to establish a balance which is the cradle of human action. "This is the reason why human beings cannot divest themselves of their motor functions and have to slide again and again into the active mode" (Plessner, op. cit.:245). This feeds back into the work of the senses; whatever can be grasped has already been seen in such a way; that which can be achieved is being distinguished from the unachievable; the manipulation of the environment is being anticipated even in the act of perception itself.

Seeing and touching complement each other in human beings in such a way that sensory experiences immediately organize themselves into action possibilities. In comparison, the sense of **smell** is less important and today less necessary as a means of orientation from a distance. Instead, it has become a means for enhancing the experience of physical closeness. For this reason it is the sense most shaped by civilization, even though among all the senses, cerebrally it is the most ancient one. Nowadays, it mainly serves to segregate "pure" nature through creating spontaneous disgust.[10]

Hearing, though, is of cardinal importance, partly because it extends our special orientation beyond that which we can see; even more so, because it adds the temporal to the spatial dimension of perception. Of course, seeing movement in itself creates a sense of time; the eye can attach itself to something immoveable, even if it is not able – nor permitted – to remain still. Sounds, though, fade and repeat themselves: time passes. Remembering sound that has faded, and listening out for a repetition, we can experience time. In this case too, we cannot separate one sense from another, cannot isolate any of them from our motor function. The unity of the senses is constitutive for the specific human organism/environment relationship. Biologist Francois Jacob writes:

> It is most likely that the pressure of natural selection for hominids favoured spatial perception through use of the ears so that sources of sound could be more easily localized. This way, an ever better and more coherent image of a spatial and temporal world emerged where moving

> objects could simultaneously be heard, seen, smelt and touched. Since the temporal continuity of these objects was certain, it was possible to store their representation in memory. The way this representation is organised has consequences, especially for two remarkable properties of the brain. In the first instance, it is possible to deconstruct these stored images into their constitutive parts, and they then can be put together again into representations and situations which are new and beyond patterns which already exist. This capacity is the precondition for our ability not just to remember images of previous situations – but also to imagine contingent events, i.e. to invent a future. Through connecting acoustic perceptions of temporal sequences with regard to changes of the sensorimotor apparatus of the voice, it also becomes possible to symbolise and coordinate cognitive representations in a completely new way.
>
> (Jacob, 1976:23)

In this way, the sensorimotor unity of orientation and manipulation eventually leads to sensual awareness. But nevertheless, it is worth the effort to look at each of the five senses separately, at first physiologically and then with regard to the formations and deformations which the senses have undergone in the process of civilization. On all these levels we would see proof of the fact that our senses do not copy the world but discover and invent it – configurate it. Gestalt psychology has made an essential contribution to this recognition. The pictures of the Gestalt psychological experiments which convincingly show the tendency of our senses toward completion, toward creating foreground/background constellations, as well as showing the contextual dependency of perception, are accessible to anybody.

These properties of our perceptual apparatus need to be understood as cerebral patterns of functioning, resulting from the *experience* of our upright walk and the coordination of the hand-eye field. The theory of the contacting process takes one more step. The process of Gestalt formation does not just rest on the *experience* of different forms, but also depends on the interest which is generated by the objects. Perceiving and reaching out – orientation and manipulation – are guided by *experience,* but *driven by need:* controlled arbitrariness.

What is true for the individual and their biography can be generalized with little modification to the species and its history. The influence which the process of civilization has exercised – and still exerts – on our senses and our motor functions rests on new needs evolving as well as on socially required restraints. Ever since perspective as a perceptual modality was discovered, ever since optical science and optical technique and more recently the visual media have strongly favoured seeing over smelling, feeling one's way, touching and handling things, tactile experiences in general have become more marginal. Spheres of privacy and intimacy have been created, the centres of which are our bodies. So now fear of contact can also be experienced as the anxiety physically to touch and be touched.

The objects of the contacting process, human beings as well as things, increasingly are kept at a distance, because the body as body is not public. This is not contradicted but confirmed by the fact that today the body, barely concealed by any veils of shame, is visually presented in the media and on nudist beaches. This in itself is a distancing process. The incomparable refinement of our sensory equipment through technical instruments nowadays stands in juxtaposition to an increase in experienced distance to objects which we can perceive and manipulate. This includes the medicalization of the body. The contacting process, though, is a process of *incorporation* – both through our senses and symbolically – of that which must satisfy our needs and interests. Frequently we are overfed with abstract and incomprehensible ideas

Let us take a brief look on the phenomenon of **touching.** Human beings need the touch of skin, and this is not only true for the survival of new-born and small children. Modern research shows that under secure conditions and applied by trusted others, stroking, gentle caressing and massages produce hormones stabilizing the immune system; improve the functions of the hippocampus; reduce stress and depressive tendencies. These are only some of the beneficial effects found by researcher Thomas Grunwald working in his laboratory at the University of Leipzig, Germany (Grunwald, 2017), and others.

There is, however, a problem inherent in the closeness of touching: it invites the exercise of power, even violence. Since our bodies are not only the haven of our pleasure and lust but also harbour weaknesses, illnesses and decay they are always easily victimized and exploited by dominant others. Hence, physical contact with the body of the other can always be either friendly and supporting or hostile and dangerous, thus creating a peculiar mixture of longing and anxiety, a fact on which a whole historical anthropology could be built. Presently it seems that in Western society the process of civilization – always characterized by a tendency of growing distance between one's body and its objects – leads to a growing scarcity of touching contacts between strangers – meaning everybody who is not an actual sexual partner. Physical contacts between family members, even parents and their adult children, seem to diminish. Never before in history did average middle class citizens claim so much space in their habitation for individual use, thus increasing the distance between their bodies. Also singles living alone in their apartments seem to grow in number everywhere in the urbanized Western world (von Thadden, 2019). More and more the body is hungry for touch while our hands remain empty.

The search for correctives to the kind of instrumental reasoning which used to govern almost every sphere of our culture before the advent of populism has led to the development of many new therapies and physical exercises focussing on our capacity for mindful sensory awareness. The problem with many of these therapies is that we easily forget how little we still know about our senses and how they function psychologically. For example – why five? We can see and hear, smell and taste and touch. We also have a sense of equilibrium. But what about those senses which do not have any specific organs outside our brains? We have a sense of place and a sense of time, and we have a sense of beauty and of harmony. And what of intuition? Or our social capacity for picking up atmospheres of friendliness, hostility, interest and authority?

Sensory experiences – which have long been used and practised in the sensory awareness work of Charlotte Selver or in the bio-energetic schools of Alexander Lowen and John Pierrakos or in the focus on subtle energetic flows in Tarthang Tulku's Tibetan Kum Nye work – are difficult to spot through the Cartesian lenses of scientific medicine. The bitter fate of the late work of Wilhelm Reich is symptomatic of this situation, especially since his case is extreme. His speculative Orgone theory was condemned, not because it was scientifically disproved (which nobody bothered to check out), but because it generated political aversion to the point that his books were even publicly burned.[11]

Even today we cannot with any degree of certainty say anything about the significance for the organism of the electro-magnetic field which surrounds the body. But since time immemorial some people have claimed to be able to see such an aura. We also know nothing certain about the fine streams of energy, which begin to flow in acupuncture and while doing bio-energetic exercises. A major obstacle arises from the difficulties presented to the natural sciences by the human brain. An example would be the current conjecture of some scientists that we respond positively to light and negatively to darkness, because quanta of light reach for the deeply hidden pineal gland.[12] This leads us to the last question regarding the senses: how useful is it to speak about perception when we are dealing with so-called "subliminal perceptions" of which we are not consciously aware? For example, not only do we react to a sexually attractive image with an extension of our own pupils but we also notice this extension in the pupils of another person, i.e. we find them attractive at this moment – all without any conscious recognition of this process (Morris, 1978).

Of course, this is very significant for the contacting process. It appears as though we do not have much conscious awareness of any of the processes involved in sensory perception. Regarding the state of scientific study of "subliminal perception" in the early 1980s, brain researcher Helmut Emrich created a graphic image:

> Our cortical system for dealing with stimuli can be compared with a correctly working civil service department, where all incoming information is dealt with and – if appropriate – answered. The chief of the department (consciousness) does not see all the letters that come in or go out. Everything is dealt with according to existing guide lines (attitudes, values). Only new cases (novelty), unusual or complicated information are handed to "him". Only if he is not too busy may he look at

> something quite unimportant. Additionally, according to request, he will look at all letters which belong to a specific category (focussed attention). Everything else is dealt with correctly and according to rule by many civil servants. If any of them go on strike or fall ill – if there was no selectivity any more – the chief would be unable to cope with the flood of letters, and the department would grind to a halt (chaotic perception).
>
> (Emrich, 1983:192)

This model dethrones consciousness from its singular position as the authority over all decisions and turns it into one factor amongst many in the data processing system. Now, this does not mean that we have to give up the principle of the unity of the senses and its indissoluble connection with that "willed" motor function characteristic for human beings where they need to touch and seek touch. Instead, it is the pre-conscious selection of information which *enables* the organism to use directed attention to press ahead with the contacting process. This is not passive "data processing", but an *action modality* which includes motor functioning. We are no longer dealing with selection of data, but with its organization. Below the level of conscious awareness, and apparently due to inherited and learned programs, selected data is bundled into units and organized in such a way, that it activates and triggers the motor functions in all unproblematic cases, thereby making it relevant for actual behaviour.

5 Consciousness and awareness

Accepting and rejecting[13]

This analysis in the last section may not be the latest state of the art in brain research today but it marked an important change of our perspective on consciousness: it was no longer seen as the power controlling every detail of our daily struggle for survival but a much more flexible agency in the centre of a highly complex network awakening to activity especially in situations of crisis. This, then, comes close to the understanding of Perls & Goodman that caused them to replace the notion of consciousness with the word "awareness". For being aware means being excited and the degree of excitement will direct the degree of its intensity. There are good reasons for this replacement because it connects the activities of our mind directly to our needs and longings and hence to the environment's promises and dangers (notwithstanding M. V. Miller's contention that we are or should be dealing in Gestalt Therapy instead of awareness rather with attention would, if elaborated, shift the emphasis again on consciousness).

The image of the brain as a civil service department with consciousness as its chief, deciding important matters, needs to be checked regarding its actual usefulness as a model of the contacting process. In the past two decades brain research has made considerable progress and made some claims which have led to great hopes for some and a lot of criticism from others.

For a start, compare Damasio's position (Damasio, 2005). The human organism is not a body equipped with a "black box" (the brain) which like a computer has an input-output relationship with its environment, but is a self-aware, flexible subject which touches and stirs up its environment through seeing and conducting itself as part of this environment. The images of "department" and "authority" are too static for an organism which perceives, moves and acts in an ever changing environment, perennially restructuring it according to need. This action modality is typical for human beings as consciousness/awareness plays its part as a function of the contacting process.

The question is: which function? The psychological concept of consciousness with its many facets offers little help. Psychology has had a hard time overcoming the black box model. Only after conducting investigations along phenomenological lines was progress made and the basic intentionality of all action was recognized and emphasized: consciousness/awareness is always directed towards objects, which indeed are part of its very being. This creates the danger that we might see the environment simply as a phenomenon of consciousness, even while the organism obviously depends on incorporating parts of it – not just on the level of consciousness but also in very physical ways. This was the trap in which Husserl found himself by insisting on a programme of pure essentialism ("reine Wesensschau" = the idealistic turn of his philosophy). Gestalt therapy's use of Phenomenology can and should remain more modest. Suffice it that the phenomenological perspective stays focused on the insight that it is always consciousness/awareness of *something* and that this something presents itself for our attention as "new". If in addition we keep in mind that the object is intended and also differentiated from what is more relevant or less, down to the space/time horizon of the situation, we are on a safe Gestalt therapeutical line of thought. This way we remain informed, as the use of phenomenology in Gestalt therapy thinking originally was and should be, by the Gestalt-psychological insights about the dynamics of the fore-ground/background relations.

It is true though, that the essential character of contact, being a *process* with a *direction*, still remains too indistinct in this phenomenological conceptualization of intentionality. For it turns experiencing, thinking, and acting into undifferentiated aspects of the field of consciousness. Due to this Carl-Friedrich Graumann, the leading German psychologist of the phenomenological tradition in the last century, considered – with reference to Maurice Merleau-Ponty – letting go of the concept of consciousness altogether:

> Unfolding the complete structure of the concept of behaviour […], i.e. behaving-in-relation-to-something would serve us better than the overused concept of consciousness.

However, this just shifts the problem into another dimension, since now everything depends on how I behave: whether reactively-impulsive or

> intentionally-planning, whether sensuously-experiencing or rationally-planning, whether with alert attention or according to dull habit.
>
> (Graumann, 1966:19)

Another problem is the question of who is the originator of the acts of consciousness? Who chooses the senses we use, makes the choice of their object and decides on the intensity of their attention? A pure philosophy of consciousness quickly loses itself in conjectures about a transcendental subject as happened to Husserl. If on the other hand we acknowledge that we are dealing with an embodied organism which as subject constitutes the field of consciousness, we quickly see that intentionality does not characterize a dynamic independent of will and independent of need, but that it is a figure-ground process whose perspective is directed towards the interesting object which one has discovered and desires. This means: the subject of conscious acts is a living organism in interaction with its environments, and its consciousness has a (limited) control function in this process.

However, the organism/environment field of human beings remains vulnerable to problems arising from the paradoxical nature of our relationship with our bodies. Since human beings can and must use the body at will, we are to some extent free to act consciously. Even in situations where automatisms normally tend take over, we have developed through evolutionary processes or cultural training the potential to act consciously, as with breathing. Yawning can be repressed, the flow of the breath can be modulated, meditation can change the necessary intake of oxygen from 15 to 5 per minute (Young, 2014), and anxiety can be overcome. In the contacting process, though, whatever is new becomes paramount: that which has not yet been incorporated. And quite frequently it is the new that leads to problems.

Awareness entails consciously experiencing while acting on what is happening at the contacting boundary, a process of being in attentive contact with what is most relevant in the organism/environment field – based on fully activated sensorimotor, cognitive and energetic powers (Yontef, 1979). Sensual awareness describes the way the self experiences itself through its senses. It is the experience of being fully present in a situation, "being here now". Mobilization of sensorimotor attention is constellated when the contacting process is rooted in the currently dominant need of the organism and is animated by it – the organism orienting itself through action and according to the actual conditions of the situation – its specific inherent possibilities and obstacles which affect the satisfaction of current need. Margherita Spagnuolo Lobb in her extensive article on the somatic experience in Gestalt therapy (Spagnuolo Lobb, 2015) states:

> The idea that somatic experience is formed at the contact boundary between therapist and client in the here-and-now of the therapy session

> emancipates us from the intra-psychic mentality that sees the body as a container of "emotions" and conflicts that the client brings to therapy.
> (op. cit.:80)

The relationship between sensual awareness and the self is similar to that between experiencing emotions and expressing emotions (see part IV of this book): The more an emotion is expressed in mime and movement, the more intensely it is experienced – the more the self experiences itself with awareness, the more fully it unfolds; the contact boundary becomes more fully active and Gestalt formation becomes richer in the contacting process. Putting it slightly differently, the more a contacting process is *experienced with awareness* the more easily it becomes a satisfying experience. This is the reason for Gestalt therapy simply relying on increasing awareness, leaving the rest to the capacity for self-regulation of the organism/environment field.

It would be wrong, though, to deduce from this that human beings can do without consciousness (as defined above), to see in it nothing but an obstacle for spontaneous self-regulation. Perhaps, with their consistent exchange of the term consciousness by awareness Perls & Goodman were too optimistic in trusting the latter for its capacity of complete concentration – and also the power of self-regulation. Even full awareness of the contacting process, requiring the mobilization of all relevant senses and a focus on what is new, does not absolve us from hesitating for a moment, pausing, and from thoughtful deliberation, which in the final analysis is rooted in the paradoxical relationship with our bodies. Of course such hesitation can be exaggerated, so that each action is obscured by too much thought and consideration, rather than being illuminated by the light of its own endeavour. But normally, the body's instrumentality and the varying potential of the environment for reorganizing its Gestalt formation demand spontaneous thinking and perhaps some planning when difficulties arise in the contacting process. We may need to make judgements regarding the possibilities and dangers entailed in this situation. Beyond our daily routines we are constantly (and in today's terms more than ever) faced with choices, accepting or rejecting objects of need satisfaction, goals and strategies. All these mental activities are properly part of the functions of consciousness. Yet it remains true, as Margherita Spagnuolo Lobb insists, that "From a Gestalt point of view, any relationship with the other is always 'embodied', lived intensely on the aesthetic level, constantly mediated and activated by the perceptual channels, by the sensory system" (op. cit.:23). The important point here is that from the phenomenological perspective of Gestalt therapy the body is not an entity separated from the mind – the old Cartesian duality – but a mind-full organism as the organism is an embodied mind. Therefore it does not make sense to therapeutically focus on the body as an independent biological *corpus* but on the speaking body, the body as an expressive medium of the human organism.

This begins with thoughtful imagining: I picture what it would be like if I did X: what is possible, what significance would this or that of my possible actions have for me and for the other participants in the situation. But this first step of running through possibilities in imagination remains stuck with the images, while it is yet constitutive for the function of consciousness that it *differentiates through naming*. That is the specific process through which thinking of a fantasy becomes thinking with imagination. The old debate, whether thinking pre-supposes language or whether there is pre-linguistic thinking, is irrelevant here. It was the American social philosopher George Herbert Mead who first pointed out that every contacting process – including those with concrete objects – is always a *social* process, a symbolically mediated interaction, rooted in the assumption that whatever is perceived and imagined can be named. This is the only way in which consciousness can integrate previous experience into the contacting process as "common sense". The stock of everyday knowledge is socially mediated and for it to function appropriately, we have to make an assumption that it is shared by others.[14] Of course, the spontaneous use of everyday knowledge is not a linguistic process, but only because it is possible to articulate it linguistically does it become shared knowledge. "To be conscious and to experience something means to communicate from within with the world, with my body and with other people – to be with them, rather than next to them", says Merleau-Ponty (1962:79).

This suggests that consciousness, as thinking about appropriate behaviour and potentially successful strategies in a confusing and problematical field of contacts, is structured *dialogically,* as communicating with oneself. But it doesn't make sense to assume that consciousness is only used for inner dialogue. On the contrary, a function of consciousness is the exchange of information, shared reflection, an exchange of experience through the medium of language and non-verbal communication. We create our world through naming and therefore differentiation, linguistic symbolization, as well as through using our senses and our motor functions. Specifically through this phenomenon, the constitution of whatever we experience as "real" is social from its inception: talking means achieving agreement about differentiations, thus creating a common world, a taken-for-granted reality which we relate to together. Speaking is the expressive mode of thinking-consciousness.

Just as the organism cannot be limited to the matter inside the skin, so consciousness is not confined to its organic substratum, the individual brain. There is no need, though, to speak about a collective consciousness. Thinking-consciousness is a function of the organism/environment field, which allows us to consider and reconsider our needs and our steps towards fulfilling them. Such reflections are processes of discovering and inventing at once, i.e. our creative intercourse with the conditions and possibilities of verbal expression, which enables us to constitute a shared world that becomes functional only through naming.

"The uniqueness of language", writes the French biologist Francois Jacob,

> … seems to be related less to its capacity to allow us to give directions for action, but rather because it enables us to symbolize, to evoke cognitive images. We create our reality through words and sentences in the same way as we create it through our visual and auditory senses.
>
> (Jacob, 1976:82)

Language offers countless possibilities for combining words, which can be understood because such combinations follow rules and thus they can be shared and comprehended. Language makes it possible to collectively devise and plan the future, anticipate with imagination and planning whatever is still embryonic, not yet realized both for the individual, for social groups, and for society as a whole. Thus we can understand why consciousness becomes most conscious of itself wherever we happen to find the biggest problem, no matter whether we deal with it in communication with real people or with their internal representations.

Summarizing what I have said so far, we can say that thinking-consciousness fulfils two functions in the contacting process. It enables *problems to be solved* and it allows the development of *tolerance of frustration*. If it seems likely that a problem could be solved within the given situation, if need satisfaction seems to be a realistic aim, then thinking-consciousness specifically has the capacity to somewhat delay action, in order to facilitate further consideration, planning and talking together. From an instrumental point of view the aim is to find the right strategy and to gain a realistic appreciation of any obstacles, while on the normative side we need to ensure that means and actions are considered legitimate through achieving consensus with relevant others. Thinking-consciousness therefore has an instrumental and a normative aspect. Both require verbal communication which duly find the attention of Perls & Goodman (part 2, VII, pp. 99–112).

If on the other hand the need remains unsatisfied, the problem unsolved, thinking-consciousness enables us to consider a quiet retreat into reflection – an action which allows us to creatively use part of the energy of our frustration. Through this we may ensure the containment of potential explosions of useless rage, and at the same time realize that there are energy implosions which may lead to paralysing resignation.

Thinking-consciousness may invent and discover alternative possibilities for the frustrated need and in the interplay of inner and outer communication, secure an anticipation of future satisfaction in new and different contacting processes with new and different others.

Tolerance of frustration is achieved through reflection and – as we shall see later – by empathy. It is not an end in itself, but the basis for and departure point of either the continuation of the contacting process in other situations or a new start and a search for satisfaction with different objects. This last, of course, is what Freud termed sublimation; except here we are not dealing with a replacement of satisfaction but with real alternatives. "Being gifted is well sublimated rage", T. W. Adorno says. In our context this means: the energy which could not be discharged in good contact, turns with unbroken strength – a strength which may even have grown through being barred from satisfaction, i.e. retroflected – towards another attempt or even another task, thereby perhaps *increasing* the drive towards mastery. The interplay of retreating into consciousness and the openness of awareness towards hitherto unnoticed possibilities in the environment generates invention and discovery which is not sublimation but creative adjustment.

A recurring problem arises though from the fact that apparently some needs can only be satisfied with this particular person or only through this particular kind of work, etc. – as if the childhood situation where we had to depend on one mother was still operative. A change of partner or a change in work situation or travel plans, the discovery of new possibilities and the invention of new strategies – all of these require reflection and dialogical conversation for fantasies to become concrete future actualities.

There is one phenomenon still missing in this exploration of the functions of consciousness and awareness that is a realm of *unconscious* mental activities. Part of it are the numerous workings of automatically functioning physical or biological processes. A close look at them immediately reveals that no strict boundary is to be found between unconscious and conscious processes: both realms are permeable with typical interfaces: As mentioned above some physical autonomously working processes can be deliberately brought into awareness, like breathing or most of our senses, while others make themselves noticed by feelings of irritation like a shortage of nourishment by hunger, or through pain as in most cases of physical dysfunctions.

However psychologically more interesting is that what seems to be sleeping in the unconscious realm are phenomena like *intuition* and *dreams*. The latter may also be called an altered state of consciousness in that dreams can be remembered – even if they usually aren't – and we can even learn to make them altogether conscious. Freud had discovered their value for psychotherapy and this insight was taken up by Perls & Goodman, even if they changed radically the way to work with them. What Perls & Goodman argued about Freud's procedure to gain access to the client's "subconscious", the so called method of "free association", was also true for their view on therapeutic work with dreams: instead of leaving the interpretation of what comes up in the clients' deliberate memory of a dream or spontaneous associations, a Gestalt therapist would help them to discover for themselves what in their contents would be meaningful for their lives by bringing them into the here-and-now of the therapeutic session through dialogue and identification methods. In Gestalt therapy the unconscious realm is not seen as a trashy pool of repressed instincts and desires which have to be brought into the light of consciousness to be controlled by the super-ego and brought to adjust to the norms of society but rather as Perls & Goodman pronounce it:

> … that something not known as his, comes from his darkness and yet is meaningful; thereby perhaps he is encouraged to explore, to regard his unawareness as terra incognita but not chaos. From this point of view he must of course be made a partner in the interpreting.
>
> (Perls & Goodman:108)

And they continue to importantly state: "The thought here is that the maxim Know Thyself, is a humane ethics; it is not something done to one in trouble, but something one does for oneself as human. The therapist's arcane attitude toward the interpretation withholding it or doling it out at the right moment, is contrary to this" (pp. 108–109). In this way the client may become aware of their autonomy to define what is meaningful for themself including their own limits, physical, intellectually, socially, whatever, and learn to value the unaware resources in themself and their powers of awareness in the here-and-now. The unconscious realm is a wonderful pond of ever-surprising creative solutions and insights if one is open and attentive to its gleams and sparkles. Without its interplay with awareness creativity would remain a mystery.

But still the question of who is the *author* of all these internal and external activities remains unanswered. The traditional answer of psychology was: "the self". The nebulous character of this concept was not much improved by the insistence of Perls & Goodman that the self is a *process* rather than a static substance phenomenon, even if this pointed in the right direction. In any case the continuing confusion among Gestalt therapists about the nature of the self was impressively illustrated by Jean Marie Robine's recent book (2016) *Self: A polyphony of Gestalt therapists*, containing a collection of 19 articles with 19 different views on this topic by 19 internationally well-known Gestalt therapists! Maybe the breakthrough is now coming from the neuro-sciences: Thomas Metzinger, a philosopher contemplating recent brain research on the nature of our consciousness clearly states that "there is no such thing as a 'self' and contrary to what most people believe nobody ever was or had a self" (Metzinger, 2010:2). It should be noted here that with this claim he is in total agreement with the mystical schools of all religious traditions with their millenniums of history! (Huxley, 1945b). This is not a small matter, given the extreme difference of their methods of getting knowledge – meditation there, scientific research here. In his theory of the "Ego-Tunnel" Metzinger describes the complex mechanism by which our brains produce the ongoing illusion of having a "self" or an "I". This has tremendous consequences for our thought as well as for any kind of social organization (see also section 10 of this chapter on "Self-identification and social anchoring"), beyond the questions it raises in regard to artificial intelligence and the attempt to replicate human brains technologically, which are Metzinger's overriding concerns. I will not discuss these developments in this book. They may entail our future, but for the practise of Gestalt therapy today it may suffice to keep a close eye on those neurotic processes which express an exaggerated blown up ego or self – a task which for the moment surely keeps us busy enough.

6 Aggression

Destruction and annihilating

There is a constant danger that this inner and outer checking process becomes an end in itself, that consideration before action turns into the deadlock of rumination; that verbal exchange with others becomes an endless pointless questioning of everything. When the contacting process is unfolding undisturbed, though, thinking-consciousness (just as our emotions) serves our orientation. We consult language like a map, whose symbols stand in for real conditions – and now we step out, enter into the landscape and go towards the places that seem interesting and promising. This stepping out and eventual grasping belongs to the next phase of the contacting process – what in the theory of Gestalt therapy is meant by aggression – the process of actively restructuring and changing the given situation.

The organism's aggression consists in its manipulation of its environment – neither concept is meant in a negative sense, but they both indicate positive functions of the contacting process. Thus the concept of aggression which is entailed in the theory of the contacting process differs from most other theories of aggression. We will see that from a Gestalt therapeutic point of view the core problem of human aggression – aggression against the environment – is not the result of a lack of self-control, but its converse: aggression follows when we inhibit the spontaneous aggressive functions in the contacting process.

According to Perls & Goodman, aggression as a mode of action contains three elements:

- the initiative of stepping out and grasping,
- destroying in the sense of de-structuring obsolete Gestalts, and then
- annihilating and disposing of those obstacles which cannot be destroyed or assimilated.

When we say somebody is taking the initiative, we mean that the organism reaches out into the environment, pushes the contact boundary towards the exciting objects of interest in the environment. There might be one which excites arousal and raises hopes of satisfaction, or perhaps there might be an obstacle in the path of action which has to be removed.

Initiative is the connection between a need with which I identify, and the motor activity which seems suitable for the occasion. I address someone (an essential part of motor function is using the voice), I open a book, I pick a fruit, or I reach out for my guitar. I introduce a topic of conversation, I ask to speak, I grasp my tools and start to work – in all these ways my body and/or my intellect becomes the instrument for contacting the environment.

The organism which reaches for something both sensori-motorically and intellectually may encounter something that is unknown, resistant. In order to be able to work on it and digest it, or to stroke and caress it, these wholes (alien because they do not belong to one's own self) must be taken apart. A Gestalt is being changed, dissolved into its parts and must be re-constituted into a new Gestalt, so that the salubrious parts with which I can identify are separated out from what is insalubrious, that which I need to reject as alien. This process of destroying – de-constructing – is a normal part of everyday activities in a myriad of ways.

The clearest example of this is taking nourishment: Everything we eat, be it bread, meat or fruit has to be peeled, cut up or broken. Specifically, it has to be broken with the teeth and chewed before we can swallow and digest it. Hands and teeth are our specific tools in this process. Their use again shows the paradox of our relationship with our body, the interplay of inner and outer aspects of being a body and having a body. The civilizing process, in the course of which many instruments and techniques were developed and which refine and multiply the destructive powers of hands and teeth, does not change this principle in any way. Whoever experiences a loss of teeth or of a hand immediately feels their self-assurance shaken – these "instruments" are not only very practical, they are also an intimate part of our identity. Nowadays most foods are cooked and baked, grated and mashed, milled and kneaded, chopped and filtered, before they are taken up to the mouth with fork and spoon: the function of our teeth – to be instruments for biting and chewing – is to some extent externalized in the civilizing process, thus again emphasizing the natural tension between the body's neediness and its instrumentality.

Other examples for de-structuring in the contacting process can be illustrated as somewhat analogous with the process of eating. The reception of intellectual materials equally demands disassembling and breaking down into constituent parts: – the process of intellectual analysis works just in this way. Each successful learning process, even if we are just dealing with imitation, requires the material to be prepared and unfolded for absorption. Didactics are to learning what cooking is to eating: the art of preparation. Whatever has been presented in this way still has to be chewed and carved up by the learner. Then, by comparing and re-constituting some parts, putting them together with what they know already, they make their own appropriate sense of what has been heard, seen or read, absorb the material and make it their own. Of course, as a rule some material is lost in this process. Some bits are rejected as insalubrious, other bits are simply forgotten. Children spontaneously forget whatever they don't understand – and just through this capacity they are extraordinarily capable of learning and if not discouraged always stay curious for what is unknown. Whatever material is lost is in fact no loss for the organism, since damage can arise through surfeit, the organism exceeding its capacity for absorption. Absorbing and eliminating are two sides of the same process. Two issues have recently gained some urgency in this context. First: the everyday use of computers with their "delete" buttons and the arrival of the internet giving access to an almost unlimited number of "facts" (true and false). This has changed the relationship between learning and forgetting. Our children must learn new techniques for quickly deciding what is to be kept in memory and what can and must (!) immediately be "deleted". And second: the more older people we have, the more pressing the question becomes of how a brain growing older can be helped to preserve its short-term memory as much and for as long as possible, essential for the management of everyday survival – instead of using up too much energy by focussing on long-term memory, which is not always pleasant but can also be painful, even terrorizing, as in traumatic memories.

Finally, even the more tender interpersonal situations require a de-structuring of what is immediately given – a change and new constitution of the present Gestalt. In touching the beloved I change her (or his) position, pull her towards me, take her in my arms, push her gently onto a cushion, undress her perhaps and excite her through my caresses. Eros and sexuality require this active element of tender-aggressive grasping, to overcome any natural awe of another alien if attractive body, to dissolve resistance into desire. In truly reciprocal situations none of this is limited to the male role: both partners are equally subjects of action and objects of intervention. There is no gender difference in this complex movement of reaching out and allowing oneself to receive, in an interweaving of activity and passivity, except where sexual roles are forced into limiting cultural frames.

The pleasurable aspect of aggression may be less obvious in argument, contention and conflict. Still, even in these situations – provided the contacting process is not interrupted – the destruction and change in the Gestalt formation is experienced as pleasurable. The reason for this is that this element of aggression is a function of appetite itself: here, too, pleasure arises from need. In experiencing needs which are about to be satisfied, the source of pleasure is in grasping and biting, chewing and working on something. Goodman calls this process identification with parts of the environment. We see it when teeth are shown in rage or in laughter. In addition, there are the many causes of dissatisfaction which call for a change. Destroying knots created through unsatisfactory habits in couple relationships; dissolving prejudices amongst friends and colleagues; political conflict around distribution of resources – all of this can be a pleasurable fight, hot quarrel or a cleansing thunder storm. Its completion creates a new situation, a more satisfactory distribution, a new Gestalt in relationships.

Apart from this "warm" grasping aspect of aggression there is the "cold" one, directed towards annihilation and removal of obstacles which interfere with my need satisfaction. Here, whatever the organism needs is usually not directly accessible; there are ever more obstacles, something stands in the way, frequently real dangers threaten. It starts out with harmless trifles: a vase disturbs the eye contact with my partner in conversation – I remove the vase. Rotting rubbish threatens my food – I remove the rubbish. An unpleasant person in a group prevents the hoped-for conversation – we ask them to shut up or remove them from the group. In most cases the removal of obstacles does not create significant difficulties. Emotionally they are accompanied by some irritation, which usually is quickly forgotten.

If, on the other hand, dangers and obstacles in the environment become too difficult to overcome in a given contacting situation, then we have circumstances where normally the organism withdraws, gets out of the way of danger, circumvents the obstacle, tries to reach the aim in a different way or at a later point in time. Almost always there are alternatives. Almost always there are many roads leading to Rome, and if there seems to be just this one way right now, there is always the question of whether really there is just this one aim, just this one object which is capable of satisfying the presenting need. The healthy organism gets itself out of the way of dangers and obstacles which it cannot manage: it is not interested in the heroism of victory or failure. It has, however, the courage to face a conflict, to destroy the old conditions which no longer satisfy, and to touch what is new, the unknown, which can only be created and discovered in and during the contacting process.

Difficulties arise when either – like a soldier compelled to serve in war – we are forced to stick with a dangerous situation rather than flee and search for need satisfaction elsewhere; or when the object of our desire is also the source of the threat, as violent parents are for their children. In both cases, the transient anger driving any process of removal and annihilation turns into cold rage focussing all the powers of the organism. It turns into despair if these powers are still insufficient to remove the source of danger or to flee from it, and this experience of frustration and powerlessness is usually at the root of violence. In an undisturbed contacting process, physical violence against other human beings is – aside from sheer sadism – never anything but a reaction of self-defence with regard to a real and present physical threat in situations one cannot leave. Therefore, the successful removal of a threat, or flight from danger successfully accomplished is not followed by the kind of happy satisfaction which follows the warm rage accompanying the destruction of resistant objects. Instead, it brings nothing but relief, ends in relaxation or exhaustion.

However, there are many pathological reasons for imagining oneself in a dangerous situation or for fixing exclusively onto the alternative of victory or defeat, which always interfere with the contacting process. The greatest danger threatening our civilization, though, is the internalized inhibition of aggression, which prevents a bad word from passing our lips but cannot prevent the unexpected punch, when pent-up rage breaks all controls. What we need to learn as pedagogues and therapists with regard to the problem of violence in our world is that flight and avoidance in real danger is a rational response, while heroism is a neurotic one – and that the de-structuring and annihilating aspects of aggression are a normal part of any contacting process. As long as this fact is denied and this denial remains introjected, the disproportion between cause and means in warfare and terrorism, and the fear of annihilation caused by it, will remain part of our lives.

If the threatening or violent person is identical with the longed for source of love, a paradoxical situation comes about: one part of the other must be negated, rejected and rendered harmless, while another part is desired, wanted and loved. In this situation the quality of the conflict becomes painful and gruelling, which is characteristic of many arguments between people living together. Of course there is always the question: why be fixed onto this *one* partner, who is supposed to fulfil all needs; why hold on to this *one* group, when there are others besides? Only for children, who are completely dependent on their relationship with their parents, can this constellation turn into a true double binding situation (Watzlawick et al., 1967). Repeatedly experienced contradiction between attention given and rejection threatened – in conjunction with the child being unable to leave the situation – can produce neurotic attitudes. The process is that at first the child learns to control the stirrings of their need and then habitualizes this mode of self-control. This contradiction, if it is repeated continually and is contained in the same communicative act – for example when words and gestures are mutually exclusive in their intention – only drives the recipient truly crazy. Aggression with its threefold function of reaching out, de-structuring and annihilation isn't just normal but is an essential part of any contacting process. A person who feels secure within their environment and secure within themself, uses their sensorimotor, emotional and cognitive abilities and the authority at hand to change that part of the environment – and *only* that part – which will lead to the satisfaction of their needs, leading to growth and development. This process of change entails the de-structuring of Gestalts presenting themselves in the given situation. Using one's ego-functions of de-structuring and annihilation by which any participant influences social arrangements, encounters and communication are made possible, If my own powers are not sufficient to confront the barriers against satisfying contact I get out of the way or leave the situation: one interrupts the contacting process in order to unfold more fully in other, new contacts. Anything else leads to resentment or even to latent hatred, which eventually destroys in the environment what may be needed in a future situation, or certainly that which nourishes other people in different ways – indirectly a condition of one's own life and survival, also.

7 Integration

Surrender and enjoyment in full contact

Only now is the way free for the self to unfold fully into the contacting process – to assume the free-floating position of full contact. To reach this platform, all intentional ego-functions have to be surrendered, just like ballast. Once the object of contact is fully in focus, grasped and fully recognized, it begins to fill up the whole background. The figure is no longer emphasized in contrast to its background but now encompasses everything which is meant by this contact. The human organism is no longer opposite to an object, but its whole energy flows into the contact. Fully integrative contact between subject and object is the merging of organism and environment into a unified experience at the point of contact, with no spare capacity for anything else. Anything planned and intentional recedes; everything is spontaneous surrender to the rhythm of the encounter, in which another "I" or rather "Thou" completely fills me – in a way which is meant for me and only me.

Prototypical experiences of this nature can again be found in functions which secure individual and collective survival: in eating and in sexuality, since in these experiences the body perceptibly becomes an independent entity of experience according to its own rules; for a moment it eludes any instrumental intention. For that moment we *are* our body rather than *having* it – a transient breakdown of the "ex-centric" mode of experience which at all other times is definitive for human beings (Plessner, 1970a). Chewing our food leads to increased production of saliva and finally to the swallowing reflex, ensuring that the food is taken in and, if there is a corresponding appetite, the process is accompanied by pronounced feelings of pleasure.

The involuntary nature of some physical reactions is even more obvious in orgasm, where "I" and "Thou" become one in unified experience. Here the self, defined as a function of the contact boundary, is most itself, receives its strongest contour, since now my entire experience is this interfusion of "I" and "Thou". As all energies accessible to the organism at this moment are wholeheartedly mobilized, all is exclusively focussed on realising You in me, thus giving such intensity to the orgiastic experience. Only by surrendering all intentionality, leaving behind all orientations and all plans and manipulation, can I completely pour myself into the other and simultaneously receive them into myself. Surrender is certainly self-forgetting, but it is not self-abandonment, instead it is letting go of all the strategic ego-functions of the self: they have fulfilled their roles. Integration, becoming one with the discovered and invented Gestalt, can only be fully achieved if it is the fulfilment and completion of a contacting process which has gone through all the preceding stages of fore-contact, orientation and re-organization. Premature integration (due to regressive desires) always remains unsatisfactory. "Each orgasm has its history", feminist author Barbara Sichtermann says (Sichtermann, 1986). It is the spontaneous and unplanned culmination of a process where we gradually approach and touch the other. Of course it is possible to reach orgasm simply as a physiological reaction through intentional stimulation, just as I can force myself to swallow something. But in such a process orgasm remains limited as a physical experience; the organism – instead of fully surrendering to another – merely wrests a reaction from the body. In the full integration of "I" and "Thou" no part of the organism continues to use another part instrumentally. Letting go of all arbitrariness is a spontaneous act of surrender to the process. You cannot plan an orgasm – but it is possible to support wholehearted surrender by creating appropriate conditions in the earlier phases of the contacting process.

The tension typical for human beings – of always being suspended between involuntary and voluntary action, between having and being a body – is the foundation of the realization that even orgiastic experiences can be of different quality. Complete self-forgetfulness does not easily come to us, especially since this experience at the essential moment requires not doing but letting go. It is as if one had to step aside in order not to stand in the way of one's own spontaneity. The spontaneity of full contact gains its own power and energy in the delight of orgasm which is balancing lack, satisfying need, and incorporating new experience. All these steps are accompanied by an arousal so intense that it burns up – as it were – anything pre-planned and anxious. With letting go of planning, the time perspective – always attached to having aims – also disappears. All delight is timeless, "wants eternity" as Nietzsche's Zarathustra says; the wish to extend this experience is the desire to become one with its boundlessness.

The phase of integration in the contacting process is not yet completed in self-surrender, but continues in the enjoyment and appreciation of a gradually noticeable sense of satisfaction which eventually dies away into the post contact. Enjoyment is at the same time an active process of approach and surrender of the senses and motor functions as well as passive absorption, allowing oneself to be filled by the other or something other. The delight of surrender is already beyond time; in enjoyment, though, we hover at the edge of time and play with the transitions between having and being as the two modes of experience associated with being embodied. This is the reason why – in spite of everything intentional now absent in the surrender to Eros – everywhere and always, there has been a culture of erotic and culinary enjoyment, which by no means ends with the arts of planning and preparation but aims to increase and extend enjoyment.

Each culture develops its own particular richness and simultaneously produces its own particular poverty in the possibilities it offers for shaping and forming surrender and sensuous pleasure. Each culture promotes and diminishes the chances for the satisfying contacting processes it offers its members living in and through it. Our own culture's weakness lies less in the breathlessness of fast food and "instant sex" than in the commercially promoted narcissism which insists on Ego-centeredness, even when we engage in pleasure; there is a wide-spread fear of losing self-control in surrender to the other. All this is the price we must pay for the rule of instrumental reason. It is true too, though, that this same culture has found its own historically fresh answers in various forms of body-psychotherapy and self-awareness explorations.

Some aspects of these reflections will become clearer when we remember that surrender and the varieties of pleasure are not limited to the erotic and culinary arena. Each uninterrupted contacting process is completed in the integration of organism and environment. Our language offers hints at this – we say "I'm all ears" when our attention and energy is fully engaged in listening or gazing at something. Whenever we concentrate perfectly the subject is absorbed into the object, merges with it, becoming one with it. Everything else is shut off – not just as irrelevant background; nothing else enters awareness. I can be so intensely immersed in considering a work of art or natural scenery, absorbed with working, thinking or reading that for a time everything else around me disappears.

And again this surrender entails permitting spontaneous interaction with experiencing the object of my interest – a process of active surrender and passive reception at once. Some people experience music so completely that it fills every fibre of their being; they become one with it. This is an experience where music is not realized until it is – as it were – embodied in every cell of the listener, who becomes a different being through the process of listening. Thus it is with the experience of merging: Rilke ends his verses about the aesthetic experience of a sculpture with the line: "You have to change your life". The philosopher Peter Sloterdijk has built a whole anthropology on this sentence (Sloterdijk, 2009). In fact, whoever had the deep experience of gazing is already changed: we have absorbed that was something different from us a moment ago, which now is still resonating, until it is gradually assimilated, and thus becomes part of our own being.

It is truly remarkable how surrender itself constitutes the moment of creativity. Always the integration of organism and environment extends beyond itself, leaving organism and environment changed, at least in experience, and often enriched by new qualities or competencies. Just as new life sometimes emerges from sexual surrender, sometimes too, from surrendering to technical or artistic or scientific tasks a new form or a clear insight opens up, a moment of seeing through, seeing the whole, described here by Dorothy Sayers when it happens to her detective hero Lord Peter Wimsey:

> And then it happened – the thing he had sort of expected. It happened suddenly, with certainty, and just as unshiftable as a sunrise. He remembered in just one moment – not this bit or that, nor the logical sequence of events, but everything together, the whole story, perfect and complete, in all its dimensions – in such a way as if he stood outside the world and

saw it floating in space with myriads of dimensions. He did not need any further reasons, he did not even think about it. He knew.

This experience of suddenly knowing the solution has been described by many people; we can find it in the commonplace "Aha!" when we finally find the missing ingredient in food; likewise "Eureka!" at a brilliant insight into the interplay of cosmic powers, at the solution of a common technical problem as well as in the experience of a "mini-Satori" – the name given to some special therapeutic insights of patients by Jim Simkin. Contacting processes are as different as are the needs which drive them and as the objects toward which they are directed. They simply share the structure of an irreversible sequence of the phases of approach, contact and finally integration with and through its objects, whether material or immaterial. Without the integration phase with its fullest unfolding of the self's capacity for experience – always dependent on who is involved, what situation it finds itself in – there can be no change. Only through surrender and in enjoyment can new experiences be worked on, worked through, ensuring growth and development.

Of course, not every contacting process guarantees such moments of full integration. Often the climax of self-unfolding consists in just enjoying the very closeness of the contact itself, the shared play of senses and movements around the contact boundary, beyond which the organism loses itself in the timelessness of pure delight. Sometimes people engage fully in brisk, purposeful exchange of thought and argument; or embrace each other whilst moving with the rhythm of the dance or in the process of co-operating and playing together. In such cases what counts is not a result but the shared activity itself. This process works in a similar way when we are alone with ourselves and make contact with material and immaterial substances: when we surrender to the water in swimming or diving, to the rock when climbing, to the wind when sailing. So also in the cognitive spheres: the surrender to a memory, a train of thought or an idea are all experiences of full contact where the organism approaches the boundary to self-forgetfulness without necessarily crossing it. And yet, this unification with whatever it is that touches us is the aim of an often unacknowledged longing.

The process of integration or full contact has a deeper significance, beyond the pleasure of surrender and becoming one with an activity. Definitely we are not concerned here with an attempt at catching hold of lust and delight for its own sake – that is the concern of addiction to self-indulgence which simply leads to empty exhaustion and is soon followed by an urge to repeat the experience. Instead, the function of savouring an experience of full contact is to allow the feeling of satisfaction to slowly grow and fill the whole human organism. Only if satisfaction can be deeply sensed and experienced is it possible to avoid satiation and surfeit. While savouring the experience the organism gently frees itself from the totality of surrender and still remains completely engaged with it. Nothing can ever be savoured with finality, but at least lack has been remedied, and gradually the motoric pleasure accompanying the enjoyment turns into the languid delight of satisfaction. Thus the process of savouring slowly initiates the last phase, post-contact, which has its own kind of sensuousness as full contact is traced again and slowly allowed to recede.

8 Post contact

Enjoying the afterglow of experience and affirming

Each event needs time for it to become an experience. The intensity of an encounter with something new does not ensure that the organism will be sufficiently satisfied and enriched in the long run; in retrospect, a passionate encounter may seem nothing special and in memory becomes empty, does not leave a permanent impression. Or it remains a singular event having nothing to do with the reality of one's everyday life; it resists being integrated and for that very reason may become an object of longing reminiscence and day dreams. As the old saying goes "Post coitum omne animale triste", depressively reducing such experiences to the point. What is lacking here, what any encounter requires in order to become an enriching experience is the time to identify what has been gained during the post contact phase. Having been found and invented, the Gestalt dissolves; the contacting boundary becomes blurred, the self loses its energy and fades; the organism is unfocussed, is at rest and the environment is beginning to be perceived again in its specificity, though remaining relatively uninteresting.

In contrast to PHG, who left out this fourth phase of the contacting process, I think that it is an important part in the whole process of the satisfying experience: Post contact has three functions in the contacting process:

1 Letting an experience sink in, enjoying its afterglow, *affirming* it. At first the organism just needs time, to allow what's been experienced to settle in order for it to take root so it can continue to have an effect. In this respect post contact is simply-it-be-as-it-is, while the organism is still open and still resonating and letting what has been touched slowly die down. It is still permeable, and therefore vulnerable, too, and in need of protection. Rest is now required – both for the senses which are still replete with what has been perceived and received, and for the spent motor functions. Being hauled out of the previous absorption too quickly can work just like an alarm clock tearing us out of deep sleep, i.e. it may inflict a psychological and even physiological injury to which we react with light-headedness, disorientation and sometimes despair. The organism here is mainly vulnerable with regard to fellow human beings, who perhaps weren't quite as involved to the degree of full contact. Or who – in a narcissistic disposition – are shocked by their ego boundaries melting in the encounter with

something new, and need to diffuse the effect of the contacting process through premature categorization, cataloguing and valuation or simply through turning their backs. It can be hugely irritating when there is immediate commentary or speedy criticism while we are still deeply moved by a play or by a film; how painful it is when the usual instant applause fastens on to the last chord of a concert which has barely finished; and how hurtful it is when the lover immediately withdraws as soon as love hunger has been appeased. Indeed, it is sufficient to allow free rein to the field of organism and environment, not interfering with one's own organism but simply allowing space for the feeling of satisfaction to unfold.

2 Even this process of surrender to the afterglow of an experience, the second function of the post contact, is not really an activity of the self, but rather a passive, almost lazy attentiveness, directed towards the changes in the organism itself; towards what is new in their experience; what abides. It has already been incorporated but not yet assimilated. Of course it is possible to boost these processes of tracking and appreciating what has been experienced with cultured finesse – in the realm of the senses as well as in the interpersonal one. For the senses, we may usefully apply the culinary arts of closure and post contact with which we are most familiar. This is the place not just for desserts ending the meal, but also those special drinks: coffee, cognac, dessert wines – and for many people that most enjoyable postprandial cigarette. In the social realm we have rituals which, at the end of the shared activity bringing people together, allow some space for a less focussed kind of togetherness: the "social" or "informal" part of the evening after work has been accomplished; at the end of a meeting or an exercise class. We exchange experiences and opinions after a shared visit to an event or talk about the visit after the last guests have gone.

3 In the social realm the third function of the post contact is of the greatest importance: *affirmation*. We have to re-assure each other that it really was that way; I have experienced it in this way, you have experienced it in that way – we both had an experience. This matters for two reasons. Firstly, through this mutual affirmation of the contacting process now about to end, we mutually constitute our social reality through interpersonal contact; through this affirmation we define something as an experience which we can (confidently) invoke in the future. Secondly, this affirmation has the function of providing a ritual of reciprocity, a standardized communication which enables us to maintain or re-constitute norms of reciprocity.

Naming the experience is part of the constitution of reality, clarifying the question of what has actually taken place. For most contacting processes this is unproblematic; ready-made labels are available for use. We already know, of course, that we went out together for a meal or took part in a conference or went to the movies. What may be lacking is an evaluation: a "good" meal, a "boring" conference, an "exciting" film. But these labels are not always are so readily to hand. Has this been a "night of love" or a "passing sexual adventure"? Was this an "educational experience" or an "unnecessary ordeal"? It is necessary to begin to find preliminary answers to these kinds of questions through reflection, re-construction, and re-investigation – and mainly through talking about it all, jointly finding labels which encompass assessment and ordering. Much of this will be clarified somewhat later, after the complete closure of the contacting process – though sometimes it will be clarified only much later, or never at all.

Rituals of reciprocity tend to take three forms, normally a regular part of the post contacting phase in the social realm: expressing thanks, arranging another meeting and saying goodbye. Each of these rituals can take very different forms, depending on the nature of the contacting process, the types of relationships involved and the semantic traditions – words and gestures belonging to the everyday culture of the social groupings concerned. The norm of reciprocity,[15] universal for all cultures, entailing a gift given being balanced by a gift given in return, can take many different forms. Saying "thank you" is but one of them, if the most common. Its function always is to maintain social balance. Arranging to meet again, however vaguely expressed ("Why don't you give me a call?" or "We should do this again soon!") has the function of fastening a personal relationship to the level which has been reached at this point. Saying goodbye serves to offer a closing ritualized evaluation of the shared contact ("What a great meal this was!" or "I am very glad you could make it!"). It also serves to mutually affirm the status of the relationship ("Bye, see you tomorrow!" or "Goodbye, Mr. Smith; I hope you have a good trip home!"). These ritualized forms should not deceive us about the fact that we are dealing with an ever fresh assessment of previous contacting processes; each of these rituals offers the possibility – through voice tone and gesture – to fine-tune it to what best fits each contacting process.

Through its functions of letting things sink in, experiencing the afterglow of the event and mutual affirmation, post contact allows the assimilation of what was taken in – a process which happens once the contacting process has been completed, largely outside awareness. Letting things sink in, through appreciating and mutual affirmation, a preliminary decision is made regarding which parts of what has been absorbed will finally be assimilated and what is going to be eliminated – what is going to be kept, becoming part of the organism, and what is pushed away or forgotten. The functions of the post contact entail a sensory-cognitive short-term memory, which begins to decide what is going to be kept in long-term memory and what may soon be forgotten. It is the post contact which ensures that the harvest of the contacting process gets into the storage barn.

9 Assimilation

Remembering and forgetting

Each contacting process leaves behind a changed organism/environment field. The organism has incorporated something from the environment, its need is satisfied for the time being; it no longer needs to be active to ensure its regeneration. At the same time as it has been enriched for the longer term, it has become something else, has grown – sometimes noticeably, sometimes imperceptibly. What does this growing consist in? It is important here to recognize that successful contacting processes are not just about reconstituting the original state through re-balancing lack and through need satisfaction, but they are also *learning processes* through which the organism *grows,* that is gains increasing competency and a refinement of its needs.

In each contacting process already existing competencies are being practised again. But gradually additional competencies are gained: perhaps I become more perceptive, move with greater agility, express myself more clearly, experience things more deeply, think more sharply, enjoy more fully, can say "no" more firmly, etc. In other words, the most significant gain of any successful contacting process is a strengthening of the ego functions, of the skills and abilities through which we attempt to satisfy our needs. It is through them that we maintain movement in the organism/environment field, and that means we keep it alive. Oddly, this particularly shows in the fact that our basic needs re-emerge again and again – and can be sensed as such. Creatures are open ("dissipative") systems that would cease to exist if they ever reached a completely balanced state.

The re-organization of the organism/environment field through contacting processes where ever-better competencies are applied also leads to ever-new needs developing. With the strengthening of the ego functions and under auspicious political and economic conditions, certainty grows that in the future, too, it will be possible to satisfy our most important needs. This security constitutes the basis for more differentiated needs developing through which the organism responds to previously unnoticed challenges coming from the environment. Another outcome of the successful contacting process may be that now I need different things and wish for new objects. As the organism's self unfolds in ever new ways in subsequent contacting processes, it does not only achieve new ego functions but also new id functions. Growth of the organism therefore initially consists in regeneration and extension of ego and id functions.

We know little about the psychological processes involved in assimilating something new: how assimilation actually takes place. On the physical level, of course, we know about the metabolism of breathing and digestion. The most important issue at this point is that the body cannot assimilate everything it takes in, for this equally applies on the psychological level. Breathing out and eliminating are life-sustaining processes. Apart from illness, when they are blocked or interrupted, we are dealing with a characteristic symptom of neurotic disturbance. On the cognitive level this corresponds to forgetting as a healthy ego function, which shares the task of protecting the organism from information overflow through selective perception. Again, we see blocking of this spontaneous function, the inability to forget, as symptomatic of a disturbance in the self-regulatory processes in the organism/environment field. The process of assimilation, starting right after the closure of the contacting process, largely happens outside awareness and is based on an unconscious capacity to differentiate between what is useful and what is not useful for the organism. It appropriates what it needs and eliminates or forgets what it doesn't.

By forgetting I mean at this point that the information has finally disappeared. Some kinds of information may be latently available and will spontaneously be brought up into consciousness, "re-membered" if and when it is needed in a later contacting process. If the organism cannot remember relevant information, we are dealing with a memory lapse which may mean that something has been repressed. Repression entails that the memory of the original need is blanked out – as well as the method of repression which was originally used. If the organism cannot *forget* irrelevant information, we are dealing with a fixation to an earlier contacting situation. In both cases the current contacting process will be impeded.

What we remember, therefore, is not always consciously present, and relatively little of what we do remember actually needs to be remembered. Other types of information will have become second nature for the organism and therefore are part of the taken-for-granted background for all following contacting processes. I no longer know when, how and from whom I learned this or that; I just know how to do it, just as I know how to walk or talk. Spontaneously remembering what I have seen before, what I have already experienced or suffered, what I have already evaluated, is a natural potential in the contact between organism and environment through which our capabilities will be enhanced, our potential extended. Without the capacity to recognize something again, each situation would – in unbearable ways – be new and alien, and complete disorientation would be the consequence. This is, for instance, the catastrophe of Alzheimer's disease.

Even today, after decades of brain research we do not know a great deal about how our memory functions (Kandel, 2007). It appears as if perceptions and experiences leave behind cerebral traces, which are more permanent the more they retain the holistic character of a process and disregard detail. Gestalt psychologists have long maintained that memory is not simply a container for holding memories but a self-actuating process which changes memory traces in order to attempt Gestalt closure, spatially and temporarily as well as emotionally.[16] Only through this process do "decisions" seem eventually to be made regarding what is to be forgotten and what will remain accessible to be remembered at a later stage.

On the cognitive level, it is quite apparent that whatever has simply been memorized without a contextualizing understanding of the organizing principles behind it persists only for a short time – this is different when material is well organized. Beyond this I think that emotionally relevant experiences which closely concern the ego will make a significant difference to the question of how well and for how long something is remembered.[17] It is amazing how tenaciously experiences of shame, frequently attached to quite banal events, can dig their claws into our memory – the more strongly, the more they concern our bodies. In any case the affective cathexis of memories – quite independently of their accuracy – has a significant influence on what we find attractive or repelling in any given environment.

Cognitively and emotionally, memories have orientating functions in the contacting process – more strongly if memory has formed a vivid Gestalt from the traces of previous experiences. This Gestalt formation can be strongly influenced by narratives within a family or other groups and by a memory being repeatedly presented as a story. Also in this epoch of photography, the memory will often be structured by photographs and video films. It is important to reckon with the fact that remembered images are not reflecting immediate experience but are based on photos, films and videos, and storytelling. We must add here that since photography became digital its claim to authenticity has gone – memory has not just lost its support, but can actively be falsified.

Through this process, reality gets transformed in many ways, which does not, though, diminish our capacity to act – indeed Gestalt formation is in itself an expression of a capability, without which we could not cope with reality. In part, the ability to form a Gestalt from unstructured separate bits of memories already takes shape in internal processes of the brain; in part formed in communication with oneself and with others, in the shape of an anecdote for example, or a horror story or a funny tale, and only through these narratives do the original memory traces gain their power to orientate action.[18]

Whether my memory is actually accurate or not is irrelevant as long as it is not socially confirmed, because this, like any other reconstruction of reality, in principle also requires social affirmation. If I stick with my memories (or other constructions of reality) outside of what counts as shared historical experience, my memory will be considered defective, possibly insane. If on the other hand I can agree with others or they with me on a shared memory, then it is socially safeguarded and can fully enter into our construction of the present. That is one of the reasons why cognitive and emotional reference groups are so important – they share my own interpretations, supporting my perception of reality. It is not too difficult to live as a member of a cognitive minority (Berger, 1969) in society as a whole, but being alone in one's cognitions will lead to psychosis. Trauma patients, for instance, need to be listened to in an accepting way by a therapist and perhaps by other victims, for only this can provide the necessary social affirmation which was not available in the solitary and uncontrollable space of remembering.

It is true, though, that in producing shared memories – a favourite activity and a very important function of couples and families – we are not just dealing with equal contributions to establishing a memory mosaic, but this activity is also a struggle for the power to define situations. This explains the phenomenon of family members and couples so often interrupting each other with "That was quite different; let me…" when telling about an event. In other words, the whole creative re-construction of what happened matters a great deal, because gradually the form of reconstruction becomes more important than what is to be reconstructed. Often we remember the highlights of a story, the drama, the tragedy or the comedy, but not that which once served as its model. Childhood memories can most easily be used to check this phenomenon: often we remember the legend which the family created from an event – not the event itself; we see the event retrospectively through the optics of presentation.

In addition the organism has an altogether different way of remembering: the *memory of the body*, which is often ignored – not merely because many psychologists think of "memory" as an exclusively cognitive and conscious achievement, but also because, at least in our culture, this kind of remembering can hardly be socially validated. Just as we spontaneously remember something we have seen before, something already experienced; suffering we have undergone, good or bad judgments we made in the past – all of this helping in the current contacting process to increase capabilities and the potentialities of the situation, so the body spontaneously remembers agonies endured, hunger suffered, lust experienced in orgasm, injuries borne. There is no need to think only about torture and deprivation; amongst surgeons there is a wide-spread belief that the body – in spite of the best anaesthetics being used – always registers and remembers the surgical intervention as traumatic. A long time ago, Otto Rank already pointed out how traumatic the birth process can be for every woman and child (Rank, 1924).

However there is an important difference in relation to other kinds of memories: under normal conditions, what the body remembers remains unconscious. Or in the case of experiences which have been physically traumatizing – car accidents for example and war experiences – body memory may be partially conscious, partly repressed and returning in dreams. Usually such body memories only become perceptible in spontaneous reactions of the body, when danger threatens or when we are suddenly startled. These days, we are able to trigger and make such body memories conscious by using specific therapeutic techniques.[19] Just as with other physical competencies, the body's capacity to remember has not attracted sufficient attention. That the body can be trained is part of everyday knowledge in our culture. That in this training (which to some extent of course is part of any process of socialization, at least in our culture) many of the more subtle capabilities of the body are repressed – which under different circumstances would unfold spontaneously – is rarely noted. We fail to take note of the body's capacity to remember, which could be very useful indeed in our understanding of and dealing with illness and health processes.

Assimilation is an internal learning process of the organism and has various facets. To start with – and outside of our awareness – what has been newly incorporated is separated out into that which can and cannot be assimilated. Whatever is insalubrious or superfluous will be spontaneously eliminated or forgotten. What is useful, though, becomes second nature. The organism is specifically regenerated and enriched in its abilities and strengths. Whatever becomes second nature needs practice, and can be lost again. Once acquired, abilities which require coordination of sequential movements like cycling or car driving apparently do not get lost, even if they remain dormant for years. But they can be lost forever through traumatic experiences like accidents. This is why doctors advise to continue driving immediately after traumatic accidents. Even the most elementary capabilities of human beings like walking or talking or crying can be unlearned, if we are prevented from using them long enough, be it through illness, violence or introjects. Nevertheless, newly practised old competencies as well as newly acquired ones – however they may be threatened by loss or diminution – are a part of the organism which cannot be disregarded. Just as the organism's needs arise afresh again and again, new ones are developed; they have become (more or less strongly) second nature for human beings, like the ability to cycle or drive a car.

Beyond this, the organism particularly stores emotional experiences which are either spontaneously used to inform action strategies in new contacting processes or are deliberately consulted by the actor in order to help their orientation. These experiences are stored as memory traces and seem to undergo Gestalt formation processes if they closely affect the ego and have an affective charge. The Gestalt process seems to form the remembered material in such a way that it is capable of powerfully supporting the actor in their orientation in the environment. Where purely cognitive memory traces are concerned, we seem to see a codification, i.e. we find that the information is transposed into a more economical version for the purpose of storage – like a map which codifies essential aspects of the territory with the help of symbols (Hörmann, 1964:267). Such memories need to be decoded again for use in the current situation. The ability to decode then is part of remembering, an ego-function. In everyday life these memories are relevant for our spatial and temporal orientation, whereas affective memories tend to play a more significant role in personal relationships.

When I speak of storage here, this must not be taken to be an invitation to imagine the brain as a kind of container for information which through coding and Gestalt formation processes gets cooked up into useable memories. Of course the brain is responsible for memory achievements; but the "computer" which does the storing must be understood as a process or a "flowing pattern" which organizes the interplay between the manifold functions of the organism. Intellectually as well as physically and emotionally, we bring some memory to mind as we are engaged in our particular activities – all functions of the organism work together in the contacting process in such a way that a creative solution for the concerns of the organism/environment field can be found. Bringing something relevant to mind is how we access this reservoir of stored experiences. This ego-function can be used spontaneously as well as intentionally. We are largely unaware of the body's spontaneous memories – the body simply reacts to the new situation according to previous experience and in this sense it is conservative. This is less apparent in spontaneous emotional and specifically in cognitively focused experiences. Memories we search for intentionally are of course always conscious – and are therefore susceptible to falsification. They can deceive other people and lead to self-delusion.

For an interactionally-oriented psychotherapy, we would have to turn to the following very interesting observation by R. Bandler and J. Grinder – that in almost everybody, eye movements indicate whether we are dealing with "constructed visual images" or "remembered (eidetic) images". In the first case the eyes move automatically up and right, in the second case they move left and up (see Bandler / Grinder, 1979:25 et al.). "Constructed images" are definitely not attempts at deception or self-delusion, but valid attempts at reconstruction. I suspect, though, that the eidetic memories have the greater affect attached to them.

What we intentionally search for is subject to an additional social reality control, whereas spontaneous memories have to try out their reality content in the contacting process straight away. In the contacting situation the reality content of a memory is fully actualized in its functional significance for the present, whereas consciously searched-for memories are concerned with the question of how it "actually" was. Another reason for a reality check of these memories is: did it take place in the presence of actual people, with imagined ones or even just with members of our reference groups we may have internalized in an abstract way. Importantly the verbal form in which these memories are couched plays a role since they may become a vehicle for meanings which can be passed on as "collective memories", and in this way may contribute to individual or group identity formation – which has, of course, social consequences.

Finally, the process of memory normally protects itself from overload, not only by quickly forgetting everything stored in short-term memory that is of significance only for the actual tasks of orientation in the present, but also by forgetting content after longer time intervals when it has lost its function. Past events and experiences only live on for as long as they have meaning for the present. What we have learned persists while we use it, and what we remember can only be spontaneously remembered if we are dealing with currently useful experiences or those which have regained significance. "It is not by inertia but by function that a form persists, and it is not by lapse of time but by lack of function that a form is forgotten" (Perls & Goodman:75).

10 Self-identification and social anchoring

Identifying oneself and taking responsibility

There is a great deal more to a successful contacting process than remembering and assimilating. It clearly makes no sense to speak about the contacting process as a learning activity without thinking about a learning subject which remains constant throughout many contacting processes. The model of the contacting process, therefore, cannot do without a concept of the subjective centre of the organism. After all, in everyday practice we associate it with core questions about our sense of identity and the continuity of the human organism. Clearly these issues are of great importance socially and psychologically. The problem is this: it is easy to get stuck in the conceptual undergrowth of personality theories. They speak of the "I" or the "self" (which I could not do without, either), about identity, personality or the character of a human being. These are concepts which in the first place only express a desire to find – behind all the roles and masks, beyond all contacting processes which everybody is involved in – a permanent being which will persist throughout life. From the perspective of our model however, human beings are just and only just that which they show themselves to be in exchange with the environment. According to a central understanding of Philosophical Anthropology we are only ever that which we embody, that with which we identify (Plessner, 1964). This reflects the knowledge that our human character is at once historical and culturally relative. This recognition has long been consolidated in the Human Sciences. In our context this means that any growth achieved through a contacting process can only be validated by the way it shows up in action and self-presentation in later contacting processes. This applies particularly to all learning, including psychotherapy.

We ask the question of the role of personal identity for our model as one regarding the significance of *personality functions* of the self in the contacting process. *How does a human being experience themself as a subject which in different contacting processes remains identically the same, as having continuity?*

We have already achieved a first answer: through the fact that *learning experiences* constitute memories. Second there is the sometimes immediate and sometimes slow realization that I am *different* from what I remember I had been yesterday, and yet in some sense the same. Which leads to the knowledge that I am somebody who has a *history*, who has gone through developmental processes, somebody who nevertheless is one and the same – somebody who was then like that and is today like this. The amazing discovery is always the ongoing process, one's development, one's growth or decay. We all share the experience of gradually changing: of physically growing fast at first and then more slowly; then developing increasing competencies, our needs expanding. All these processes provide the basis for the certainty that I have continuity.

This certainty of my continuity is the assumed background of my contacts with the environment: my special competencies, my specific needs and my personal experiences together make up what we usually call personality. While something new takes shape in the foreground of an encounter between organism and environment "the continuities of personality are mainly present in the background as the basis of the Gestalt taking shape" (Latner, 1984a, p. 102). Perls & Goodman formulated a basic principle of Gestalt therapeutic personality theory, when they maintained that the healthy personality has little character (compare the considerations in Perls & Goodman, p. 144). This means that the competencies, needs and memories in the background of contacting processes are themselves fluid. It is simply not the experience of remaining the same, but the experience of change which endows me with the certainty of my continuity. Our character on the other hand can be said to be the sum of our rigid introjections.

When somebody's character traits move into the foreground and interfere with whatever is interesting in the environment, or colour what goes on, the contacting process is disturbed; perception of the environment and access to interesting objects of need satisfaction are now limited by preconceived notions, rigid strategies and – as Wilhelm Reich showed – physical "character armour" (Reich, 1945). In this way we could say, that Robert Musil's "Man without Properties" (Musil, 2017) is the ideal subject of contacting processes: he has many competencies, but is not fixated on certain ways of perceiving or behaving. In him, too, the certainty of his own continuity is rooted in the ever-renewed experience of change.

But the knowledge of growth and impermanence of one's person out of which grows this sense of our own continuity is not yet sufficient for answering the question of how we experience ourselves as the identical subject of contacting processes. Here is the second answer: we know about our continuity through *identifications.* Apart from the memory of our former self, we have our identifications with parts of our natural and social environment which help us and others answer the question: Who are you? And we don't use ontological definitions but define ourselves through identification with our own groups and through demarcations from others ("I'm a man like you" or "Unlike you, I'm a woman"). Identifications are of central importance, because they always already contain demarcations; while demarcations reduce the range of possible identifications, they do not fix them. Genetically, though, demarcations seem to be primary and the identifications may build upon them, for instance under the pressures of racism.

As we are using a concept of identity whose content is contingent and can no longer be distinctly defined, the focus moves to the formal level of identifying ourselves as such-and-such. The new perspective of Gestalt therapy theory was to replace our substantive and systematic concepts of the self with an understanding of the self as "active potential and resource which is capable of generating contingent aims, values, roles and identities" (it is interesting that this formulation comes from a sociologist [Gebhardt, 1975]). This contingency, however, has limits: Our identifications are always socially determined. Not only do they need affirmation by others but by definition they are socially constructed. This connection has been explicated by George Herbert Mead (1934). Mead's famous distinction between the "I" and the "Me" anticipates the differentiation between id functions and personality functions of the self in Gestalt theory: "I" refers to the drives with which human beings are equipped – as well as our capacity for being spontaneous and being creative; "Me" at first arises as an idea of the image the other has of me, and is therefore the reflection of an internalized "significant other" (Mead, op. cit.). In identifying with the perception of the other ("taking the role of the other") I take up their standards and values which now channel and structure the spontaneity with which the "I" seeks to satisfy their needs. But this process of taking up the other's perspective is only to start with an undifferentiated, uncritical process of absorption. According to Hans Joas' work on Mead's social psychology, the most important factor is that the child is gradually confronted by *different* "significant others", so that incompatible internalizations develop.

> In order for any kind of consistent behaviour to be possible these internalizations will have to be synthesized into a consistent self-image. If this synthesization is successful … Ego identity develops as a unified – as well as an open and flexible – self-valuation and action orientation, increasingly oriented towards accommodating different partners. At the same time a stable personality structure develops, which is certain about its needs.
>
> (Joas, 1980:117)

Therefore, according to George Herbert Mead identification does not mean undifferentiated acceptance of parental models and norms as assumed by Freud's model of a Superego, but as the necessarily always new, creatively achieved outcome of the individual's synthesizing activity. Frederick Perls – in a different context – achieved the same insight. He thought that Freud had overlooked the importance of teeth in the process of psychological development. As they grow there is no longer a need to swallow the food whole, without chewing, as is the case with babies. Analogous to chewing, Perls recognized the child's gradually increasing capacity for critically analyzing what it absorbs intellectually. The condition of the possibility for synthesizing a range of influences coming from different significant others is firstly, then, the ability to say no, to reject, to refuse; and secondly, the ability to disassemble (de-construct) into component parts whatever has been taken in, to differentiate what fits together and what does not. Therefore, it is our reflexive and aggressive competencies which allow us to grapple with the normative expectations of others, and access, as Hans Joas has it, "the social norms of communicative exchange, where instinctual impulses can increasingly be adapted according to insight – voluntarily, because such re-orientation brings satisfaction" (Joas, op. cit.:117).

Essential for Mead's theory of the personality is its dialogical character; self-valuation and action orientation, as well as clarity regarding one's own needs, are constitutive elements of personality. They arise from the encounter between "I" and "Thou". Over and over again in the course of life, these elements have to prove themselves flexible and capable of creative modification in relation to very different significant others – individuals as well as groups. Identifications do not arise through one-sided decision making, but stem from the dialogical structure of contacting processes between the individual and their social environment. Not only do I adopt the position of the other, but I present myself and my position towards them as well: identifications are the outcome of reciprocal processes of identification.

When and if this dialogical structure of identifications as they emerge and change is understood, we could define the personality or Ego-identity of a human being as the sum of their current identifications. Anselm Strauss pointed out quite some time ago, that:

> Since the concept of the self has been used as a noun, the existence of a related entity or object is implied. But this is a wrong concept. [...] The concept of the self, if it is to be useful at all, has to be formulated as the organization of activities.
>
> (Strauss / Gebhardt, 1975:25)

This is exactly the concept of self in Perls & Goodman – a theoretical tradition which I am following here. But then the idea of a stable Ego-identity, or personality is obsolete. The self is the contact boundary at work; it is nothing substantial but an on-going process. As such it has certain functions: id functions, ego functions and personality functions. These personality functions then can be seen as expressions of identifications achieved – the result of many successful or frustrating contacting processes. Even such results, though, are never permanent but fluid and provisional.

In this we have another piece of evidence for the self-reflexive character of the human organism: we are not just whatever has been accumulated in the experience of contacting processes. Through assuming the perspective of the other we always must affirm our being by identifying once again with what we have grown into, in order to be able to stand on our own ground: "Only by taking a detour via the other are human beings sure of themselves" ("Nur auf dem Umweg über andere hat sich der Mensch": the often-repeated formulation from Philosophical Anthropology, especially H. Plessner).

Trying to answer the question “Who are you?” – which in the final analysis is unanswerable – will automatically transformed into answerable questions like “What is your name?”, “Which side you on?” or “For whom or for what do you stand?” In identifying with a role, a social position, a group, I make sure of my social anchoring – and thereby create a measure of predictability of my own behaviour and of those others who are involved in the contacting processes that I participate in. This is one of the functions of social identifications: *self-reassurance through social anchoring.*

The other function is the emergence of *responsibility.* In response to the question, “Where do you stand?”, I make myself known as the relevant subject of my actions – in responding I become responsible, and only now can I not just stand by my actions, but be answerable for them. “Personality is essentially a verbal duplicate of the self”, as Perls & Goodman succinctly express it (p. 130). We summarize what we think is relevant and interesting to know for the other and since that has to be formulated, the self now has to put itself into words. That means that human beings as personalities are completely transparent; our personality only exists in the modus of consciousness, in contrast to the self which is aware of itself mainly through sensual awareness. At the same time, personality is relatively enduring because it is the system of identifications we hold on to and which we have to hold on to when asked, when our response-ability is in demand. I describe myself in a particular way and become the one who is responsible and can be made accountable. And only now agreements and contracts, commitments and loyalties become a possibility. This shows that the shared constitution of a responsible subject is the indispensable condition for solidarity to function in our social world. Personality as the system of responsible identifications is the basic element of our social framework through which spontaneous contacting processes are possible – even if we sometimes step out of the frame.[20]

Yet contacts are only complied with, agreements will only be honoured, and loyalties only come alive in contacting processes where the driving power is real needs. Take an obvious example: couple relationships. According to the perspective I am developing here, these relationships are built on an action-motivating expectation – that I will have satisfying contacting processes with this person right into the future. And of course, such expectations are often enough disappointed. In such situations loyalty helps, an attitude where I identify as part of a relationship and stand by it, especially when my needs remain unsatisfied for a while. Not only the sense that a relationship will provide mutual satisfaction in the future will be sustaining, but loyalty may grow from difficult situations, far beyond currently frustrated needs through an insight that neither partner is perfect; that nobody can satisfy all the needs of another; from the knowledge that it is worthwhile to be patient, because there still is a lot to discover in the other. Such knowledge is a personality function; to be loyal means to stick to the agreed continuity of the enterprise in order to ensure eventual success by developing greater tolerance of frustration.

But the personality functions must not take on too much of a life of their own with respect to the needs, because they might coagulate into rigid character structures which could prevent creative adjustments with new possibilities for satisfaction. Good relationships grow from satisfying contacting processes – just as organizations live through the actual contacting processes of their members. Articles, contracts, agreements and even simple loyalties provide relief from pressure in that they protect in times of crisis, and if crises occur they help to manage them better, bridging difficulties. The function of institutions is one of exoneration, as philosopher Arnold Gehlen convincingly argued in his "Man, his Nature and his Place in the World" (Gehlen, 1958).

To be a responsible subject means to stand up for each other in such situations. We are here dealing less with the moral dimension of the personality – however somebody conceives their morality – but with the moral *personality functions* of the self in specific contacting processes. These are spontaneously and intuitively guided by the knowledge that each and every dialogue – however fierce – needs a shared ground on which we stand and must not endanger. The rest regulates itself through spontaneous adaptation of the order of priorities of our needs to that which is necessary in view of the prevailing conditions.

The ground on which we stand now is not just the social world. The background – against which each newly discovered and created Gestalt emerges – has four dimensions in which we human beings have to anchor ourselves by individually or collectively identifying ourselves: *nature, society, individuality, transcendence.* Only through these background dimensions of the respective organism/environment field could we possibly describe the full breadth of our potential identifications and how we achieve them.

To summarize: we can identify ourselves

1 **In relation to myself as nature**: Through having a body, that I am this body; through having been born and the realization that I will die; that I have been born as a man or a woman; with the fact that I'm in need, and have needs; that my body has strengths and weaknesses, is young or old, goes through processes of illness and health.
2 **In relation to myself as society**: Through having relationships and loyalties, through having entered into obligations and having signed contracts; through belonging to specific groups; that I am involved with some and not with others; through embodying social roles and thereby having ownership of social norms and social interests.
3 **In relation to my individuality**: Through acknowledging that I am unique and that I express this through my personal style – in my gestures, my language, in my presentation, etc.; through having a specific biography and through living it. This means that I also have a unique past and a

future horizon exclusive to me; through having specific characteristics and habits, some of which are virtues, some guilty pleasures; finally through the fact that I have developed a personal mode of stigma management (Goffman, 1967); and through presenting myself as a self-quoting figure in narratives (Goffman, 1974:553).

4 **In relation to myself as source and embodiment of transcendence**: That I am part of an encompassing whole, whose dimensions absolutely transcend that which is comprehensible to human beings – and which therefore push us towards humility and modesty, whether I experience this dimension as meaningless or as meaningful; and also through the fact that I am a part of the cosmos, and that especially through being a self-aware being I, too, am an unfathomable source of creative processes.

The sequence of nature – society – individuality – transcendence contains an order corresponding to the hierarchy of needs: first come the elementary needs of survival (nature), then those related to the survival of the species and of social connectivity (society), and only then follow the needs for self-presentation (individuality) and union (transcendence). In general, we will probably accept a person as being psychologically healthy when the basic identifications with their own nature and their own society can be achieved. But the so-called "therapy scene" nowadays offers many opportunities which go beyond these basic requirements of psychological survival. They offer personal development and transcendent experience. If the purpose of these offerings is to allow new kinds of shared experiences to people who are already capable of attending to their natural needs and are taking care of their social attachments, we can quite easily accept this phenomenon of present-day culture – new in its extent! – as enriching us. But here, too, the order of priority is often turned upside down. Whenever we do not attend first to what we need, neglecting or even despising it, something goes wrong; whenever we forget to take care of our bodies and our natural environment we endanger our existence; whenever we avoid working for our own and our fellow beings' survival, or waste our capacities for creative adjustment and development of our culture, we miss out on the human potential with which we are all endowed.

When finally we can responsibly identify ourselves as someone who in varying situations is capable of a dialogically flexible and open response, thus participating in nature and in society; when, according to our capacities, we take part in culturally developed possibilities for expressing our personality; and when we have even learned to accept modestly our ignorance of the cosmos of which we are evidently and surprisingly a part – then perhaps we will have attained some degree of maturity. This then would not be the result of effortful striving for self-control, but the result of many valuable contacting processes turned into satisfying experiences.

Notes

1 For the theory of autopoetic systems see Jantsch (1975). Jantsch gives a resumé of various approaches, including those that have become important for biology. They are concerned with organisms as evolving – or dissipative – systems, which are not organized according to homeostatic principles. In this way, the organism is a dissipative or autopoetic, i.e. self-referential system embedded in its respective environment. Jantsch shows the properties of systems which maintain their structure vs. evolving systems for comparative purposes. An overview of the hierarchies of the specific aspects of the system clarifies the difference between two fundamentally different classes of systems. Systems which maintain their structures are either in homeostasis or irreversibly move towards such a state. Evolving systems are far from homeostatic and evolve by an open sequence of structuring. Heik Portele (1989a:5) has shown the relevance for and connection of these models with Gestalt Therapy. Compare his book: *Autonomie, Macht, Liebe* (1989b).

2 Karl Marx developed the concept of the *conditions of production*. It describes the class structure arising from the distribution of capital and labour, which has developed historically in a given society. Included in the conditions of labour are the relative distribution of workers in agriculture, industry, commerce and the service sector; the way industrial disputes are conducted and the existence of hierarchies of employees and Civil Servants.

3 This concept from phenomenological sociology describes the factual differentiation of all conditions of a situation with regard to their significance or importance to the acting person, as soon as they focus clearly on the object of their need satisfaction or the concern of a social situation. Compare specifically: H. P. Dreitzel (1980), Chapter II, p. 3.

4 With regard to the concept of the self, compare part I, II in this book, as well as part V, 2 in H.P. Dreitzel (2004). Perls & Goodman differentiate between "self" as the complex system of necessary contacts which are required for adapting to a difficult field, and the three "aspects" or "structures" of the self – "id", "ego" and "personality", which represent the major stages of creative adaptation in the contacting process. "The id is the given background, which dissolves into its possibilities; it contains organic arousal, unresolved former situations which we become aware of, the vaguely perceived environment and the unexpressed emotions which connect the organism with the environment. The Ego is the ongoing process of identification and de-identification of possibilities, the process of increasing or decreasing the current contact. It entails physical movement, aggression, orientation and reaching out towards reality. Personality is the figure created from the self, which assimilates it to the organism, in combination with the results of earlier developments. Of course, this is nothing but the process of figure/ground itself" (Perls & Goodman:156–157). The most significant difference from other concepts of "ego" and "ego-identity" is that in this context the subject in its different aspects is exclusively seen as a function of the organism/environment field.

5 "Handling" (German: Handhabung) – is the original meaning of "manipulation" (from the Latin manus = hand), the way Perls & Goodman uses it. Manipulation of the environment here does not have the usual negative connotation of using underhand strategies and deception, but implies the process of physically and intellectually grasping what is needed to influence and adapt the natural and social environment according to need.

6 The fact that the model of the contacting process can do without constructing a position like the "super-ego" does not of course mean that the contacting process between organism and environment isn't normatively structured. Recognizing, adapting and taking ownership of norms and values is in fact a task of the

contacting process, achieved though the core ego function of identification with other close reference figures and groups. Later however, Frederick Perls implicitly re-introduced the "super-ego" when he talked about "top dog" and "underdog". More correctly we should here speak of introjects which are always recognisable in the organism's partial rebellion against them. For a critique of this development see the corrections in Isadore From (1984), – best summarized by Bertram Müller (1996). For orientation of behaviour to reference groups see the classical presentation by Robert K. Merton (1957).

7 Of course only some of the ego functions are blocked; to speak of a complete loss of ego functions would only make sense in a case of complete catatonia.

8 Whether psychotherapy still helps in such a situation or whether it might even contribute to hide the true conditions of their suffering from the patient – i.e. the political and economic circumstances – are questions difficult to decide. The ethos of the psychotherapist obliges them to work towards a higher level of awareness in the patient, even if that means suffering. It is important to respect the patient or client as a responsibly acting individual, and this entails acceptance of refusals. The therapist's working hypothesis is that the client in spite of everything still has more room to manoeuvre than he/she perceives and uses. But the therapist must also be prepared to have this hypothesis rebutted, and must be careful not to generate guilt feelings in the client for not being happier.

9 "Willpower is the drive which awareness has lifted into the Ego sphere, which can manifest itself freely and creatively within the personality." Thus formulates Otto Rank, who taught Goodman and Perls a great deal. From: Rank (1929:28). Quoted from Mueller (1988)

10 The distance we have come in a very short historical sequence from "pestilential smell and flowery perfume" is shown by Alain Corbin in his book *Le Miasme et la Jonquille* (1988). For our sense of smell and reactions of disgust, questions pertaining to their modification in the process of civilization are particularly significant. Compare chapter IV, section 3.

11 For the tragic history of the late Wilhelm Reich being branded as a heretic in the USA see the biography by David Boadella (1973). In 1956 the US Food and Drug Administration demanded – and had it confirmed by the courts – that all accessible copies of sixteen works of Wilhelm Reich (including his famous "Character Analysis", 1933) and four volumes of a journal which he had edited, were to be destroyed in a New York incinerator. Reich himself was condemned and died in prison after he had disregarded a judicial injunction against spreading the word regarding his Orgone Energy generator.

12 According to "Der Spiegel", Nr. 6, Band 38, Edition 6.2.1984:24, Article: "*Forschung Drittes Auge*" Compare: Hess (1975).

13 Perls & Goodman use the term Identification and Alienation, which I think are full of unnecessary philosophical baggage. Therefore I prefer Accepting and Rejecting.

14 Re "common sense" compare: Clifford Geertz, *Common Sense as a Cultural System*, in Geertz (1973). It is part of the phenomenon of everyday knowledge that it is assumed without question. It is always naturally presupposed, it is always shared, so that it is often expressed only in hints. Since we are dealing here with cultural and sub-cultural systems, as therapists we need to know the cultural or social system of whoever we are working with. For an introduction into the issues regarding everyday knowledge – today a central term in phenomenologically oriented social research, compare Berger and Luckmann (1966).

15 Regarding the universality of this norm of reciprocity compare: Marcel Mauss (1966) (French original *Le don* 1924), and Alvin Gouldner (1960). Also see: Hans Peter Dreitzel (1980).

16 "What remains in the memory, the psychological 'engram', should not therefore be thought of as an unchangeable impression becoming fainter as time goes on, like an image scored into a cobble stone. In fact the engram suffers changes according to Gestalt psychological rules" (Wulf, 1922, quoted from Hörmann, 1964). In these publications further information regarding Gestalt psychological explorations of memory function can be found.

17 This is very important for psychotherapy of patients who have suffered sexual abuse during their childhood. See particularly Hans Crombag & Harald Merkelbach, (1996). Generally for Gestalt therapeutic work the cognitive aspect of the material which is reproduced has less significance than the emotions which are attached to the memory, since we are concerned with working on the method of repression, of the block, *in the present situation.* This emphasis on the present experience of emotional memories of past experiences has another advantage: recent brain research seems to indicate more and more that auto-biographical memory is extremely unreliable. See Hans J. Markowitsch and Harald Welzer (2009).

18 Compare Konrad Ehlich (1980). In this volume there are some contributions from psychoanalysis to the topic of telling stories. For the expressive aspect of telling stories compare Erving Goffman, *Frame Analysis* (1974), chapter 13 "Frame Analysis of Conversation".

19 In the new body therapies, some regression techniques are used which are capable of making conscious body memories extend right back to pre-natal experience. For instance, even more impressive than Stanislav Grof's school of Transpersonal Psychology is the technique developed by English psychiatrist Frank Lake, who uses the group to help clients remember their own birth and to re-experience it (Lake, 1986).

20 Erving Goffman talks about social situations whose meanings are intersubjectively constituted as "frames", a concept he borrowed from Gregory Bateson. Frames are organizational principles of social experience; we move in social situations already meaningfully organized by everyday rituals and conventions, etc. Frames make sure that we all know what is going on or should go on, e.g. in normal conversation or therapy, teaching situations, practice, dramas, etc. Social situations therefore are meaning-frames and in them contacting processes unfold – and of course overlap and interpenetrate each other in many ways. Basic elements of such social frames are identifications of the participants as actors or audience members, as role players and even as individuals (Goffman, 1974). For "definition of the situation through role play" compare the relevant section IV, 1 in Dreitzel (1980).

Chapter IV

Emotional orientation

Considering the significance of emotions in the contacting process

Our senses tell us about the world outside of our body, they are the elements from which the "reality" of the world around us is constructed. Only what is available to our eyes, ears, tastes, smells, and our senses of touch and gravity count as tests for what we experience as real, even if we use instruments as tools to help them. In Buddhist psychology the activities of the mind are seen as a sense, too, and if we include these we can also account for mathematics as another building block of our construction of "reality". We must add, though, one important factor, which is communication, or rather *language,* to enable agreement among the members of our species about what to consider as real.

The problem with this notion is that we also experience sensations which originate *inside* our body-mind, even though they may cause voluntary or involuntary external expressions. To these belongs a whole world of what makes up our "inner life" usually referred to as our subjectivity. This consists of our thoughts and other cognitive processes caused by all kinds of bodily excitations and urges, and last but not least our *emotions.* Thus our senses in complex ways also reach inside our bodies and help to construct some sort of "inner reality". In this process our emotions are of particular importance; they have to be taken into account if we are to understand the complexity of human interaction with the environmental field. In a way it could be said that the notion of "inner" and "outer" perceptions is misleading because both can be experienced as given phenomena being part of the field rather than of the organism. But that is an old topic of philosophical debate which we may leave aside here. In any case emotions in the sense of affects are usually experienced as part of one's own subjective experience of what goes on in the outside world. Not that each encounter with the environment is necessarily connected with significant emotions, but obviously whenever our emotions spontaneously emerge they have an important function in allowing satisfactory contacting processes, or avoiding dangers for the organism, and therefore the emotional experience of the client rightly receives special attention in the practice of Gestalt therapy.

There are numerous biological and spiritual connections between external and internal perceptions. But before we can tackle this book`s second major topic we need to take some time to consider the nature of human suffering. After all people seek therapy because they suffer and are convinced or have been persuaded that medical or psychological therapy might help them to overcome or at least alleviate their unhappy condition. Hence even Gestalt therapists with their optimistic view of human nature need a deeper understanding about what drives our patients when they are seeking help from us and what indeed we all share as an existential experience.

Hence I will begin this chapter dedicated to the role of emotions in the contacting process by considering the phenomenology of physical pain as a paradigm for human suffering as such.

1 On physical pain and the nature of suffering

What then is this suffering of ours? Psychic suffering clearly is not an affect, although we feel it. We take it for granted that we know what suffering is, and still the concept immediately eludes any clear identification, as soon as we approach it with analytic intent. Neither can its opposite be reliably defined – happiness, blessedness? Bliss? Yet in contrast to its opposite, suffering is always its own evidence, at least in the experience of the person who suffers. Suffering is a burden, diminishing our vitality, oppressing our *joie de vivre.* With this kind of "psychological strain" ("Leidensdruck") people come into therapy, hoping to shed this burden. At the same time, suffering from psychological strain is on the whole the only motivation sufficient for engaging in this unknown and therefore frightening adventure of getting involved in a therapeutic relationship. Therefore it is important for psychotherapy not only to develop hypotheses about the causes of specific symptoms, but also to develop a deeper comprehension of the nature of suffering as such: to establish that it is an existential constant which cannot be cancelled out through psychotherapy. Neurotic suffering can be alleviated and sometimes even made to vanish; other kinds of suffering can be diminished through economic, political, medical and other means – human suffering per se, though, is immune against all efforts since it is part of human life itself.

This may require exemplification. For a closer look we need to do a phenomenological analysis – as always when we are concerned with fundamental human experience where subjectivity plays a crucial role – followed by a historic-sociological perspective.

Some general remarks

That human beings are suffering beings is so evident that it has never been questioned. This special mentality of suffering is caused by the dual positioning of human beings between nature and culture. In human beings the four Horsemen of the Apocalypse – death, illness, war, and hunger – are so closely yoked together that suffering as natural beings and suffering as social beings turn us into beings who suffer each in our own individual way. Human beings are aware of their suffering and therefore always have to question its meaning – and as this question remains unanswerable, simultaneously its significance increases. The connection between meaning and suffering also entails the possibility that sometimes within the suffering person nature and culture mutually negate each other. So it is in death that a martyr and a stoic hero may defy nature, whereas for victims of torture or people who suffer from a progressive dementing process leading to extreme infirmity, anything social is extinguished and nature prevails.

All forms of suffering have their shared root in our individuation, in our separateness, our isolation from a containing whole, since we must be embodied in two different ways: in becoming incarnated in this particular body, which we cannot leave; and in assuming the mask, which I use and must use in order to fashion myself as an individual, becoming recognisable to others. I *am* this body into which I am born, so that I can live this individual life, and I *have* this body – have it at my disposal – in order to survive this separateness and to invest my individuality with significance through gaining social distinction. So, for example, what in lovesickness is quite harmlessly experienced as pain at the absence of the other or from their reticence, when we feel the agonies of passion they turn into an abysmal burning pain about the reality, that individuation separates us irredeemably, cannot be overcome, can never be bridged.

Etymologically, the German words for pain and suffering ("Leid" and "Leiden") indicate their origin in separateness. Old German "lidan" as a noun means "foreigner", "enemy", sometimes simply "pirate" – and as a verb it means "going into foreign lands", "having to endure foreign lands". All these imply separation and displacement from one's own community, from one's family and tribe, house and home country. Indeed, over and over again loneliness and isolation are major themes in psychotherapy.

In the fact of our being embodied, our suffering has the same root as have our cravings for life. Living and suffering are inextricably linked and so it is no paradox that all attempts at conquering suffering are potentially hostile to life itself.

Attempting anthropologically to distinguish suffering related to our physical existence from suffering based on our social existence leads us astray, as does trying to differentiate psychic, physical and social suffering. It is true that sociology has been able – at a very high level of abstraction – to map two social sources at the root of individual suffering: *alienation* and *anomie* (Dreitzel, 1980). Alienation here means a situation where an individual's creative self-determination ("ego functions" in Gestalt therapy terms) is curtailed by an over-tight, potentially totalitarian web of norms and thus is dispossessed. Forms of alienation range from slavery and various methods of economic exploitation to enforced military service, and it also encompasses everyday suffering through being controlled by others, subjected to anonymous forces. Anomie, however, describes a situation of low orientation, lacking connection through lack of regulating norms and orientating values. This extends from the homelessness of refugees, emigrants and other marginalized groups to the suffering arising from being segregated in any way – to the subtle damage inflicted by the pressure to consume, addictions promoted by the media and the destruction of the family and other groups with whom one has bonds of solidarity. Socially conditioned suffering I would suggest is a more or less significant deviation from a mid-point between anomie and alienation; between social chaos and social order, as measured against subjective suffering, and therefore it remains highly variable both historically and culturally. The source of suffering, especially in our industrial capitalism, tends to result in exclusion – subjectively experienced as suffering – of the exploited and marginalized from participating in the processes of social self-organization.

However, subjective experience is objectively manifested instantly in our bodies, and this can easily be seen in health and death statistics. Being excluded from participating in the *inter-subjective practice* of creating a meaningful form of living for the species, powerfully foregrounds the fact of our isolation through our bodies and thus strengthens the suffering which is already pre-structured into our being bodies. Therefore, individuation which is given with our bodies also resonates with any socially induced suffering.

> All pain and negativity, engines of dialectic thought, are the multiply mediated, sometimes unrecognisable forms of something physical, just as happiness aims towards sensuous realization and thus gains objectivity. Unhappy consciousness is no blind vanity of the spirit, but inherent in it, is the sole authentic dignity it receives through the separation from the body. It reminds itself negatively of its embodied aspect.
>
> (Adorno, 1966:200)

In this way all social suffering is suffering which pre-supposes bodily suffering and also refers back to it. Only when suffering again becomes embodied is it serious suffering in the sense that it has that immovable, objective reality status, which in subjective experience exclusively belongs to physical suffering.

> Somatic experience if formed in contacting the environment, through the feeling of being recognized and contained by the other and the feeling of being free to move in the world. It is clear that the different forms of relational discomforts all involve some sort of suffering.
>
> (Spagnuolo Lobb, 2015:25)

Thus psychic suffering always searches for appropriate physical forms of expression. And for this reason physical pain can serve as a paradigm for all kinds of human suffering. Indeed any anthropology of suffering has to take the experience of bodily *pain* as its starting point.

The concern with *meaning* is intrinsically tied to suffering. In so far as life means suffering, suffering manifests the question of the meaning of our existence. Ever since Job's experience it has been obvious that this question has no answer and still the question remains. Pain always cries out for meaning, and in a way we might say that it only exists "when for better or worse it surrounds itself with meaning" (Morris, 1978:327). Nietzsche, on the other hand, maintains with his own emphatic heroism "It was the meaninglessness of our suffering, not the suffering which was the curse" (Nietzsche, 1883:27). In other words, meaningless suffering increases the pain, which in turn can be relieved either through raging against one's suffering, or surrendering to what one has to endure. The question of what actually has primary importance is impossible to decide.

If living means suffering, then suffering has as many aspects as has life itself, and just like life it will historically show itself in ever different disguises. "Anywhere in the spheres of vital, aesthetic and ethical values one can find oneself happy or touched with pain, suffer", Buytendijk says in what is still the best study of the phenomenology of pain (Buytendijk, 1962). We could begin – as a first step – by distinguishing between physical, psychological, social and spiritual suffering. Physically, we would be concerned with pain in its basic form; psychologically with depression and anxiety; socially with loneliness and care; and spiritually, we would be concerned with what Kierkegaard calls "the sickness unto death", the anguish of not-being-oneself and not-being-wanted-by-God (Kierkegaard, 1983). Such a classification offers a first overview of the realms of suffering and the Gestalts it might take in these areas, and that is a real advantage. Looking at the phenomenology of human suffering in much greater detail would lead to as differentiated a tableau of suffering as there are realms of life itself – which means the epistemological value of such a classification would be lost.

Instead, in order to grasp the anthropological core of suffering it is advisable to start with a focus on pain per se. Looking at physical pain we gain insights which also apply to those kinds of suffering which are not directly physical.

- In the first instance pain *happens*: it comes over us, it befalls us, is – from the beginning – part of the precariousness of our physical existence, always threatening us as a danger in exactly the same way that psychological suffering once seemed to be a burden inflicted by fate. Therefore our lives largely consist in fending it off: in our bodily lives we do this by taking material and medical precautions, more recently also through mechanising our bodies; psychologically we use defence mechanisms, as studied by depth psychology; in the social realm we keep it contained through the norms of social contact, and in the spiritual realm we confront it through sacrifice, ritual and prayer. But when physical pain cannot be warded off, it just befalls us – has to be *suffered.* The same kind of relationship between suffering and defence can be found in psychological pain too.

- Also, pain can be *accepted* ("erdulden") and *borne* ("ertragen"), for example with stoic equanimity, through religious enhancement and immersion in the Passion, and finally through mystical absorption in love. Equanimity, passion and love are human potentialities for enhancing and deepening what dwells at the heart of any suffering as something we must undergo. The same is true in psychological and social suffering. Margherita Spagnuolo Lobb adds:

> Unfinished gestures and incomplete movements tell the relational history of each person. Each body bears the marks of incomplete gestures, and at the same time each incomplete gesture speaks about non-spontaneous contacts, about interruptions in intentionality of contact. Anything that does not find closure is perpetuated. In this case somatic experience may take the form of psychosomatic disorder.
>
> (Spagnuolo Lobb, op. cit.:25)

- Beyond all this, pain is *inflicted* and always a *threat*. This means that pain has a political dimension: through war and the threat of war, through punishment and the threat of punishment and specifically through torture, pain becomes a constitutive element of power. On a psychological level withdrawal of love and attention is one of the most frequently threatened and applied instruments for inflicting pain.
- In addition, pain can be *eased* and thus offers departure points for moral, medical, and psycho-therapeutical discourses and practices each with their own history.
- Finally, pain can be *cultivated* as an instrument of an intentional and sought-after state of de-individuation. Paradoxically, the suffering owed to individuation can – through intentional cultivation and enhancement – serve as a desperate attempt at undoing it.

The phenomenology of pain

Physiologically, pain is generated by an electrical and chemical stimulation of nerve fibres which transfer these stimuli to the brain. But what is it that is generated in this way? It seems that pain is composed from *perceptions* and affects; there is no such thing as pure pain. It cannot be compared to sensations of pressure and temperature which can be measured as physical sensations. It also seems to lack the proprioceptive character of other sensory perceptions. "Pain is given: most of our sensory experience is taken" (Wall,

1977:363). We create our sensory world through perceptual actions. Pain is suffered, is a passive experience. Pain belongs rather more to the class of thirst and hunger, since – as they do – it appears independently of context, has its own urgency, and we don't get habituated to it. In this way, purely physical pain is *different* from psychological suffering, which indeed is co-determined by its social, cultural and economic contexts. It comes as no great surprise that recent psychological research has found that positive emotions have a relieving effect and negative emotions have an aggravating effect on the experience of pain (compare Lumley et al., 2012).

Pain tolerance does not mark a perceptual threshold but indicates the degree to which we are inured to pain. But in contrast pain tolerance is not a function of our needs; the way it moves is not attraction, but aversion. And although it isn't an extreme form of sensing pressure, still it is closest to the sense of touch. The senses which are tuned to distant stimuli – seeing and hearing – can only mediate pain in intangible, immaterial ways. Pain is a kind of core condition of our neural organization (Vincent, 1990:253pp). On the whole, part of this core condition which also applies to psychic pain is made up of perception plus one's current mental state plus personal experiences from the past. It is this combination which makes it hard to understand pain from a biological perspective. The pain researcher Patrick Wall offers the following formulation: "If each stimulus changes the pattern of activity by adding memory and recall, the code is a shift code which is un-crackable – we have a problem" (Wall, 1977:368). This problem is repeated on the levels of psychic and social pain: the experience of pain apparently is endlessly variable.

Pain is a physical experience of pure negation. Pain is pure being-against-it. Something in me is against me, and I'm against it. I and this "Something" are irreconcilably opposed to each other, each side attempting to extinguish the other. In this way, chronic pain is perennial warfare. Pain as such is never chosen. It can be put up with and even cultivated for the sake of other kinds of aims, but in itself it is never attractive. That is true even for masochists, who are after liberating their fettered delight in living, and are not seeking suffering per se. This can be seen in fantasies of rape: lust which has been jailed is projected onto the aggressor, who forces the jail open. In reality any rape is a catastrophic experience, since the aggressor no longer represents one's own desired self, but an alien force destroying both jail and the house of desire at once.

In our dual constitution as human beings both having and being a body, pain creates a regression to being nothing but a body. It represents being defencelessly thrown back into a form of existence where we are no more than barely alive. Pain always tends to be total. It starts with the experience that we can no longer concentrate; we are distracted, and it ends with being unable to stay with oneself – I am nothing but pain. Pain dissolves the content of our consciousness.

> Pain is being thrown back on to one's body without any defence and in such a way that we can no longer be in relationship with it. The pain-ridden region appears to have hugely extended itself, overlaying everything else, seeming to eliminate everything else completely. I only consist of tooth, forehead, or stomach. Burning, gnawing, cutting, piercing, pounding, pulling, digging, shivering pain appears like a forced entry, destruction, disorientation, a force whirling us into a bottomless pit.
>
> (Plessner, 1970b:152)

Buytendijk developed an important distinction between two modes of pain: sudden acute pain when one is *being injured* ("verletzt werden") and the chronic pain of *injuredness* ("Verletzt-Sein"). In acute pain gestures and movements are those of panicked flight – pulling away, turning away, etc., with no chance to face up to this pain, to relate to it. In other kinds of pain which occur suddenly – unexpected loss or the experience of an extraordinarily embarrassing transgression of shame thresholds – reactions are quite similar: One is "stunned" or "wants to become invisible". In injuredness, though, a relationship with one's self is re-established, albeit with a great deal of effort, and it is like a battle, the agonia with – mostly helpless – rage.

> The first type is demonstrated when the person cries "ouch" or "ai"; pulls a face; pulls in his extremities, or if he has been hit in the head or in the body, reaches out towards the place of injury with his hand. In injuredness (chronic suffering) we see a different picture. He sighs, groans, laments, moans in distress and howls. He turns and contorts his body, moves the head to and fro, makes fists and grits his teeth. The eyes are tightly shut or stare with an empty gaze into space.
>
> (Buytendijk, 1948:123)

The differentiation our language makes between pain and suffering has its root, as we can see here, in the phenomenology of our physicality, in different modes of expressive motor activity according to different types of physical pain.

In pain we no longer experience the difference between "inner" and "outer"; it is dissolved. A knife entering the body is experienced not as a knife, but as body. Merely being shown instruments of torture not only generates anxiety and fright, but can actually be experienced as real physical pain. Conversely, we often cannot describe pains originating within the body but experience them as inflicted from outside; and in any case, we can only describe them as such. The only way we can organize our inner experiences of pain is in the modus of understanding the nature of the world of objects opposing us. Thus, when we make an effort to describe our pain experience, we have to resort to experiences we have undergone in the outside world: it burns *like fire*, it pricks *like needles*, it pierces *like a dagger*, is sudden *like the lash of a whip*, and so on. In this is rooted our tendency towards projection.

The intertwining of "outer" and "inner" in pain is further complicated when perceptual and emotional capacity become extremely sensitized in strong continuous pain – all our senses now become entry doors for further torture: slight vibrations are experienced as an earthquake; friendly light becomes painful glaring; harmless sounds become additional burdens. The traditional village community in Greece had a custom where immediately after the death of a spouse the widowed person would shut themselves away in a darkened room for a fortnight, only receiving food through the barely opened door. Psychologists now call this "sensory deprivation" – as if generally there was too little sensory information coming our way, rather than too much. In psychic pain, too, there is a need to withdraw – rarely accepted by society – corresponding to a tendency to experience any situational demand as an added source of pain. If for instance a beloved person dies, the widow or widower is often unable to organize the practical and ceremonial tasks of burial and needs the help of relatives and professional undertakers.

Pain is a-social – this is the departure point for any social-psychology of pain. The reason for this is that pain resists empathic understanding. There is no emotional memory of pain (we would probably not survive if we had such a memory), which would make us suffer in harmony with the sufferer, as is the case with pure emotions. Other than with those emotions whose uninhibited expression evokes the same emotions in the other, the person who suffers physical pain remains alone in their hell, even if giving free rein to the expressive forms belonging to pain – whining, howling, and crying out loud. For even the witnessed pain of the other, despite not feeling it ourselves, instantly triggers an aversive reaction: we want them to disappear, even fall back on denial. "To suffer strong pain entails intuitive certainty; to hear that somebody suffers from pain triggers doubt in us" (Scarry, 1987:16). And this doubt inflicts double pain on the sufferer, coming also from their communicative impotence.

We say that shared suffering is suffering halved. That is true as long as pain remains communicable, which is only the case when we are concerned with the meaning of pain and suffering. Of course there is a lot we can share with each other about preventing and alleviating suffering. But shared suffering itself is suffering to which we can together attribute meaning and therefore question it. Suffering and pain cannot be shared per se; only by jointly constructing the meaning of suffering can it become a social fact. In this way, when all is said and done, psychotherapy is an enterprise always dealing with existential questions. Indeed, talking – overcoming the wordlessness both attached to and a part of purely physical suffering – will have a healing effect on patients, particularly those who have been traumatized.

The loneliness of people who suffer also consists in the fact that pain undermines our *ability to communicate*. It eventually destroys it. Initially, in psychic suffering language is reduced to the language of grievance and complaint. With growing intensity, suffering demands one's full attention; we can talk about nothing else, and even silence has to be wrested from the organism. Physical pain, though, eludes objectification through being worded and eventually – when it reaches high degrees of intensity – it destroys our very capacity to objectify, to distance ourselves from it. The body in extreme pain is no longer a body I "have" but I "am" that body, and even that experiencing "I" is reduced to sheer pain excluding all other perceptions.

Gotthold Ephraim Lessing already recognized that "shouting is a natural expression of physical pain" (Lessing, 1901). The sound of pain, though, is pre-verbal, ambiguous, of uncertain meaning. "Our first response to the world is an outcry. We've no sooner taken in a little air that we expel it with a complaint, a long cry of pain, which having heard it, nobody ever forgets. What it communicates is ambiguous: 'I'm here', it seems to say, 'I am alive. I don't like it'" (von Matt, 1995). The cry of pain is an imposition which in turn can inflict pain. It is eerie, since in it something extra-human, demonic, seems to break out from the body. Therefore, it is not surprising that shouting became an object of the civilizing process. At the outer reaches of Europe there are still memories of professional mourners, whose task it was to take up the cries of the people who were immediately concerned and turn them into a communal lament. Lessing remarks, already anticipating Norbert Elias,

> I realise, we more refined Europeans of later ages know better how to rule over our mouths and our eyes [than the Greek Gods]. Politeness and manners prohibit shouting and tears. Active valour of the first unrefined age has evolved with us into a suffering mode.
>
> (Lessing, op. cit.:144)

This also means that a person who refrains from using this one and only modality for expressing strong pains, will doubly suffer.

Looking at all this from Elias' perspective, it is not really surprising that shouting was cultivated just before suffering became silent. Even today we can read in acting handbooks about the so-called *Wolter-shout,* that special art of Charlotte Wolter, star actress at Vienna's Burgtheater in the 1890s, when she pushed the art of demonizing women – fashionable on the stage at that time – to ever greater heights (von Matt, op. cit.:104). Nietzsche in his essay on lying and truth had already celebrated the shouting human as a being still free from all attachment to reason. But in reality the project of the "Übermensch" came to grief with pain: at the very time Charlotte Wolter stylized and cultivated shouting, Edvard Munch's famous picture "The Scream" was painted (1893), and this has a strange sense of soundlessness about it. All this takes place four years after Nietzsche's breakdown in Turin and at a time when a contemporary of Nietzsche's – sick and sunk in regression – reported in Weimar of the "long, rough, groaning sounds, with which he cried out into the night" (von Matt, 1995:104). These are stages in a process which could be described as the disappearance of the shout. I recall nobody mentioning any shouting being heard from inside the trains travelling to Auschwitz. But perhaps there was nobody there then who was able to hear it.

The most mysterious aspect of pain – and the one we find hardest to come to terms with – is that there is no unambiguous relationship between pain and physical injury. Even Buytendijk's differentiation between "pain of being injured" and the "pain of injuredness" only describes a difference in how it is experienced and therefore in expression, which does not necessarily have to have an equivalent in the actual condition of the body. In other words, pain does not always have a warning function and neither does the intensity of the pain necessarily indicate the severity of an injury. Early in life we all learn that those very painful injuries of the fingertip – owing to a very dense network of nerves – are not as serious as they feel. Later in life we have to learn to pay attention to the health of inner organs necessary for our survival, which do not always send out pain signals. Pain does not in itself have biological meaning.

I will illustrate this point with three cases. Firstly, some *injuries* have no *pain attached to them*. In the state of injuredness we are mostly dealing with internal illnesses, which cannot be recognized through pain from the afflicted organs, like most kinds of cancer, liver problems and life-threatening weaknesses of the immune system. If there is pain in such cases it means that several organs are already affected and often it is already too late. In suddenly being injured, too, there are cases of stupor following being wounded, phenomena without which we can barely imagine the wars (and medicines) of a time prior to the discovery of analgesics. Stupor happens in borderline situations of our existence, when we dip below the always precarious balance between being-a-body and having-a-body, as in conditions of fright and shock or complete exhaustion and deep depression; or when we rise above and beyond it as in situations of heightened intellectual activity, experiencing the ecstasy of complete surrender; or psycho-pathologically, in mania.

> When a human being is – for whatever reason – transported beyond himself, he cannot experience pain. For then, his body has become alienated from him and the digging and burning in him no longer conveys a sense of being-affected in his own body
>
> (Buytendijk, op. cit.:137)

Apparently, we must be hurt in our sense of Self to feel pain at all. Following similar reflections, Maurice Merleau-Ponty concluded that the unity of body and soul is not a deliberately concocted external connection between subject and object. "It actually happens from moment to moment in the movement of existence itself" (Merleau-Ponty, 1962). Pain comes in waves, generated through this movement in the body.

Secondly, there is *pain without injury.* Two well-known cases of this are migraine and phantom pains. Migraine often comes with a particularly severe kind of physical pain which belongs to both of Buytendijk's modalities, but which has no organic correlative. And even phantom pains, occurring in the empty place where limbs have been amputated – can be extremely painful. Merleau-Ponty made an important contribution to analysing this phenomenon (Merleau-Ponty, 1962:102pp).

And finally, a third example is *birthing pain.* Its intensity stands in strange contrast to the life-giving function of the birthing process. Buytendijk assumes that the meaning of birthing pains

> … exclusively consists in the possibility – since they arise with it – that the woman as she suffers may participate directly and consciously in the objective developmental process of a new life emerging, which separates itself out from the old one thus generating devotion and true surrender of the old life for the new.
>
> (Buytendijk, 1948:164)

In this way we can understand why some women – and decidedly not for the sake of masochism or regressive love of nature, but for the sake of existential participation – fiercely object to the project of painless birth (compare, e.g. Bergmann, 1989).

But this should be left in the realm of their own sovereign decision as long as the lives of mother and child are not in danger. For women easily become victims of religious convictions as for instance that expressed by philosopher Max Scheler, who was inspired by Catholicism: "The same dark pressure of all living beings – to reach beyond itself, seeking ever more life – which shows itself in collective association as much as in reproduction, is just the ontological precondition of suffering" (Scheler, 1923:57). Translated into political praxis this would make women vessels of suffering, if for ontological reasons.

This leads us to a differentiation between suffering and pain as illness which we have to heal or at least alleviate – and pain and suffering as existential afflictions to which we must respond as whole persons. Ever since the Age of Enlightenment, Modernity has banked on an understanding of illness – including the naïvely enlightening project of a "Sociology of Suffering" (Müller-Lyer, 1914) and the not altogether naïve attempts at mechanising life itself in reproductive medicine and gene technology, trying to eliminate pain altogether. In contrast to this position there has always been the experience

> … that there is a personal need to experience unhappiness; that for me fear, deprivation, impoverishment, midnights, adventures, perils, mistakes were as necessary as their opposites; yes, to express myself mystically the path to my personal heaven always had to lead through the lusts of my own hell.
>
> (Nietzsche, 1976)

Thus suffering and even the most devilish pain would turn out to be learning experiences if nothing else. This then leads – via the New Age principle, that there is no such thing as coincidence – to the question "What does this teach me?" which is indeed helpful in constructing meaning *ex post*, but may not serve as an *a priori* for action. Using pain and suffering as pedagogical means relates them to torture and deprives the individuals – whom it is pretending to teach – something of their sovereignty, which alone would allow them to be subjects of insight and awareness. Suffering is never annulled by other kinds of suffering. It is important here for psychotherapy to realize that an enduring threat of pain and suffering can be internalized and may narcissistically be claimed as heroic self-control. However, nowadays it is the threat of love being withdrawn in the family rather than physical punishment; the threat of identity loss through loss of work, rather than loss of freedom in one's working conditions which may create such situations. In any case, the possibility that we experience external pressure as an inner straightjacket of potential introjections at least partly explains the extraordinary inertia with which the powerful and the powerless equally regard environmental catastrophe, even though they do not suffer equally from it.

Most importantly, an anthropological inquiry which does not prematurely leap over the boundaries into metaphysics needs to ask which function is fulfilled by the fact that we are able to experience pain, although strong non-painful *stimuli* could do a sufficiently good job as warning signs of biological dangers. Gehlen (1958:73 ff.) and also Buytendijk (1948:98ff) referred to the French philosopher Maurice Pradines (1934), who starts out from the observation that only the higher-functioning animals, especially those mammals dependent on touch in bringing up their young, develop a capacity to experience pain in the classical sense. Pradines concluded from this observation – as well as from research into their sense of pain conducted with people with an intellectual handicap – that there is a positive correlation between intelligence and sensitivity to pain. This is not surprising when we realize that pain is not just a reaction to stimuli but that it also gives rise to specific complex experiential Gestalts which integrate various neuronal, affective, cognitive and social components. When considering pain as a function of intelligence, this concept should not be limited to the cognitive dimension and must not be misunderstood as that which can be measured by tests. Instead it may be useful to understand pain as a function of a higher and broader consciousness.

That pain might indeed be connected to higher intelligence or more acute awareness is proved in a different way by the fact that a disturbance in aesthetic order can also create pain. Whenever we encounter sounds which are not tuneful or colours which clash – and we cannot intervene to change them – we experience mild displeasure or actual pain, depending on intensity. Everybody has their own physiological limit with regard to unbearable sounds; sometimes even thinking about them will make us shudder. Here the transition between physical and emotional pain is particularly clear:

compared to less musical people, musical people are more likely to experience as pain the perennial sound pollution we encounter in the public sphere, and the same is true for other kinds of aesthetic experience. Essentially, when all is said and done, we are children of our own time and culture. For a person from the 17th century the monstrous noise we create with our machines and loudspeakers would probably be as intolerable as would be to us the smells of those 17th century cities. It is neither the kind nor the extent, the duration nor the intensity of stimuli which explains such pain reactions, but our specific subjective sensitivity about disturbed aesthetic orders, which – according to an observation made by Erwin Strauss (1980:143) – is stronger when we are removed from our own milieu, when we are in foreign places. Whether we choose to correlate a subjectively higher degree of sensitivity with greater intelligence – quite different from a low tolerance for pain – completely depends on how we define intelligence.

Pain endured

Right at the beginning of the Odyssey, Homer introduces a distinction rich in consequence: the difference between destinies as imposed by the Gods, and human responsibility. "No!" he has Zeus say. "How those humans blame the Gods! From us, they say, comes everything bad: though they create, through their own outrageous behaviour, more than their own share of pain"! We have not been able to go back since this: from that point onward, it has been impossible to lay all the blame onto the gods. Indeed, the Greeks had already developed a very acute sense of how blind human beings are regarding the consequences of their actions. This blindness is at the heart of Greek tragedy. Over and over again their protagonists cannot read the signs, fail to comprehend the utterances of the oracle and blindly grope for their fate whose cruelty is confirmed by its extraordinary painfulness. More than in the better-known Greek tragedies, this is shown by Sophocles' *Philoctetes*, who enters a holy grove unawares and immediately has to pay for this transgression by being bitten by a snake. Philoctetes' wound festers and suppurates and pains him. Incapacitated, he is left behind on Lemnos by the fleet on their way to Troy and limps across the stage wailing, groaning and shouting and finding no peace. Even nine years later, when Ulysses cunningly manages after all to persuade the embittered man to come with him to Troy, where his Heraclean bow is required for the final victory, his wound has not healed.

The inescapability and pure negativity of pain together constitute the reason why pain always throws up the question of its meaning. And for this reason the history of pain is not identical with the history of the fight against it. Perhaps another story started even earlier: the story of enduring it and justifying, yes, even celebrating it. In antiquity there was no real answer to the question of the meaning of pain; what was needed was to endure it and to undergo it – and if possible, in such a way as to preserve one's dignity. "Do you believe you are achieving nothing, when you show self-control in your illness"? Seneca writes to Lucilius.

> You are proving that illness can be conquered, or at least endured. […] Believe me, a good and courageous composure of soul has a chance to be affirmed, even on the sickbed […] If it does not conquer you, does not make you fall apart, you are a shining example.
>
> (Seneca, 1928)

In the Stoic teaching of virtuously enduring pain we find the defiantly courageous attitude of nomadic cultures coming to fruition, quite specific to advanced civilizations – in Modern times still to be seen in Native American culture. Chiron, though, wise centaur from the Pelion mountain, preferred death to the unending pain which Heracles' poisoned arrow had inflicted on him when he was hunting wild centaurs in the mountains. Immortality had been gifted to him as son of a Titan just like Prometheus: the loss of dignity which often comes with pain has sometimes been feared more than death. Today much of this is mirrored in discussions of assisted suicide.

Every religion has to deal with the problem of reconciling God's benevolence and justice with the facts of suffering, pain and generally of evil. Christianity, more than any other religion, has focussed on suffering per se and specifically on physical suffering, on pain. It was Augustine's achievement in the first place to liberate God – not partially but altogether – from responsibility for the evil of suffering. Augustine`s reception of Gnosis in the shape of Manichaeism subsequently generated an ethics of suffering. Being capable of making decisions, human beings as subjects produce moral pain through their sinful lives and therefore draw physical suffering on themselves as God's pedagogical mode of punishing them. The teaching of Original Sin exonerates God once and for all and puts human beings on permanent trial.

Furthermore, Christianity interprets the death and martyrdom of Jesus as redemptive, his death having been suffered vicariously for humanity. That does not mean, though, that human beings are freed from pain. If anything, it is only the soul which is reprieved: the body still has to carry its own specific cross until the Day of Judgment. In this way, all life is life in a vale of tears which, dependent on God's grace, cannot be escaped until death. A Christian theology of suffering is summarized by Thomas Aquinas in the formula: "Flesh conceived in sin is forced to endure pain not just according to the principles of nature, but also through the bondage arising from our sinful transgressions" (quoted from Buytendijk, 1948:171). Through this argument, once it achieved power, the church was able to firmly establish the social status quo to which ideologically it still adheres.

Beyond this, Christianity demands commitment to a system of beliefs, similar to the demands Judaism makes, maintaining an exclusive truth claim, demanding complete surrender, as otherwise only Islam requires. Therefore, in

Christian belief we find a special form of hypostatization of martyrdom which in which the threat of death and torture did not resolve in renunciation. Undergoing extreme pain was seen as proof and highest profession of one's Christian belief. On the other hand, Islamic martyrs are mostly soldiers killed in religious wars or Jihads and there are similarities to Jewish victims of pogroms and the campaigns of Christian conversion. Augustine had already postulated that it mattered not *what* somebody suffered, but *how* he endured suffering. In this way, reaching beyond Thomas Aquinas, suffering itself could become a path of redemption. "Whosoever bears his suffering with patience, he has Paradise: whosoever fails in this is in Hell", Philip of Neri claimed (quoted from Huxley, 1945). Eventually the church was able to develop a politics of pain based on this philosophy, where suffering bodies could even be misused as instruments for celebrating the power of the church. But the obsession with professing one's faith also opened up the possibility of testifying – through the pain of one's own body – to one's own true faith, even against the power of the church. This becomes apparent not just in the endless history of the persecution of heretics, but also by the testament of flagellantism, which Clement IV was forced to forbid in the plague year of 1349 – while significantly and simultaneously extending the powers of the Inquisition.

The church has always had great difficulties with mystical traditions. Celebrating pain as a vehicle of profession easily opened the door to personal experience, where in fact the aim was to transcend precisely this experiencing self. Christian mystics searched for love in suffering. "Whoever suffers for love does not in fact suffer and his suffering is fruitful before God" says Meister Eckhart (quoted from Huxley, 1945:292). This experiential possibility survived even in some corners of Modernity – to which it was essentially alien – and was even enhanced into a metaphysics of pain. Thomas Macho, in his study of Simone Weil (Macho, 1993:502) showed this in an exemplary way. "Evil", Simone Weil says, "is the shape God's compassion takes in this world". This statement goes far beyond any sentimentality regarding pain, much of which can be found in trivial Catholic literature of the present time. But Simone Weil is not alone in her position – surprisingly, Buytendijk himself ends his penetrating investigations with applying a positive Christian charge to suffering, which called "The royal road of the cross":

> All natural attitudes and reasonable reflections may finally help to prepare the way which in the end the person himself has to take to find meaning in his own pain – and thereby at best fulfil the meaning of his existence. Not just thinking about this path, but entering into it – since it cannot be shortened nor circumvented, not through psychological techniques, which can do no more than ease the sharpness and bitterness of pain, the only way forward is that of blissful suffering and of redemption, which happens through suffering itself and with the help of God's compassionate love.
>
> (Buytendijk, 1948:171pp)

However much the role of the psychotherapist has been compared with that of the pastor, here we see a limit of psychotherapy, which is never permitted to make pain and suffering seem better than they actually are – not even for the sake of spiritual comfort.

But there is also Liberation theology, which understands liberation very much as a matter of this world – specifically, the liberation of poor people from their collective suffering. Liberation theology is attempting to understand human suffering in relation to the fact that most who suffer are in fact victims of organized exploitation and repression. Peruvian theologian Gustavo Gutiérrez, who initiated "Liberation theology," has done much work on the story of Job (Gutiérrez, 1987). According to Gutiérrez, Job eventually recognizes that the injustice of his suffering is related to the injustice suffered by those to whom he had devoted his energy: "I have been the eyes of the blind and foot for the lame / I was father to the poor" (Gutiérrez, 1987:16–17). The question of why God permits Job's current sufferings as well as those of the poor, remains as dark for Gutiérrez as it does for Job. He draws not the quietest conclusion from Job's encounter with Yahweh, but rather the revolting one of active love. From an anthropological perspective T. W. Adorno comments: "This moment incarnate flags up a recognition that suffering should not be, that things should be different. 'Woe says: Be gone!'" (Adorno, 1966:201). Suffering *moves* the world in that it wants to disappear, and therefore there will be history as long as there is suffering. The nightmare of post-histoire, the possibly that delight may become insipid, isn't worth one word in praise of suffering, since all by itself it already cries, "Be gone!"

> Abolishing pain or alleviating it to an extent which cannot theoretically be anticipated, whose limits cannot be enforced, is not the task of the individual experiencing suffering, but of the species to whom it still belongs – even where subjectively he renounces it and objectively is pushed into the absolute loneliness of a helpless object.
>
> (Adorno, 1966:201)

In this age of environmental destruction – fast turning into the destruction of the whole of civilization – in order to alleviate suffering, the species needs to perform what ancient Buddhist experience points to: We have abundant evidence of the extent to which our *greed* for consumption – driven by economic production mechanisms – is mainly responsible for those catastrophic developmental processes worldwide. Buddhism has always insisted that the basic source of human suffering is to be found in our greed. From this perspective it seems that suffering is indeed part of human experience as is our ineradicable need to take from our environments whatever our psycho-physical organism demands for its survival. But this can be alleviated according to our willingness to reduce the extent of our desire to our elementary needs. There is, however, a danger of overstretching this view: the path to ascetism leads yet again into pain. Greed may be tamed by moderation; health food does not involve starvation.

Buddhist experience values increased awareness of our needs as well as of our suffering. Through this, some kind of inner distancing becomes possible, not to be confused with what psychology describes as dissociation, a splitting-off – where pain sensation, with bad results, would just be extinguished from consciousness. In his research with victims of the Holocaust and war criminals Robert Jay Lifton has observed "that the core of our human attempt to cope with pain is our damaged ability to feel, a psychic deadening" (Lifton, 1979:173). Here however we are concerned with increased awareness, where the affective part of pain is replaced by an attitude of noticing more objectively. "Thus we find in the essence of pain a separation between subject and body, to which he still remains helplessly attached, that in the misery of suffering which it gives rise to can be found the possibility of its 'gnostic' dissolution" (Buytendijk, 1948:185). Another possibility may be a stoic rather than a gnostic attitude.

Pain inflicted

A martyr can become such a powerful figure for identification because they set the limits of power. Dying is a more powerful testament than pain. Death offers a final and most radical form of asserting one's identity, in that by being self-precipitated, it becomes a social fact. This is true for Islamist suicide bombers as well as suicide protesters as in the case of Tibetan monks etc. who set themselves on fire.

In pain, though, the person is reduced to being nothing but a body. The path of pain leads from losing one's ability to speak, to losing one's perceptual capacities, to losing consciousness. Pain is pure negation in that we are indeed able to repress its expression, but we cannot find an identity through it. Many researchers have wondered why those who are the most severely oppressed – slaves and mercenaries; peons and factory proletarians – only rarely revolt and have not often achieved a successful revolution from within their ranks alone. They are chained to their suffering through their daily drudgery, condemning them to having no effective voice. Mostly their actions are nothing but short-lived avoidance reactions to their situation.

Here too from the start, the possibility or impossibility of giving meaning to suffering is part of the equation. When pain is inflicted in battle, something is always at stake, even if it was just the saving of one's life. There are victories and defeats and of course the distress of the wounded. This kind of suffering is never as profound as that of victims of torture and of the oppressed, whose suffering allows no meaning to be generated from it; nor does it allow people to *actively* exert themselves to create such meaning – whereas in the misery and humiliation of defeat there may still be a sense of "having given one's best". It is no coincidence, therefore, that etymologically pain has been more frequently connected with punishment than with battle. The Latin word *poena* in French becomes *peine;* in English *pain* and *punishment*; and in German *peinsam, peinlich,* as in "*peinliche Befragung*", which means being questioned under torture. In some trauma patients – especially those with a Christian upbringing – the (human) pressure to attribute meaning to what we experience leads to a temptation to understand what has been suffered as something that they themselves have brought about – an attitude which does not aid their recovery.

The fact that pain is so easily inflicted but so hard to empathize with makes the pain of torture into a ubiquitously available instrument of power. Michel Foucault and others have shown (Foucault, 1977) that those cruel festivals of inflicting pain which initially found their climax in the inquisition of the church, during Absolutism, were expressions of an economy of power. They were not really meant to act as deterrents; public martyrdom, painful punishments, blinding and racking, bone-breaking and tearing apart, dismembering and fragmenting, burning and annealing functioned as a power ritual, in which the dis-embodiment of whoever had dared to deny the ruling power was visibly and obviously celebrated through lengthening the time of the torture. In a similar vein, Norbert Elias remarked that a religion whose basis is the fear of God's omnipotence does not exactly serve any civilizing purpose. He described the process of strengthening internal thresholds of shame and embarrassment and how only once this was achieved did torture as such become less interesting, even if it was the discourse of Enlightenment which made torture topical. Later bodily punishment was more or less abolished and now it is banned from the public sphere altogether. Yet even in the middle of the 19th century the Mayor of London invited guests for breakfast and to see a public hanging, something which would sicken later generations.

Fascism pointed up how much Elias' description of the civilizing process was in urgent need of being extended to the problem of legitimization of power. The horrendous torture practices of the Nazis were only gradually allowed to enter public awareness through the totalization of the war which dulled public consciousness. Torture by now has lost any last shred of legitimacy, but nevertheless still operates in the shadows. It is kept secret, although a widely-known element of all those state apparatuses whose democratic constitutional legitimization stands on feet of clay; sometimes legitimacy is not even claimed. Once upon a time torture attested a legitimate claim to power: today its existence attests illegitimacy. The fact it lives on proves how rare and precarious legitimate rule actually is in our world today. Nothing has done more damage to the claim of the US government that its actions are legitimate – even outside the territory of the USA itself – than the existence of Guantánamo and Abu Ghraib. "The decisive characteristic of pain is its presence. … The decisive characteristic of torture is that it exists" (Scarry, 1987:51ff).

The effect of torture is not just based on pain per se, but particularly and additionally on the experience of total impotence. This indeed epitomizes the experience of pain, but is not complete until the ability to move is lost through being shackled and imprisoned. An exact analysis of torture – whose scenarios have remained astonishingly similar in spite of different instruments being used – shows that its effectiveness rests in a combination of factors which aim to completely destroy the identity of the victim:

- The utter immediacy of pain disallows any form of avoidance.
- The dwelling place, clothing and human relations are themselves turned into instruments of torture: any possibility to withdraw is destroyed.
- Ritualized self-betrayal by confessing what the torturers frequently already know serves – just as the practice of making victims inflict pain on themselves through their own body movements and postures – to destroy psychic and physical identity.
- Taking away any shred of privacy to attend to the most intimate needs and requirements of the body – pain, hunger, sickness, sexual arousal, defecation – leads to a complete collapse of any capacity to be separate, to maintain distance.
- Pain – in this process of becoming total and overwhelming – is objectified in the instruments of torture, turning them into an embodiment of one's own impotence and the other's power, so that the destruction of identity is initiated or promoted just by the showing of such instruments.

The current proliferation of torture is based on its being both pre-modern and post-modern, in that the state's power fills and occupies the private sphere right into the most intimate corners. In this, it documents the insidious destruction of the difference between private and public life on which our civic world used to rest. Only through this phenomenon can we explain why it is not just in states poised at the threshold of Modern times that we find torture. In one aspect, though, it remains as primitive and simultaneously modern as is Fascism, in whose recesses it always thrives best: and that is in its abhorrence of all forms of weakness (Heinsohn, 1995).

> Inhumanity needs more than an average capacity to be cold, rarely based on an inborn or milieu-specific atrophy of affectivity [...] but on the will to destroy any form of weakness. And the devil would not have his hand in this process if the destruction had not also been insisted upon in the name of the Highest.
>
> (Plessner, 1956:228)

Pain alleviated

In parallel to the celebration of pain there has of course always been the fight against it. Pain itself aims at its own disappearance: it wants its own negation. But strangely, in the West this fight was a secret one for a long time, and sometimes it was even persecuted. It may have been difficult enough to find more effective agents in nature to alleviate pain than the bite sticks which had been used from times immemorial: even brandy was invented quite late (around 1100). But the Christian apologia of pain with its idea that pain is divinely ordained hindered the search for new materials; and above all it interfered with experimentation in a way that we will never be able to fully illuminate. This is even more astounding as there must have been a misery of pain barely even imaginable today. There weren't just those excesses of martyrdom and torture but wars and assaults, illnesses and epidemics, too. And there was surgery without anaesthetics.

Besides the use of biting sticks and alcohol, there was widespread use of flames for local anaesthesia and knocking people out to produce black-out as the only available means of creating full anaesthesia. All this in spite of the fact that although datura and opium had been known since antiquity, they were rarely applied since their use in witchcraft was suspected and if they were used at all, it was in the form of so-called sleeping sponges. Ether, too, had already been discovered around 1200 and was manufactured in 1546; Paracelsus instantly recommended its use, but another 300 years had to pass until it was first used medicinally. Even laughing gas, discovered in 1772, took another 72 years before it was first used. Doctors – given a lot of leeway to get things wrong – stood under threat of severe punishment for using it. Added to this is the fact that since the Enlightenment, self-control increasingly has become a bourgeois virtue, especially for men. The civilising process generates a new *disciplining thrust* which was primarily enforced in the military, in schools, in sport, but also in hospitals and factory halls – demanding that bodies be disciplined to bear pain.

This disciplining thrust also represented a step on the as-yet incomplete pathway towards the sole reign of men, in that complaining and tears were defamed as being womanly, expressing a wicked sense of justification since birth pains were definitely considered to be divinely ordained. Fascism, still alive in some nooks of health care services, completed this development through making the victims themselves – women in the shape of mothers and nurses – into the most important agency for mediating this kind of repressive heroism.

Nevertheless, there has been a revolution in the fight against pain. In the 19th century we see the application of inhalable anaesthetics, ether and laughing gas, as well as a generous use of opium and hashish; in the 20th century a large group of new analgesics were synthesized, some working peripherally, others centrally. It is due to them that the recent decades' delusional war against opium and hashish as intoxicants was even made possible. They became the condition for enabling a great extension of surgical practice and democratizing the fight against pain.

Still, we are far removed from the leading of pain-free lives, which always remains a Utopia, since with the possibility of fighting pain, pain tolerance is diminished. At present there are about 10 to 15 percent of the population who are *regularly* taking pain killers. An unknown number of people suffer from chronic pains, especially muscular and joint pains, headaches, tumour-related and gynaecological pains. But continuous use of analgesics leads either to pain-killer dependency or to worse damage – as in the catastrophe of thousands of victims of opiate dependency by medically prescribed pills in the US. The question keeps arising why so-called "side effects" so often overshadow intended effects. There are millions of people who suffer from pain as their primary diagnosis, i.e. people for whom pain cannot be shifted even after many years of treatment with various therapeutic agents. Tragically, in itself the misuse of analgesics is one of the major reasons for conditions where pain is the only symptom. Any chronic pain represents a very personal life history, where physical, psychological, social and cultural circumstances make up a biographical Gestalt (DelVecchio et al., 1992) demanding psychotherapeutic attention.

Just as in other large experiments for alleviating suffering and pain – for example in development aid or more generally when muscle power is replaced by machines – it seems that there is a dialectic at work which ensures that the means of alleviating pain in the end leads to an increase in pain or just shifts it in some way. The phenomenon that unexpected and often unwanted consequences follow planned social action shows that life is indissolubly interlinked with suffering. It is consistent therefore that the project of a pain-free life today has found a much more radical path towards success, and that is the gradual abolition of the body through organ substitution and neural networking. "The acute question about the meaning of suffering touches on the gnostic experience of the unity between living and suffering, on the existential harmony between Weltschmerzen and jubilant redemption rhetoric" (Macho, 1993:500). But this is our current, mainly Western experience; Eastern cultures have always lived with a far less dramatic understanding of "existential harmony." And what if it were true, that developing sensitivity to pain had a functional relationship to the development of intelligence? Could we then interpret this lowering of the pain threshold as a sign of growing intelligence? In any case one challenges the other in that there is a need for ever new and more differentiated pain killers, which have to be discovered and invented through scientific intelligence.

Pain cultivated

We never seek out pain as such – but it can be cultivated as a means for achieving other purposes. Historically, the connection between pain and eroticism comes to mind which is represented – unsurpassed – by the name *de Sade*. In an age of mass production of violent pornography and horror videos it is hard to understand the 18th century's fascination with the works of de Sade. It must have been a concurrence of two civilising currents which created such a receptive climate – the removal of the taboo regarding sexuality through what Foucault described as the "discoursization" of sexuality (Foucault, 1979) and a tendency towards mechanising and disciplining all life processes. Neurologically it is known today that pain and pleasure receptors are situated quite close to each other, and one can easily tilt over into the other, depending on personal sensibility and tolerance. Through the work of psychoanalysis, we now know a lot about the historic role of masochistic and sadistic impulses in the complex household of drives and instincts in human beings. Through discoveries made by evolutionary biology we know how strongly power and submission as archaic dimensions are still alive and operative in human sexuality – not necessarily overt but covert and certainly in fantasies as demonstrated in the bestselling success of E. L. James' *Fifty Shades of Grey*.

For quite a long time now, a particular behaviour has attracted the attention of psychotherapists (Sachsse, 1994) – the intentional "cutting" of arms and legs, which can go as far as scalding and burning parts of the breast and belly; and systematic poisoning. Here we are concerned with people who escalate their auto-aggression into a war, obsessionally enacted against their own body with the paradoxical aim of breaking out of the prison of numbness erected against what they experience as the unbearable pain of their biography. This mad attempt at driving out suffering through pain is usually conducted in secret. Here we are dealing with a pathological border-line case of cultivating pain, which nevertheless is symptomatic for our culture (consider for example the popularity of films by and with Mel Gibson).

Culturally though, what sticks out about the relationship between pain and eroticism, of violence and sexuality, is its predominantly voyeuristic quality: child pornography, bought and sold worldwide, is a historical first and simultaneously a symptom of a general, always morbid-erotically coloured fascination with imagined violence. A flood of images revolves around the threshold values of life: death and sexuality. It is as if our culture needs to remind itself in just this drastic fashion of what secretly seems to lose value: the certainty of a body capable of suffering, the very source and centre of our experience of the world. The problem is that even the most extreme images in a visualized world no longer suffice to assure us of our bodies.

This is why – beyond images – in this culture many people are perennially in search of ever-new extreme physical experiences, where overstepping pain limits is accepted and even consciously intended. With regard to the dialectic of having-a-body and being-a-body, here people are looking for a state of total *being* – in contrast to the prevailing tendency towards an alienated sense of the body having to be available, under all circumstances, even in infirmity and unconsciousness, of which people can be ashamed. Paradoxically, a personally self-determined form of having-a-body is carried to extremes. When the body is under extreme control, in controlled peak performance a state of being is sought where control turns into pure being-a-body. At the limit of death and in extremes of pain life clearly eludes any inclination towards virtualization and regains its old certainty. Control seems to emancipate itself from the will and becomes independent; identity is lost and the boundary between subject and object begins to dissolve. This state is desired by some as an opening into the world; others are seeking relief from the pressures of (self-)identification through a *peak experience*. This borderline zone, this experiential realm between this peak experience and one's normal state is physically characterized by pain and psychologically by anxiety, which step-by-step begins to be experienced as painful bliss and excitement fired by fear. We now know that the body's own substances, similar to opiates, are set free and contribute to the experience. Yet those in search of such experiences are not just addicts of their own body's self-produced drugs nor only depending economically and/or psychologically on the public of their spectators but looking for an increase in their awareness of being alive with the aid of self-discipline which they stick to alone and in the face of pain. They are not trying to plumb the depths and limits of sociality, but the depth and limit of their own individual capacity. Extreme physical experience is an apotheosis of individualism. There are indeed milieu differences between "smart" sailors and extreme climbers and those countless numbers who undergo strange exertions to prove their quantitative body power by achieving a record regularly noted in the Guinness Book of Records. What they have in common and what is at stake here is the desire to enhance one's sense of individuality and uniqueness.

But we cannot separate a secure sense of individuality from a secure sense of reality. Ontogenetically Ego identity develops with and through the discovery of external reality as a physical and social Not-I. Being sure of one's identity and of one's reality is always inter-connected. And this connection is in danger of being torn apart in the stream of images; permanently threatened by the virtualization of the world. This, too, seems to provide a reason for people to search out physical violence: in pain inflicted and in pain suffered – although barely verbalized or truly imagined – the body reconstructs itself as the first and last evidence-base of all experience. Whether one inflicts pain on oneself as secretly as possible, common in more socially elevated milieus, or whether one looks for it in the gang which exclusively lives for the confrontation with its opponents – created for just this experience, as it happens in youthful violent milieus: these are issues of social status and one's outlook on life, which, though, do nothing but cover up the central theme. Philosopher Dietmar Kamper pointed out that our culture tends to expropriate our bodies through imagery:

> The body's becoming-a-picture is continued through the dis-embodiment of images. The process is accelerating so much that images in the new

> media already fade as they appear [...]. It is possible, that as the civilizing process continues in this direction of ex-carnation, all flesh will become word and image; desire may just get lost.
>
> (Kamper, 1989:309)

The search for extreme physical experiences is already a way of taking counter measures, an attempt at restoring the body to its rightful place, and this re-incarnation leads easily into and comes about through pain.

Evidence for this can be seen in the mediated content of the pictures themselves. They are about extreme carnality, with scenes of violence, faces torn by pain and bodies smashed; they also show sexuality in all conceivable forms. In the shape of reality television, they even show actual birth, illness and death, as well as a vast range of intense emotional expressions – all extreme situations of our physicality. But there is also an increase in images of extreme experiences in sports, long a part of advertising – images of tough encounters with mountains, the sea, and ice – those specifically chosen opponents to whom the actors are addicted with something like a love-hate bond. The imaginary aspect of these images is the dream of liberation from images, which the average customer wishes for when watching football, working-out in a fitness club or when jogging – a dream which a minority pursue in the Sahara, in the Himalayas or in Antarctica.

Simultaneously the desire for re-incarnation is fed by a spiritual longing for overcoming individuality, for dissolution of our existential separateness, the root of all suffering. It is significant that in the search for extreme physical experiences the longing orients itself again by choosing the Western pathway of increasing *performance* via body control, through the border-line realms of anxiety, excitement and bliss; through pain towards transcendental liberation.

Eastern traditions in contrast seek to silence the body not only by suffocating all sensual and emotional expression but by controlling all body movements in the strict discipline of a Zazen Sesshin or in cultivating movements in yoga and martial arts. The overall aim here is increased awareness. Severe suffering, however, diminishes and disables awareness, as does severe pain. But just as analgesics can alleviate physical pain to the extent that a reflexive relationship with it becomes possible again, in the same way psychic suffering can be alleviated through empathy and verbal exchange to a point where awareness can grow again. For a diagnosis, doctors need very specific descriptions of their painful experiences from their patients, because there is no objective measuring of pain. And psychotherapists need to teach their patients to again sense their repressed sufferings before they can work through them together. The utterly human desire to be rid of one's pain must not lead to a phobia regarding pain, since radical de-sensitization of pain – as we know from our experiences with drugs and intoxicants – is always followed by an *emotional* de-sensitization. Pain and suffering are not just related to each other, but identical in that they are inextricably connected to the body, in that they are an expression of life itself, proving that life always defines itself also through its negation: from the start it is not just defined by growth, but also by its transience and death. Awareness as embodied mindfulness is a modality of consciousness through which this dialectic relationship can be emotionally experienced, denying itself to both growth euphoria and pain phobia, as well as to an apathetic acceptance of supposedly God-given or fate-inflicted states of pain and suffering.

Only by *abolishing* the body could we realize a pain-free life which then no longer could be called life. Therefore, the question is not whether human life will always be connected to suffering, but why the role of joy in human experience has been given very little attention. For as with laughter and crying, desire and pain are twins, and so are joy and suffering; none can exist without the other. This is the reason why Gestalt therapy does not promise happiness to its practitioners and patients; its promise is to make life livelier, to increase our zest of life through embodied mindfulness.

2 Emotional expression and emotional experience

On the anthropology of the emotions

It is perhaps astonishing that in spite of a growing body of empirical research in psychology and the new field of neuro-psychology, Gestalt therapy has so far not produced a theory of the emotions congruent with its theory of the contacting process – a theory which does justice to their role in the practice of Gestalt therapy. The reason, I suspect, is to be found in the unfortunate survival of a deep alienation between a psychology dominated by operational empirical work in the behaviourist tradition and European *phenomenological philosophy*, and the German school of *Gestalt Psychology.* The theory and practice of Gestalt therapy is deeply rooted in both these frames as well as drawing from other sources like American Pragmatism. This lack is all the more astonishing since around the year 2000, a sudden proliferation of interest in the subject of the emotions occurred labelled the *Emotional Turn* in social sciences. This led to an extraordinary increase of academic as well as popular literature about the nature of emotions.[1] But a closer look at this literature reveals that very little research has emerged which would really help to understand the importance of emotions in our everyday life, in our culture, and specifically in Gestalt therapy. In the following explorations I will attempt to formulate such an approach towards understanding the existential significance of human emotions generally – and for the process of Gestalt therapy.

When I began to work on the first edition of this book (Dreitzel, 1992) there was still little interest in this topic. Emotions were not considered a serious object of reputable philosophical or scientific study. The Cartesian *cogito ergo sum* still served as a barrier towards taking a closer look at what was considered to be irrational impulses. There were notable exceptions, though; practitioners and theoreticians who had the courage to ignore this paradigm, in search of enhancing the creativity of their studies. Most of them were inspired by Husserl's Phenomenology (such as Max Scheler and Maurice Merleau-Ponty) or biology (Charles Darwin and Paul Ekman) or both (like Helmuth Plessner). Others were inspired by Sartre's and Heidegger's Existentialist philosophy (such as Ludwig Binswanger). Another significant exception is the ingenious Australian musician and engineer Manfred Clynes who developed a highly original approach to the empirical study of emotions. He combined a phenomenological view with a scientific methodology and arrived at what, in my judgment, is the best theoretical model for understanding their role in Gestalt therapy.

I should mention here that there have been notable attempts as early as the 1970s at approaching the topic of emotions by some researchers into motivational psychology. The American author of the most comprehensive presentation of these studies, Carroll Izard, was – unsurprisingly – also working as a psychotherapist, particularly with children (Izard, 1977). All these contributions have influenced my own enquiry into the nature of our emotions and their meaning for Gestalt oriented psychotherapy.

Emotions have great significance in the contacting process in general and specifically for the practice of psychotherapy for two reasons: anthropologically speaking, emotions have a powerful action orientation; and they have great significance in helping us to understand how psychopathology reflects culture-specific channelling or repression of emotional expression. Ever since Darwin's famous study *The Expression of the Emotions in Man and Animals* (Darwin, 1872) these two aspects of our human emotionality have been polarized and used to challenge one another; biological ideas about the universality of human emotional expression have been used to trump culture-specific relativistic ideas of the purely social determination of emotional life (Darwin, 1852; Ekman 1980). Due to the valuable work of a few outsiders amongst the scientists researching emotions, we can now consider the controversy between universalists and relativists as resolved. We now have studies enabling us to take account of the interactive significance of the emotions.

The philosopher Agnes Heller in her *A Theory of Feelings* provided us with an analysis of the importance of emotions for our everyday life (Heller, 1980a). She dispenses with the false and unfruitful polarization of the emotions and the mind, returning the emotions to a place of philosophical exploration of issues worthy of questioning – as they already had been in Spinoza's ethics for example. Thomas Scheff, well-known through his sociological analyses of psychopathological labelling processes ("labelling theory"), with his analysis of the experience of emotional catharsis (Scheff, 2007) has re-awakened the interest of interactional sociology in the problem of emotions. Of greatest significance in our current context are explorations into the functioning of emotional communication conducted by Manfred Clynes. It is through his investigations that it has become possible to consider the role of the emotions in the contacting process in a way which can be empirically validated (Clynes, 1976; 1980a).

Before looking at these investigations in greater detail, some conceptual clarifications are necessary since neither scientific nor everyday language is really clear and unambiguous with regard to emotions. In the social sciences the meaning of concepts like emotion, sensation, affect, mood, passion depend on an author's theoretical position, whereas our everyday language either makes distinctions of feelings or disregards phenomena depending on their culture of origin. For example, some Western languages distinguish different degrees of intensity in one and the same emotion, as in "anger" and "rage", while not having even a single word for others. For instance, Clynes reports that Balinese people have a word for our reaction when we suddenly see something overwhelmingly beautiful. And even closely related languages carry untranslatable nuances when naming a range of emotions. For example, the English word "reverence" is neither adequately translated (into German) by "humility" ("Demut") nor by "awe" ("Ehrfurcht"). Everyday language, therefore, is essentially an unreliable guide through the psychological domain of the emotions. On the other hand, sometimes everyday expressions can be quite revealing, showing the significance of a specific emotion within the tradition and present situation of a culture, and for the process of setting and maintaining social norms to which the expression of feelings and emotions are subjected. The word "Angst" (fear/anxiety) for example seems to have its indefinable undertone only in German, motivating the French to differentiate "le Angst" from "l'angoisse" and the English-speaking world to talk about the "German Angst". Some other terms for emotions are class- or gender-related: vulgar expressions especially – usually connected with sexual arousal or body secrets – are typically avoided in upper-middle-class talk and often would not have even been *known* in puritanical circles.

Before attempting an enquiry into the social nature of emotions, we need to clarify what the subject to be explored actually is. I will establish some definitions, a terminology I will use in the following exploration. Let us be clear that from a phenomenological perspective such terms are not to be confused with facts in the material world but taken as linguistic agreements or conventions which have emerged historically and point to subjectively experienced states of consciousness. For the sake of clarity, I ask the reader to follow my linguistic suggestions throughout this enquiry.

Firstly, I would like to distinguish emotions from *bodily sensations, moods* and *passions.* Bodily sensations are always part of any emotion, but they can also appear without emotion, lacking the emotions' evaluative, relational character regarding the environment. Sensing hunger and thirst informs us about our bodies lacking something, though not how to assuage it. Physical pain often does not offer an assessment of what is wrong with us. It does not tell us from what ailment the pain arises and neither its intensity nor its locality offer unambiguous indicators (see this chapter, section 1).

Moods indicate dispositions towards a specific emotional orientation, becoming relevant for action as soon as a concrete contacting situation is as when a man coming home frustrated and exhausted by a long working day greets his joyously barking dog with a kick. The whole of the environment then takes on a specific emotional colouring; everybody knows the phenomenon of the same environment seeming grey today and rosy tomorrow, depending on one's mood. Moods are generated either by subjectively irrefutable environmental influences (for example by the weather) or from overspill: emotional residues from other satisfactory or unsatisfactory contacting processes as particularly in dreams. Moods also have a completely physical side, as shown in the way they can be influenced by drugs. The disposition towards certain moods, such as inclining towards a "depressive prevailing mood", can also be influenced by psychological and social factors; for example, through strengthening an individual's competencies for dealing with difficult environmental factors and an increasing ability to achieve nurturing experiences, as well as through directly changing the environment. In the first case we are dealing with pedagogy and therapy, whereas the second is dealt with through technology and politics and also through art. Moods are different from emotions in that they are lacking emotions' cognitive function; as opposed to emotions, moods disregard the specifics of a particular contacting situation, don't take account of the special new quality of phenomena but instead – in the form of emotional prejudices – colour each new situation in such a way that everything appears in the same light as before.

Like moods, *passions* also have a quality of persistence not belonging to emotions, arising spontaneously in contacting processes. Unlike moods they arise from a conjunction of individual deficits regarding the *culture* of the environment: passions are culturally enabled and symbolically enhanced fixations on either desired or hated objects of past or future contacting processes. Love, for example, can become a consuming passion – especially in a situation where the desired person is socially or physically unreachable, such as in a fixation of cultural significance (Luhmann, 1989). Even hate can become a passion, if or when one is forced into a social unit with the hated person, for example a marriage or a village community; or in response to persecution, interrogation or torture by the hated person, particularly when revengeful action achieves a special cultural significance, as for example in a manhunt.[2]

Perhaps it is a response to the deep conditioning of our behavioural orientations by our consumerist habits that passions as a cultural phenomenon have gone out of fashion – at least in the form of an emotional clinging to desired or hated objects or persons. But there is also a way of holding on to excitement without a human being as "object" and this kind of passion seems to fit better with our wasteful, throw-away society.

Here we also have to consider the multitude of activities accompanied by the thrill of pleasurable anxiety ("Angstlust" is the appropriate German expression) when undertaken with the kind of obsession characteristic of passionate behaviour. They are usually tainted with a physical or economic risk – and only undertaken voluntarily by the well-to-do, one would assume. Mountain-climbing and motor racing are modern examples; gambling and hunting more traditional varieties of passion whose aim is not satisfaction but excitement. Today we see more and more high-risk varieties of sport and adventure with people looking for the experience of meeting limits ("Grenzerlebnis") which they hope will extend their Ego consciousness and transcend it. Here we also find our culture's fascination with speed and acceleration. Raised blood pressure and adrenaline in these experiences operate as anti-depressants which can create dependencies. But without realising it, we are always in search of a goal – some kind of happiness, a satisfaction, peace at the end of the road – and the more speedily we proceed the sooner we seem to get there. This explains why we love the car for leisure activities: it enables us to disregard our disappointment at reaching the end of the road and not finding whatever we were unconsciously seeking: we just set off on further journeys, disregarding our disillusionment.

In comparison, *emotions* proper (some authors here speak of affects!) arise spontaneously in the immediate context of particular contacting situations. They have their specific place in this process and either promote or impede it. And they can also arise – as we will see below – in a distorted form as backlogs of earlier incomplete contacting processes, residues from over-controlled expression and from processes of repression. Otherwise, *emotions are situational evaluations by the organism of the current state of affairs in the organism/environment field and are experienced through the body and spontaneously expressed in body postures and facial expressions.* Initially this definition asserts the evaluative function of emotions particularly emphasized by cognitive psychology. Emotions are not "irrational". The polarization of "clear reason" vs. "clouded emotion" has long been overcome by the humanities: in fact, emotions always contain a "rational" evaluation of the respective balance of power between subject and object in the contacting field – as realistic or unrealistic as the perceptive potential of the individual is sharpened or dulled. I feel secure or threatened, attracted or repelled, loved or hated, and through these emotions I evaluate my relationship with my current environment. This assessment happens spontaneously, immediately, without conscious intention but with full engagement, not at all like an evaluation by the intellect, which presupposes distance and intentionality. It also differs from simple reflexes, which impulsively by-pass perceptual functions, missing the object and failing to exercise an orienting function.

"To feel something means to be involved with something", as Agnes Heller says (Heller, 1980:19). At the contacting boundary the feeling human organism is directly and committedly participating in their environment.

Each emotion pushes us towards a direction for action; towards the object, keeping close to the object, away from the object, and towards a particular action modus – to destroy, to preserve, or to avoid. In this way we experience emotionally the situation in the current organism/environment field, gaining motivation for action in and through our bodies. The reason for the embodied nature ("Leibhaftigkeit") of this experience is that normally the emotions are driven by need, which in the form of lack tends to be the driving force of the contacting process. It is this elementary embodied connection with need which gives to the judgement of the heart so much more power to motivate action than the more distanced judgment of the intellect. It has to be conceded, though, that this modality produces a lower level of differentiation. Therefore, emotions are strongly motivating evaluations of the environment but with relatively low discriminatory power – the reverse is true of the intellect.

The embodied nature of emotions finds immediate physiological expression. Each emotion is accompanied by a range of physical processes apparently arising in specific combinations and varying according to the intensity of the emotional situation: changes may be experienced in the rhythm of breath, the pulse, sometimes blood accumulating in certain areas of the body (in the head when blushing, in the genitals in sexual arousal, or turning pale with fear or rage); also, there are sensations of cold or heat or we may sweat excessively. Most important though are hormonal excretions. We know most about the role of the sexual hormones and that of adrenaline (Vincent, 1990). There is a plethora of literature online on recent research findings regarding the relationships between hormones and emotions.

Some authors distinguish emotions from affects thus separating their physical aspects from their orientational functions (among others, recently Seyd, 2016. From a phenomenological point of view, this does not make sense: the *experience* of an emotion is always that of a *unity* of physical sensations and motivational judgements. Indeed, it is this unity which constitutes the extraordinary power which unrestrained emotions may develop.

There have been many definitions of emotions as bodily conditions on the part of a psychology which modelled itself on the natural sciences, understanding the subjective experience of emotions as a simple derivative of physiological processes. But laboratory experiments studying this assumption have not delivered the desired outcomes – feeling something implies being involved; emotions are phenomena of the organism/environment field, which also but not only seek to express themselves through the body. Their embodied nature ("Leiblichkeit") accounts for their overwhelming presence; like needs, they cannot just be repressed but they can be blocked, inhibited, channelled and controlled – a fact rooted in the significance of emotions for human survival.

But emotions are not just spontaneously-experienced bodily phenomena: they are also cognitions, being spontaneously and mimetically expressed. This is the defining fact allowing us to decipher the other important function of emotions apart from their orientating function: they also serve to *signal and communicate;* they do not just inform the organism but also its environment. Just how this happens in detail is the subject of two very different research orientations which together have finally confirmed the thesis of the universality of human emotionality and the modes of its expression; I refer to the research studies of Ekman and Friesen (regarding the mimetic expression of emotions) and Clynes' studies regarding the nature of the forms of emotional expression.

Based on decades of study, Ekman and Friesen have been able to show (in both of their books Ekman / Friesen, 1972) that at least seven emotions are accompanied by distinctive facial expressions recognized across cultures, independently of race and level of civilization. These seven emotions are *surprise, anger, hate, fear, happiness, contempt* and *disgust*. Importantly – largely by exaggeration – human beings are born actors, capable of intentionally reproducing the relevant facial expression so that these come close to being convincing approximations of the spontaneous expression of the emotion. We will see that this capacity for mimetic reproduction of emotional expressions has immense significance for the functioning of social interaction. How does it happen that the muscular facial movements (and bodily postures not studied by Ekman and Friesen) universally expressing certain emotions coincide in all humans? Must they be considered with reference to the theory of evolution as the result of species-specific learning processes? Ekman / Friesen maintain they are fairly sure that there is a "face-affect programme, which is located in the nerve system of all human beings and which connects specific facial muscle movements to specific emotions" (Ekman / Friesen, 1972:138). But the triggers for this programme and their subsequent action patterns are socially learned and culturally variable; emotional expression can also to some extent be repressed. Yet to achieve living together peacefully in societies with mixed ethnic populations and diverse identity cultures, the discovery of the universality of emotional expressions is of immense importance.

* * *

For the understanding of therapeutic processes, the creative studies done by Manfred Clynes are of even greater significance. It is unfortunate that their reception has been somewhat limited, most likely because they extend beyond commonly accepted academic boundaries. Clynes starts with a question which is significant for him as an artist: how is it that music has the power to evoke emotions, and why do some kinds of music apparently do this more effectively than others? Here again, questioning what we take for granted is the first step of a fruitful scientific enquiry.

Doubtlessly motivated by his experiences as a practising musician, Clynes acted on his observation that initially an emotion is always expressed in *movement* which lasts for a certain time.[3] Microanalysis led him to discover that each elementary emotion has a specific spatial-temporal form of expressive movement belonging to it. Clynes calls these the "essentic form" of an emotion.

> Essentic forms now show themselves to be the basis of any emotion, no matter in what modality; in this way an expressive musical movement, the sound of a voice, a dance step and an expressive touch can partake of the same essentic form, when they intend to express a specific quality [...]. The nervous system seems programmed to be able to produce these forms precisely as well as to recognize them precisely [...]. In this way they are windows, bridging the gap between individuals, allowing communication of emotions and thus permitting emotional understanding between them.
>
> (Clynes, 1980a, in Plutchik / Kellerman, 1980:273)

This extract contains his most important finding: emotions are based on universally biologically-determined "essentic forms" (a similar assumption had already been suggested by Izard) which can however express themselves in very different media or "modalities". The more a medium is culturally specific and/or sophisticated, the more learning and experience is required to understand it. The anatomy of the human face is the same everywhere; this is why the "essentic forms" expressed in facial movements can be universally recognized. Also, everywhere we recognize the angry or loving tone of a human voice, no matter whether we are familiar with the language. Dance and music are examples of media pre-supposing a more specific learning experience – it is necessary to gain some understanding by attuning ourselves to the dance and music traditions of a different culture.

But even here emotional contact can be made which transcends all cultural boundaries – the reception of classical Indian music in Europe or the great significance of European music in Japan and China are proof of this contention.

Communicating emotions is subject to specific genetically determined organizational principles which, of course, are very important for the role of emotions in the contacting process. Therefore, I will discuss now in detail the six organizational principles or in his words: "basic biological design properties that appear to govern the dynamic communication of emotions" which Clynes discovered (Clynes, 1976:18, 25, 43, 53).

They are:

- Exclusivity
- Coherence
- Equivalence
- Complementarity
- Increasing intensity
- Objectless emotion

1 **Exclusivity**: Only one emotional state can be expressed at any given time. This does not mean that so-called mixed emotions cannot be expressed, where what is being expressed is the condition of the mixture. It is not possible though to express tenderness with one part of the body while expressing anger with another, as in so-called paradoxical invitations to action and other contradictory communications, discovered by studying communication patterns of schizophrenogenic families (Chaney, 2017). We are not dealing here with the contradiction between two simultaneously expressed emotions, but with contradictions between emotional and semantic levels – when, for example, something negative is expressed with a smile, or some positive content occurs in an angry voice.

2 **Equivalence**: It is quite possible to express an emotional state in very different "output modalities". Beginning with the body, Clynes used nothing but the pressure of a single finger in his studies; but of course, the *face* has special communicative significance due to its frontal position in the body and its extraordinary richness of expressive possibilities (see also Plessner, 1953). The role played by *body posture* is also important in the therapeutic context. There are postures emphasizing and reinforcing the expression of some emotions; some that contradict the emotion and interfere with its expression and some that have no impact at all. Leaning back, for example, will check the expression of anger while a bent position or crossed arms and legs might interfere with the expression of joy. In this we can easily see how chronic postures can impede the vitality of emotional communication between people. There is no need to further emphasize the importance of the voice in the expression of emotions, since much work is being done on the voice in Gestalt therapeutic practice. The voice comes close to music – especially in singing – as a medium of emotional expression. The principle of equivalence goes further, though: just as a word has the same connotations whether spoken or written, it is even possible to replace the sound of the voice speaking that word with modulations of the hands used in sign language.

3 **Coherence**: Independently of the chosen expressive medium, the expression of a specific emotion is determined by a brain programme. It ensures that inner experience and the expression of emotions are more or less in accord. "There is a connection between the physiological appearances – the character of the movement and the corresponding psychic experience. The nature of this connection is one of the most remarkable phenomena in nature", Clynes concludes. Epistemologically it may be considered as an explanatory principle in the phenomenological analysis of emotions. It remains to be seen whether brain research will one day be able to use it as a viable hypothesis. Indeed, Clynes' discovery of "essentic forms" has major implications. Significantly, it explains how our sensory capacity serves to help us recognize whether an emotional expression is genuine.

> When an emotion – in whatever medium – is coherently expressed, that is in relatively close harmony with its "essentic form", then the person expressing it experiences an *increase in the quality of their emotional expression,* while the audience or addressee experiences what they hear/see/"feel" as *authentic.*

The "essentic form" seems to create its own power of attraction independent of socially prescribed behaviours or inveterate inhibitions: apparently, an expression of emotion through the body always tends towards authenticity. To recognize the truth of this contention, just observe children: it is not because they are small and sweet that we are so easily touched by their pain or swept along by their joy; it is due to the authenticity of their emotional expression, not yet socially restrained. Emotional expression has the power to embody the "essentic form" and thus communicate it, just as the quality of such embodiment gives satisfaction to the person expressing the emotion. And what is true for the body also holds true for other media where approximation to the "essentic form" must be *practised.* The more the expression succeeds in being authentic, the greater the satisfaction experienced in the visual arts, in music, in dance, in the theatre; a good artist will not give up until they have achieved optimal approximation to the "essentic form" of whatever they want to express. This, indeed, is the mark of a great artist.

4 **Complementarity**: Both expression and recognition of an "essentic form" are regulated in the central nervous system in the same way, so that a clearly expressed form is equally clearly received. This perception is not only cognitive, but the perception of authentic emotional expression triggers an appropriate emotional condition in the person perceiving the expression. Clynes explains this as *resonance,* by contending that as a species we share the same biological programme of "essentic forms". Therefore, there cannot be an emotional resonance between bees and human beings for example. But between human beings and dogs there does seem to exist a weak complementarity, since dogs seem to respond to expressions of anger, fear, grief or joy in human beings – probably due to the smell of minimal secretions of sweat and through their hearing.

5 **Increasing intensity**: The intensity of an emotional state is increased – within certain limits – when the "essentic form" of the emotion in question is a-rhythmically but repeatedly expressed. When we study the spatial/temporal units of movement constituting an emotional expression, we can understand how this kind of intensification comes about. It appears that the experience of an emotional state gradually comes closer to its "essentic form" as it is repeated. At the same time, these repetitions are also experienced as an energetic relief through their correspondence with specific physiological processes, reaching a point of

satisfaction or saturation after a period of time. If the repetition of the expression of an "essentic form" is interrupted for neurotic or social reasons before this point of satisfaction has been reached, one achieves a less than satisfying degree of intensity of the emotional experience (i.e. the interactional relationship of need and object). Consequently, frustration is experienced, and emotional residues remain. Everybody knows this from experiencing premature interruption when sexually excited. Incidentally, Clynes also found that there is some variation in the duration of specific "essentic forms", just as the different emotions vary in the length of time before reaching their highest degree of intensity (Clynes, 1976:156–7). Between the expression of one "essentic form" and the next, there is a short pause whose duration also varies, and which cannot be omitted or extended without doing damage. During this pause we experience some degree of satisfaction from the recently completed expression of an "essentic form" and a sense of preparation and anticipation of the next, pressing towards expression.

In this context Clynes established an important finding: if there is a mechanical – that is an intentional – attempt at reproducing an arbitrary rhythm in the rate of repetition, an increase in intensity does not happen. In this form of mechanical repetition therapists will recognize a form of defence used unconsciously by some patients when they are asked to repeat a particular form of expressive gesture. In this way the therapist's intention – to enable a patient to achieve increased emotional awareness through experiencing an emotion expressed with greater intensity – easily gets aborted.

6 **Objectless emotion**: Emotional states can be experienced and expressed without there being any connection in the experience itself between the experiencing subject and an object. Normally we think about emotions in connection with human relationships. But the very fact that the "essentic form" expressed in a piece of music can move us into similar emotional states shows that there is a direct access route to those dormant pure emotional qualities. I would call these experiences "sentic" contacting processes. When I actually *listen* to music (rather than just noticing it in the background) of course it is the object of my desire; but the emotional quality which it transmits is not the result of a spontaneous assessment of my relationship to it. It is an essential part of the object with which I'm in contact, a contact with a special "sentic" quality.

Clyne's observation even goes beyond the possibility of sentic contacting processes: It is possible to project oneself into an emotional state without any external prompt by a-rhythmically repeating an expressive movement as closely as possible to its "sentic form". The reader can easily experience this. Make a fist and hit the air several times whilst shouting "Ha!" as you breathe out and you will experience a feeling between anger and rage rising within you. This is often used in political demonstrations or in the demagogical use of slogans in political speech. Another example: sharply pull down the corners of your slightly open mouth, simultaneously turning up your nose as much as possible, and then think about a dirty toilet – many people will experience a gag reflex associated with intense experiences of disgust. With a little practice it is even possible to dispense with imagining an object and still experience the emotion quite clearly. This is for instance practised in Tibetan meditations: the complete withdrawal of the emotion from its object in our consciousness while at the same time focusing our awareness on the *pure experience* of our present emotion is a useful method to control rising anger and an urge to submit to violent impulses. This capacity to produce objectless emotions is important, since it is the foundation of our ability to empathize with others.

The experience of such generalized emotional states has two aspects: firstly, the experience contains a whole Gestalt of bodily sensations specific to an emotion, which can be quite subtle. When we experience joy the body always feels light, whereas in sadness it feels heavy. Each emotion is accompanied by tensions in specific parts of the body. The phenomenology of these experiences has not been investigated much,[4] but of course they are important for clinical practice. Significantly, instead of being embedded in a complete experiential Gestalt, vanishing once the Gestalt fades, bodily stresses can easily solidify and turn into symptoms if the emotional experience is interrupted prematurely and not allowed to develop until such time as it is saturated. This, for example, happens when an important emotion like mourning the loss of a loved person is repressed.

Secondly, these objectless emotional states have a kind of "knowledge" about the relational constellations and attitudes belonging to them. Attitudes of helplessness and hopelessness are aspects of sadness, which in contrast to grief is a *mood* bordering on depression, which may at first be experienced as objectless, because it was caused by forgotten dreams of the night, or a drop in the air pressure related to the weather, or a lack of light during the winter season. But such sadness tends to generate a kind of memory connected with parting, loss, separation, helplessness and despair. These memories and fantasies show how our consciousness has an immanent tendency towards seeking objects, or even to create objects. Phenomenology has termed this tendency the *intentionality* of consciousness. This is shown by the fact that our brain, deprived of sensory stimuli, normally reacts by creating hallucinations. So the possibility of experiencing objectless emotions extends to moods and therein has its specific dangers, while in emotions they are, as we shall see later, the precondition for empathy.

The above illustrations do not exhaust Manfred Clyne's investigations into the role of emotions in human experience. They have further implications. But with this sketch I have created the basis for a much more detailed description of emotions in the context of the contacting process.

At this point let me briefly summarize what can most importantly be said about emotions from a phenomenological point of view:

1 Contact emotions (affects in some psychological terminology) are physically experienced states, containing in both actual and imagined contacting processes judgements regarding the actual situation of the organism/environment field and providing the motivation for action.
2 The potential for experiencing certain elementary emotions is genetically determined through our central nervous system.
3 Each of these emotions has a specific constant "essentic form", which remains the same no matter which mode of expression we choose.
4 To each emotion belongs a specific combination of physiological phenomena, which in experience are condensed into specific physical Gestalts of the relevant emotions.
5 Apart from the psychic experience and the physiological event, a third element is part of every emotional state and that is a series of expressive movements a-rhythmically following each other.
6 The quality of emotional expression is less dependent on the chosen medium of expression, but rather depends on how close the emotional expression is to its "essentic form", and whether it has come close to the saturation point of intensity, thus determining to what extent others involved or watching are also moved.
7 Emotions do not necessarily require an object, if they are expressed coherently. The function of generalized (objectless) emotional states is to allow empathic reaction.

Of course, human beings are what they are only ever as potentiality. They may or may not realise their potential. Which of these anthropological potentials can unfold and flourish and which will be blocked or choked off depends on the cultural context of the society in which we live. On a micro level, Clynes was able to show the same expressive movements for the same emotions in US Americans, Mexican Indians, Balinese people and Japanese Zen monks. Ekman and Friesen were able to demonstrate the same play of facial muscles in Americans and in Japanese people when confronted with horror movies – as long as their subjects felt unobserved. In a social situation, though, the Japanese exercised a high degree of expressive control, allowing them to watch horror scenes and still produce a polite smile. (Smiling is not, as we shall see, the expression of a contact-emotion but rather a gesture). At present, our own (Western) society shows two discrepant tendencies: a relatively high degree of expressive control and a simultaneous informalization of everyday modes of behaviour. Repressing emotions, however, has a significant effect on whether we can cognitively encompass the emotional experience, because *without expression an emotion cannot get close to its "essentic form", nor can it achieve intensity.* Lack of information about what is going on in the organism/environment field is the unavoidable consequence.

3 The fore-contact emotions

Aversion and attraction

Not every contacting process per se begins with strong emotions. In Gestalt therapy practice I often experience that once there is a loosening-up of introjected expressive controls and clients gradually become more sensitized to subtle emotions, they display a surprising degree of emotional vitality. But when emotions arise in *unobstructed contacting processes* and when they do not, remains a question.

In his interesting exploration of the commercialization of human emotions, Arlie Hochschild (1983) argues that emotions do not appear until a newly perceived reality collides with our expectations – as if emotions were always connected to a moment of surprise. In my opinion, this is true for many emotions but definitely not all: I mention this hypothesis because it is useful in therapeutic practice. In any case, it is safe to say that authentic emotions always break routines; they leave behind the known, loosen up habitualized territory. This does not necessarily follow from a surprising new experience or object but it can be a deepening of what we are familiar with, as we gradually discover new perspectives and dimensions, as in gratitude, or love, or with some aesthetic experiences.

But how many basic emotions do human beings actually have? How many elementary emotions does our central nervous system have as experiential possibilities? And which of those emotions, for which our language provides us with a name, have an "essentic form"? We do not know yet. For instance, the emotions the mimetical expression of which Ekman and Friesen studied, as mentioned above in Section 2, *Emotional expression and emotional experience,* have been differently selected than those in Clynes experiments. There is no unanimity about the number of emotions in human beings. We can only count those for which Clynes provided empirical evidence: anger, joy, sexuality, love, hate, mourning, humility, gratitude and bliss.[5] This list in itself will raise questions. Sexuality? Perhaps it is less surprising that sexual arousal is a specific, distinctive emotion (quite different from love!) and not just a bodily sensation, since it is obviously directed towards an object in the environment; yet we do not have a name for this emotion. On the other hand, there are language problems usually neglected in merely behavioural research designs. For instance "awe" ("Ehrfurcht") and "bliss" ("Seligkeit") have completely different meanings in the German language rendering adequate translation almost impossible, which is not to say that they or similar emotions do not exist in this culture. Yet, if people do not have an experiential knowledge of these words – which their culture may neglect – this does not mean that they are lacking the disposition for these emotions. After all gratitude, too, can be an *emotion*, not just a social convention, which is rarely experienced in an authentic way; and rumour has it that there are people who have never loved anyone!

According to the research done by Ekman and Friesen (Ekman / Friesen, 1972), some of the emotions Clynes investigated have genetically-determined mimetic expressions, while others seem to lack such anchoring. Perhaps mimetic expressive modes only developed for those emotions whose communicative function was of paramount importance for survival and human evolution. The mimetic expressions of joy, anger (rage) and sadness are unambiguous. Surprise, fear, disgust – emotions having a clearly corresponding facial expression – were not investigated by Clynes. Possibly aversive feelings like fear, disgust and surprise – when related to fright – cannot be investigated using a method based on touch.[6]

In any case, I believe that we are dealing here with emotions which also have an "essentic form". And not just these three: in the following reflections I take as my departure point the notion that all the feelings spontaneously emerging in contacting processes are variations and shades of basic emotions with specific "essentic forms". Admittedly this notion has to be proved by further research. In any case it is important to differentiate these from composite emotions like jealousy (consisting of anger and fear) and emotional attitudes like motherliness or meanness: these are the results of individual and cultural socialization processes and can be significant psychopathological reaction formations. I will consider these below.

Having to some extent clarified the character of contact emotions (affects) as opposed to bodily sensations, moods, passions and emotional attitudes, we may now proceed to find some order in the confusingly complex landscape of emotions by connecting them with the phases of the contacting process. We can differentiate between five groups of emotions which have specific functions in this process: some of them belong to the fore-contact phase, others to the phase of orientation and manipulation. Some are characteristic of the full contact stage of integration, while others belong to the post-contact phase. Only anxiety ("Angst") and emotions of shame constitute a special case; unlike other emotions, they block or inhibit the whole contacting process instead of supporting it or avoiding it altogether. They can emerge at any point of the contacting process. We must therefore differentiate between:

1 Emotions of aversion and attraction (fore-contact);
2 The aggressive emotions (orientation and manipulation)
3 Relational emotions (integration)
4 Appreciative emotions (post-contact)
5 Inhibiting emotions

Let's start with the emotions related to the fore-contacting phase. These emotions motivate the organism to either turn away from the object, leave the field or even take flight – or alternatively to proceed into the environment, approach the desired object more closely and thus to change the environment or what is experienced as foreground in it. They create a more or less significant aversion or attraction in the organism/environment field.

Anything capable of remedying lack in an organism comes from the environment. Some things we are already familiar with; others remain somewhat strange and yet others are completely new to us. When we allow our senses and our intellect to open up and be stimulated by this specific environment, we become aware of an appetite we barely noticed before and simultaneously an interest arises, guided by our appetite. An organism which is too hungry knows nothing about curiosity; it grasps whatever is available. **Curiosity** arises from the gap between need and surprise; a certain distance from one's need allows an intellectual to develop interest which is an attitude of mind; but here, in the moment of the contacting process, it arises as a feeling which can be described as burning. As children, we all knew what it meant to burn with curiosity. What is in this bag? What is behind this curtain, this closed door, the garden fence?

The need for something new, the root of our curiosity, is universal. It motivates us to playfully try something out: *let's see what this is; let's find out how this works.* It is a kind of "interest-less" interest because it does not at first narrow our horizon with an attitude of searching guided by wishing; instead, it opens itself to the emerging world of the new – whatever that may bring. In curiosity we see the specifically human intertwining of dependency on our environment and our openness crystallized into emotion. Curious interest is the fore-contact emotion per se, and an incapacity to experience it will always constrict the soul in a particularly repressive way. Hence M. V. Miller even claimed that curiosity is to Gestalt therapy what *libido* used to be for psychoanalysis, the driving force of our creativity (Miller, 1987: 18–22; See also Dreitzel, 2018, Part 1, 1).

The excitement experienced when we are expecting something new is of course always permeated by some fear of the unknown, and this fear can colour the whole emotion when we are challenging ourselves or intending to present ourselves to others. **Arousal** as a part of curiosity has many variations, from the nervous and sleep-interrupting anxiety before a journey to the much "hotter" arousal when we harness our capacity before an exam or any other special challenge; or the fever of **stage fright** which only paralyses if one tries to repress it. The burning (pre-) desire to look behind the curtain easily turns into agitated shivering before the performance. It is important to note that the similarity of stage fright to the debilitating emotion of anxiety (or excitement) which limits our contacting ability must not be confused, either theoretically or practically. Stage fright is an important vehicle for contacting the audience and connecting the content or form of one's own presentation; it mobilizes energy, stimulating the senses and giving a special vitality to one's motor functions, allowing the performance to be a real success. Shivering before the entrance is energy, already vibrating with the activated emotions. However unpleasant the symptoms of arousal may be, they must not be anxiously strangled since they are necessary for discovering again and again that relaxation is experienced only in moments after entering the stage – a discovery only made retrospectively since all the energies which only moments ago were manifested in stage fright are now absorbed by the action on stage, leaving no room for self-conscious reflection.

Sometimes curiosity is satisfied; sometimes whatever we have discovered wakens our interest even more. This now is no longer an "interest-less" phenomenon but we are completely engaged with one object, one person or group, one problem or idea. Something in the environment has aroused our special interest; we feel irresistibly, magically attracted; again and again, we look in the relevant direction; we eavesdrop, and wishes take shape in our thoughts. The underlying feeling is *being-spontaneously-attracted,* for which we do not have a useful word in our language.

Of course, much has been written on feelings related to **erotic attraction.** But this is not the same as *being* or *falling in love,* which is less an emotion than a mood, and – provided it lasts for a while – easily condenses into passion. Being in love can develop from the feeling of attraction but usually we notice it only next morning, when the world looks rosy and thoughts start circling around. Then, being in love easily intensifies and becomes an obsession, considering nothing real other than itself. In our era of the subject, this is experienced and often accepted as a source of legitimization *sui generis.* This state of heavenly madness no longer has anything to do with the original experience of being attracted (Peele / Brodsky, 1975), except that it creates a permanent readiness to keep on surrendering to this feeling. The emotion of attraction informs us that here is something or somebody who will not just satisfy our needs in general but will come very close to our particular wishes and dispositions. Being in-love though makes us truly blind, in that through the gross selectivity of our perception, we are fixated onto a single person. The expression "love at first sight" more accurately hits the mark regarding spontaneous attraction – in that talking about "love" is a retrospective interpretation. But the expression clarifies the fact that spontaneous attraction is not confined to things erotic but can easily be applied to other aspects of human beings as well as to objects, landscapes or artefacts.

A third essential emotion of attraction is **longing** ("Sehnsucht"). The German word and its association with "addiction" ("Sucht") already indicates how easily longing can become a passion or at least a mood. Yet we must not overlook the fact that longing is also a contact emotion, which sometimes bubbles up with the sudden vehemence of pain. Longing is the connection between a strong need with the recognition that it is unrealisable here and now. Here we are dealing less with survival and more with higher-ranking needs. When we need food, we speak about hunger and not about longing for food; and when we are dealing with sexual need, we only speak about longing when we are concerned with a specific and beloved person whom we wish to make love to. This is probably related to the fact that basic needs announce themselves through the body whereas the higher needs require the intercession of the soul, something we find in longing. Longing therefore informs the organism twice: that it is dealing with a strong need which should not be under-estimated, and that it is moving in an environment unable to satisfy this need as currently presented. This is why longing motivates us to move elsewhere or gets us to manipulate the present environment in such a way as to make it more satisfactory. Not that this attempt is always successful, as Goethe's Werther proved. To become entrenched in longing is an act of masochism, though.

These three emotions of attraction – curiosity, erotic attraction, and longing in fore-contact are juxtaposed with three kinds of aversive emotions: *fright, fear* and *disgust*.

To be **frightened** is part of the context of surprise. As with disgust, it is unclear whether these reactions are proper emotions (with an "essentic form") though surprise definitely creates a specific facial expression: open mouth, eyes wide and eyebrows raised. If all this is accompanied by a sharp intake of breath, we have a full description of the so-called "startle reflex" to which some authors attribute a key role in the whole system of emotional excitement (Chance, 1980). Our language does not have an unambiguous word for this; fright unavoidably describes a negative surprise, and fright quickly turns into fear and dread.

But of course, there are positive surprises too, like bad ones leading to short term paralysis of the motor function and accompanied by sharpened sensory perception. It is as if the whole body remains still for a brief eternity, uncertain where to go, to turn back or to approach. Positive fright generates curiosity, while negative fright turns pausing into freezing. A threatening surprise sets off a kind of pretend-I'm-dead reflex, as victims of rape often describe their experience. In some people this freezing with fright has become chronic: they don't move much and stare at others with wide open eyes – a reaction formation (See my discussion of reaction formations in Dreitzel, 2004, Part IV, 1). This expression corresponds to the sensory experience of feeling cold and numb, as if one had received a blow. These sensations can persist for some time if the fright was serious, even if the occasion has already passed. Fright, therefore, mobilizes the senses but numbs the limbs and especially the mind, so at first there is no chance of a clear orientation. Sometimes there is a kind of blind, impulsive motor reaction: one jumps aside to avoid something surprising without considering where one leaps; or automatically lashes out at the spectre.

Fear is much more observant. Unlike fright, fear is an emotion looming slowly before it fully unfolds, only to recede when danger has passed, or flight has been successful. I use fear to denote the emotion which arises when there is real and concrete (or imagined) danger, as opposed to anxiety which is an emotion of vague, non-specific threat. Although in everyday parlance, the words fear and anxiety are often used synonymously, it is important to distinguish these two emotions. What I call fear is an emotion of aversion in fore-contact; whereas anxiety is an inhibiting emotion (compare Section III, 6), blocking internal arousal. Fear – as opposed to fright – does not lead to a freezing of motor functions; instead, it mobilizes energy for flight or avoidance. Faced with great danger to life and limb, people are capable of extraordinary physical achievements: fear opens up dormant energy resources. Fear also sharpens the senses; perception is wide awake and intent. "Blind with fear" only applies to people who block their sense of danger because they are frightened of arousal, something which in real danger can lead to "headless flight" rather than looking for cover and a safer hiding place. Fear has an important orientating function, even in the relatively peaceful territories of modern civilization, and we don't repress it without damage. Fearlessness is characteristic of psychopaths unable to experience their fear – this does not just lead to self-damage but also to unnecessary environmental violations.

In our civilization, the real problem with fear is related to the abstract nature of our most significant dangers. We cannot picture the reality of atomic warfare; our social and political imagination is over-stretched to fully grasp the ongoing ecological destruction of the planet; we cannot imagine what tripling of the world population, or the advent of digital capitalism really mean – and yet these are real dangers which we should all fear as the possible consequences of an age of surveying capitalism (Zuboff, 2018). Other appropriate examples are the nuclear catastrophes at Chernobyl and Fukushima. The fact that radiation cannot be experienced through the senses became the real cause of confusion regarding the source of danger; fear with a clear object turned into anxiety seeking an object by fantasizing and speculating about the meaning of vague notions leading to uncanny dread. Such events and processes must be made tangible so fear can retain its orientating function. The question though is how people can be emotionally mobilized regarding a *permanent threat.* Contact emotions do not persist for long; they quickly reach their saturation point and then decrease in intensity. And they cannot be perennially re-stimulated; the organism defends itself against depletion through emotional over-stimulation by becoming blunted. Everybody eventually reacted to Chernobyl and Fukushima by using the defence mechanisms which best suited their character.

This process could be observed everywhere, not least in politicians as well as in the experts responsible for generating information. And yet, emotional responsiveness towards those extraordinary dangers threatening humanity at this point in our history is very important, for emotions are the living substratum of moral attitudes, which become empty gestures without them. Still, it is likely that new and even greater catastrophes will *not* have an emotionally stirring effect. Instead, we need well-regulated documentation to generate engagement because it also allows distancing and creative forms of enlightenment in conjunction with the discovery and revitalization of old, as well as new, expressive modes of fear. What makes fear such a "rational" emotion is that it doesn't invite us to flee when it is too late but advises us in time to cleverly avoid unnecessary risks. In order to be able to play this role, it needs to be felt, and must be expressed. That requires the kind of courage lacking in "anxious" behaviour, which in reality is nothing but worrying from a position of habitual security. Fear is an uncomfortable emotion – it certainly does not feel good. Therefore people tend to avoid it by denying facts and calling them "fake news" or taking flight in paranoid fantasies, or blaming "them", those "up there" (recently named "elites" – a subconscious admission of one's own lack of education) or the immigrants or the blacks or Jews or gays or whatever minority is close to hand for racial discrimination in one's culture. This demonstrates the importance of cultivating emotional sensitivity, which may also encompass a certain amount of courage or capacity for endurance.

Even more directly than fear, **disgust** – the third aversive emotion – pushes us towards avoidance. Just as elementary as fear and fright, disgust is deeply engrained into our biological destiny. Everybody knows emotions of disgust and we can universally recognize and empathize with its mimetic signs. But this emotion seems to be particularly susceptible to idiosyncratic formations and cultural re-organization. The universality of disgust appears to have an ontogenetic and a phylogenetic aspect. It seems that disgust is alien to babies: spontaneously and without gagging they spit out what they do not like or what they feel is unwholesome and they do not feel uncomfortable with the excretions of their bodies. Only slowly – and not just through the socialising hand of the mother – *emotions* of disgust develop, which indicate the gradual development of firmer ego boundaries on the level of the body; that food is Not-I and the excretion No-longer-I is not experienced as such to begin with. We are dealing here with an early learning process which seems to be particularly sensitive: if separation from this cosy confluence of milk and faeces is forced upon the child too early, it can be permanently formative – just a slight interference with these functions of separation can have consequences. Milk and faeces therefore are always two significant triggers for disgust.

The phylogenetic root of emotions of disgust is its survival-related significance in warning us away from decaying matter. It wasn't until the Enlightenment that our sense of smell was called a "lower sense" and discredited – and yet it is of paramount importance. Before something decaying might be eaten, its bad smell warns the nose through "this most intimate intaking" ("innigste Einvernehmung"), as Kant formulated with his usual precision (Kant, 1907) of the finest particles and substances. The resulting emotion of disgust is an almost insurmountable barrier against assimilating that substance. And just as disgust has a particular history for everybody, leading to specific individual aversions and irritabilities, in the same way disgust has a cultural and civilizing history in every society, lending very diverse forms to triggers and coping mechanisms in spite of its universality. It is well known that with our current standards of disgust we would barely have survived a visit to a medieval city without perennially gagging, and even Enlightenment Paris is described by Corbin, historian of smells (Corbin, 1988) in very similar terms. Or, to choose a very different example: not so long ago, spittoons were a civilising achievement;[7] today the threshold for disgust is much higher, spittoons themselves arousing disgust and spitting itself is deemed to be in bad taste.

Culture and society exert extraordinary pressure on the occasions for and modes of expressing emotions and this particularly shows when disgust is not just avoided by the canalization of bodily excretions,[8] but also in the cultural transformation of the boundary of decomposition in the art of cooking. Gastronomic culture has truly managed to make all sorts of decaying foods palatable – cheese and wine are just the most significant examples. But here, just as in the civilising arena of hygiene, it is true that it does not only require collective learning processes but also individual ones to catch up with specific cultural standards. Children have no time for culinary delights and what they consider favourite foods quite often arouses disgust in those with a refined taste.

In view of these complexities it is not easy to determine when such emotions of disgust should be considered "healthy" or even "natural", and when they assume a phobic character. Altogether, it seems that raising the threshold of disgust serves the organism; after all a sharpened sense of disgust would not just be beneficial in bulimia but useful perhaps even in view of our standard "hamburger". Again – at least at our stage of the civilizing process – the greater danger does not come from emotions that are too strong, but from repressing and avoiding them. The potential to experience disgust is an original part of our psycho-physical equipment; avoiding feelings of disgust can for example lead to the gag reflex getting rusty and becoming incapable of immediately expelling damaging food. Childhood memories may be strongly experienced in this realm but truly it is the influence of the culture into which the child is socialized. So Muslims might feel severe disgust when served pork in Western countries, while visitors from the West might feel similarly put off when confronted with dog meat in China. Conversely, we also find an avoidance of emotions of disgust within our own culture – when instead of it being experienced as a quickly passing sensation, it becomes chronic and produces a phobic attitude. Then and only then is disgust damaging – in fact it is disgust of disgust – and especially damaging when this emotional *position* is fixated onto something for which the organism has a natural need. The classical example of course would be neurotic disgust in the context of sexuality.

Occasionally, a generalized attribution of emotions of attraction and aversion may be problematic and it should not be taken as dogma. It is important not to forget that we are working here with an ideal, typically simplified model, which does not take all specifics into account.

These considerations of the fore-contact emotions may not do enough justice to the fact that contacting processes are complexly intertwined. In actual interaction processes between human beings there often is a lot of to-ing and fro-ing so that overlapping is normal – especially between the first two phases of the contacting process. For instance, frequently it is only after getting in closer contact and thus obtaining more information that erotic attraction arises or even feelings of love may emerge. Of course, the opposite may also happen: more experience generating more information may also lead to sudden aversion. Still, it is important to recognize that the emotions I have been discussing up to this point belong to the fore-contact phase. If they appear in the second contacting phase, usually something has been overlooked. This "something" is often one's needs and that usually has difficult consequences. Neglecting the fore-contact and jumping immediately into the second phase of the contacting process – symptomatic of a hysterical neurotic process (Dreitzel, 2004) – usually leads to frustrations and disappointment.

Emotions of attraction or aversion often decide whether and how further contact happens or not. If however such contact has a permanent basis, as for instance in marriage, the fore-contact is even more important – not only in sex, but even more consequentially for honestly sharing one's real needs, urges and dreams.

4 Aggression

The differences between aggression and assertiveness

Systematically following on from the fore-contact emotions, I will consider the aggressive emotions belonging to the phase of orientation and manipulation. In describing the contacting process in chapter III, I have already talked about warm anger and cold hate and about the delight in taking the initiative, in grasping, in pure action, when we grapple with our environment. I also indicated that sexuality is part of this context. In fact, here we can clearly differentiate three emotions – **rage, hate** and **sex**. The delight in initiative is not really an emotion per se; it is more a bodily delight which accompanies the energetic expansion of the organism into the environment, when we throw ourselves body and soul into contact. But as soon as we meet an obstacle, there is **anger**. The different forms of anger we experience are simply less intense forms of rage and hate, easily sensed once we pay attention to these differences in the subtler variations of anger.

Like all emotions, aggressive emotions seek physical expression. Rage "rises up", and will out; we feel hot, the face turns red, the eyes are slightly contracted and glare without properly perceiving (it is possible to be "blind" with rage); the mouth is slightly open and the lips curl away from the teeth. This snarling facial expression is not a phylogenetic remainder of a threatening gesture observed in many animals (Lorenz, 1980), but the expression of an oral desire to fragment whatever resists, a desire to bite, familiar to us from sexuality. Particularly the muscles involved in voice production are stimulated. Even with the slightest experience of anger, we inadvertently raise our voice and a person wild with rage wants to yell out and thereby get rid of their rage.

In contrast, the voice of **cold hate** as an emotion (in contrast to hatred as a passion) is not so much sonorous as cutting and sharp. There is no oral – or any other – desire in hate; motor energy tends to be held back, only to hit out suddenly and abruptly. Correspondingly, blood is drained from the face (pale with "rage" or hatred), and the lips are pressed together. Whereas rage surges against the resistance of the object – which often is desired and loved – in order to de-structure and refashion it, hate looks for a way to *annihilate* it; tries to remove it altogether. Anger, then, can soon be reconciled, even if de-structuring has not been fully accomplished. Hate on the other hand easily turns into a passion, wanting to sink its claws into an opponent it cannot remove – and thus eating itself up. In the political arena this kind of strain shows up in loss of rational orientation; a recent example may be observed in the behaviour of the US President, Donald Trump.

That we rate **sex** amongst the aggressive emotions isn't just due to the systematic order of the contacting process. It is interesting to note that amongst the emotions Clynes investigated, the "essentic form" of sex as an emotion is most similar to anger, whereas the "essentic form" of love resembles that of mourning (see Figure 4.1) – and both these latter emotions belong to *full contact*, the third phase in the contacting process.

Sex and rage have the same appearance, except that in sex the blood rises not to the face but into the genitals. There is the same almost irresistible urge towards motor expression, including using the voice; a delightful sensation of heat and – more clearly than in rage – hard and intermittent breathing. Completely different in sex of course is its culmination in orgasm, indicating (at least on a physical level) satisfaction, and as a physical experience of full contact providing a bridge for a transition between a purely sexual experience and an emotion of love. Up to this point, sex is an aggressive emotion: arousal is triggered by sexual stimuli in the environment, creating a need-related orientation and unfolding of emotions, while an encounter is shaped into erotic contact. If desire is a fore-contact emotion, sexual arousal is a feeling of the second stage of the contacting process: orientation and manipulation.

But is it not rather an instinct than an emotion? This is true for the sexual urge, of course. The fully inflamed sexual desire however has all the characteristics of an affect or, as I call them in this context, a "contact emotion". The expression "to fall in love" is a euphemism for this longing and desire to possess and be possessed physically as well as psychically and while the mind is busy figuring out the possibilities of seduction, the body seeks to express its desire in all kinds of movement from stroking to kissing, from dancing to intercourse. Sex is an aggressive emotion situated in the contacting process

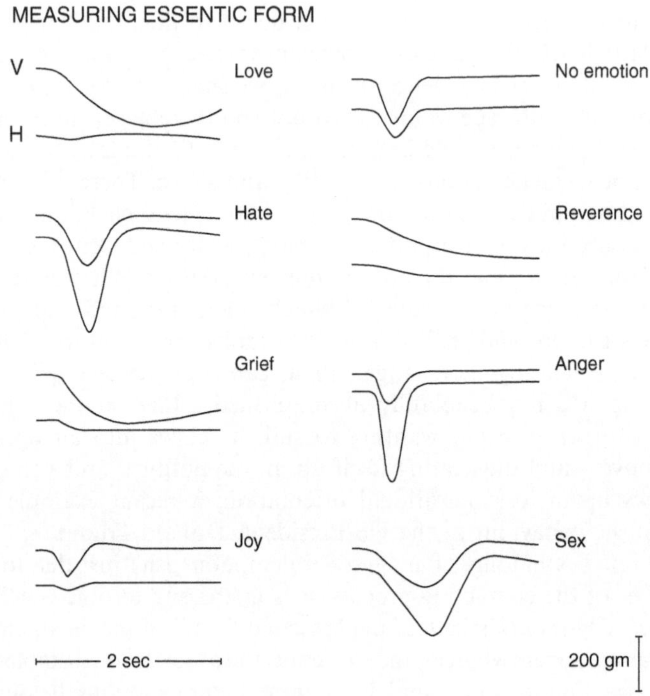

Figure 4.1 Measuring essentic form

between the longing of fore-contact and the satisfaction of full contact with its typical bodily expression of feelings of internal burning, the heart beating and other sensations of hormonal arousal together with all the symptoms of grasping part of our environment in order to integrate it into our own organism.

Aggressive emotions have a quality of disruptiveness, of anarchy; they are about changing things. These qualities make them suspect to those engaged in the civilizing task. Indeed, a certain fierceness characterizes their essential motoric expression, making them appear uncivilized. Therefore, aggressive emotions are typical victims of internalized affective controls. In societies advanced in their civilizing process, disturbances of aggressive functions and repression of aggressive emotions are part of the normal neurotic make-up of the population. Maybe this does not immediately make sense, considering the amount of conflict and violence in families, the readiness for (and incidence of) quick sex outside them, and the pervasive spread of pornography in modern culture.

But it is just the inability to properly *experience* anger and the (mostly social) impossibility to fully *express* it which leads to violent outbreaks in the private realm and to public violence when street demonstrations get out of control.

There are helpful exceptions though, like many kinds of sport – especially football and baseball – which provide a civilized outlet for aggressive energies; civilized because the need to follow rules is more or less strictly controlled and these rules are themselves a product of an ongoing civilizing processes. (It is reported that in Ancient Greece during the Olympic Games, a wrestler was once disqualified for biting off the testicles of his opponent…) The search for modes of expressing aggressive feelings without resorting to violence is always an important task of the civilizing process because the internalization of inhibitions against their expression shows that anger which is actually expressed may also indicate the return of the repressed. Whoever does not *express* their emotions cannot experience them in a genuine way. We sense the pent-up energy now looking for an outlet (and men too often finding one in a wife or child) against which we have to build ever stronger barriers. "Silent anger" and "held back rage" – like held back sex – do not lead to affective energies being guided into "more productive" channels, as a simplistic version of sublimation theory stipulates. Instead, they remain stuck with the incomplete situation and again and again divert attention from new tasks. The power of retroflected energy is never to be underestimated, especially in therapy.

5 Smiling, laughing and crying

Emotional gestures and emotional expressions

As we have seen, human modes of emotional expression are not tied to specific modalities of speech, bodily postures or mimetic expressions. One can search for an approximation to the "essentic form" of a specific authentic emotion in the facial expression of a person or equally well in a poem. Wordsworth described poetry as "emotion recollected in tranquillity" (quoted from Miller, 1980:80). But of course, in direct interaction the body is the medium of emotional communication and is of primary importance (Dreitzel, 1983b:179). And the human body is singularly well equipped for this task. A perpendicular backbone facilitates the subtly expressive potential of the human posture; sitting, walking or standing frees the arms and hands not just for the use of tools but also for speech and gesture. We can move the plane arrangement of eyes and mouth with the help of hundreds of very fine muscles, allowing for the incomparable polymorphism of the human face. And finally, only human beings can laugh and cry, thus possessing two expressive modalities of such singular experiential and expressive power that we must specially focus on their role in the contacting process.

But before that, I shall say something about **smiling,** this distinctively human expressive gesture which – beyond the undirected cry – is actually the baby's first medium of communication. Even before laughing and crying are differentiated from simple bawling and develop in their own ways, the child is able to smile. Until recently this was thought to occur at about five weeks but according to new insights, smiling occurs at the latest from day three. Initially functioning as a recognizing reflex, very soon this gesture is used intentionally. Smiling is the Ur-gesture of human beings: promising peacefulness and friendliness. Whilst remaining inscrutable, it reveals and conceals. Smiling is at the opposite pole to raging. We enter this world crying; with smiles we conquer it. Crying brings mother; the smile keeps her there. A person who no longer smiles believes that there is no more to gain, or that everything has been won already. In no other expressive gesture can we see the specific relationship we have to our body, its "ex-centric positionality" (Plessner, 1970), which allows us to use our bodies in both in an instrumental and an expressive way in relation to our world.

Smiling therefore is not the expression of emotion; it is in fact rather useful for hiding it. The gesture of smiling indeed needs to be distinguished from a flash of laughter which has many nuances and shades of intensity. When we say "I had to smile", we mean more accurately "I had to laugh a little", since laughter arises suddenly. We can repress it (with some effort), but only at the expense of authenticity. The gesture of smiling can, with some practice, be produced at any time as long as we are in control of our senses or better still, in control of our gestures. As opposed to laughing, which expresses a momentary emotional state in the organism/environment field, it designates an *attitude* and an *intention*. The attitude is that of inner balance, of being at peace with oneself and the world as is conveyed by the Buddha's smile (which nevertheless is somewhat replicated in our "satisfied smile"). The intention is to signal one's own peacefulness and to secure that of the other – an intention habitualized in our smiles when we greet somebody. And of course, inner attitude and outer intention do not have to coincide; for that reason, smiling, more than other expressive gestures, can become an instrument of deception and concealment, a weapon in the artful game of social masques.

Just because it is possible to learn to smile without mirroring an inner attitude, smiling easily connects with introjects. "Keep smiling" as an injunction, particularly for people in service sector jobs, can easily turn into the mask of a frozen "social smile" not easily dropped. This was analysed with great perceptiveness by Arlene Hochschild, using the example of American air hostesses (Hochschild, 1983). Even more frequently (and significant for Gestalt therapeutic work on inhibitions of aggression) it can be observed in the inveterate reflex of the smile that says: "Don't be angry with me!" just after uttering a critical remark, working as a reaction formation to repress the excitement anxiety (Dreitzel, 2004). This embodies our early experience that very few people are impervious to a smile. As a reflex however, this smile merely takes the sharpness out of a critical remark, making it blunt and not very effective. Nevertheless, with its thousands of nuances, smiling is the hardest to read of all expressive gestures. While it is surprising how many variants we can accurately assess instantly, there is also a great deal of scope for astonishing discoveries regarding our own expressive possibilities, as well as when observing other people's facial expressions.

In smiling, human beings control themselves; in **laughing** and **crying** they lose control. Laughing and crying after all are modalities of emotional expression and not expressive gestures; they have something involuntary about them. We are taken over by them because emotion finds an expressive outlet through them. It is possible to smile without emotion, but it is quite impossible to laugh or cry without it. In smiling we signify something; in laughing and crying we simply are. In extreme cases, sobbing or uncontrollable laughter reduces us to shaking. In laughter and crying we do not really express a specific emotion, although there is no question about the close affinity of laughing to joy and crying to mourning. But joy and grief do not necessarily express themselves in this way nor are laughter and crying fixed to them; we can laugh with love or gratitude during sex, when relieved of a burden or simply about a joke. And perhaps more tears are shed in longing or in being touched by the fate of another than in mourning; and after all there are tears of joy and gratitude.

It is strange that crying has been even less investigated than laughter. For Freud, the involuntary nature of laughing signified an energetic discharge arising from the fact that a joke bypasses the censoring unconscious – a theory which indicates a history of mostly painful experiences with norms of propriety. Bergson saw in laughter the sudden flow of "élan vital" "mechanically" brought to a halt by humour. But today we can appreciate the funny robot-like movements of an assembly-line worker in Chaplin's film "Modern Times" crying with one eye and laughing with the other.

In his classic study on "Laughing and Crying" (Plessner, 1970) Helmuth Plessner was the first to see both phenomena together and to develop a phenomenology of these expressive behaviours of relevance for therapists, too. Plessner was able to show that in both laughing and crying we see a breakdown of the "ex-centric positionality": our insurmountable condition of having and being a body – which also explains why only human beings are capable of laughing and crying. The triggers can be very different but apparently we always experience a breakdown of our normal experience, the subject playing to the gallery coinciding with itself. The "I" and the "Me" in George Herbert Mead's terminology become identical and no longer allow the individual to take a position vis-à-vis the world.

In laughing, one's personality is taken out of the equation: it just disappears. The "I" has vanished into the rupture of the world. Though Plessner thinks that there is something superficial about "even the heartiest, most humorous laughter despite its arising from the depth of emotion", this can be seen differently. "Human beings respond in this way with immediacy, without including themselves in the response. Thus, they become anonymous, a reason for the infectious power inherent in it" (Plessner, 1970:125). Only if one assumes that depth dwells in an isolated individual does laughter become superficial.

On the other hand, we easily have the impression of depth when we seem to plunge deeply into ourselves and the world around us is lost in the maelstrom of our own self. Just as we are beside ourselves in laughing, so we withdraw into ourselves in crying and the desire to hide (ideally in mother's lap) is greater and qualitatively different from social bashfulness and consideration. In laughing, we do not lose ourselves; it overcomes us too explosively, and frequently we are safe in the laughter of others and supported by it. In crying though, ego boundaries are gradually dissolved; we tumble into a sea of tears, the nose is running, the face swells, the body seems to dissolve. So we cuddle or curl up, protect and cover ourselves in this position of defencelessness, securing outer boundaries even as inside everything is dissolving. But here we come to the next section; the emotions belonging to the phase of full contact.

It remains to mention that laughter, like crying, can be used defensively. As well as the strategically-used crocodile tears which some people can activate, there is the especially neurotic crying which mostly expresses feelings of impotence and resignation and therefore of hidden aggression. Crying can deteriorate into *howling*, just as laughing can become inane: both are reaction formations. At least as remarkable as neurotic crying is the fact that in our society many people can no longer cry. Perhaps it is also true of laughing but that there are men who have not been able to cry since childhood is an established fact and proves the extraordinary power of culture-specific affective controls. Just because it is the inner life which pushes outward in crying, crying is more subject to cultural shaping than is laughing. This attitude towards crying is symptomatic of the social significance we attribute to the public presentation of interiority. The history of howling (Berkenbusch, 1985) has discovered that in the 18th century it was fashionable for men to cry. Now, it is conventional for men to refrain from tears in public and to feel ashamed if unable to do so.

In crying it is particularly easy to force or repress that which, if uncontrolled, always represents a strong emotion. In this case too we have a very fine sensorium for what is authentic. Plessner claimed that true crying has its own unmistakable expressive form, and Clynes showed that laughter has its own "essentic form", as if it were an emotion[9]. People who live in a culture of restrictive emotional expression need to re-sharpen their sensorium through observation and experience when they are confronted by strong emotions – in Gestalt therapy for example.

The most important thing we can learn from Plessner's analysis is that laughing and crying embody a specific conditionality of emotional expression – specifically the collapse of inner distance resembling a transitory Ego-loss (more accurately in Gestalt theory, a loss of the ego functions of the Self). Their authenticity and intensity can be observed directly in the loss of self-control. It is therefore quite possible that laughing and crying appear with emotions not usually considered in this context: in extreme fear perhaps or in embarrassment. And they don't have to be an emotional expression, as long as we experience the fragility of our reality, as in confrontation with a paradox. Even beyond emotions we laugh about a joke and cry with pain when reality suspends all our ego functions. In laughing and crying we react to the contact boundary – in Gestalt therapy terms the only reality we psychologically experience – and it presents itself to us as a Zen kōan: no answer can be grasped from within the system, but only beyond the boundary.

In the context of aggressive emotions laughing and crying can also appear, expressing experiences of absurdity and helplessness; we laugh about other people when their behaviour is both typical for them and "out of context", not fitting the situation; but we can also cry about another person, when momentarily we are in despair about their inertia. In this case laughing and crying turn into aggression, they are directed towards change. More frequently, in this contacting phase they contract themselves into reaction formations and – in the form of cheeky or flippant laughter or in the shape of compassion-craving wailing – in that case they interfere with a sensibility for the emotions of aggression as they arise, as well as with their expression.

6 Beyond the moment

Timeless emotions

Laughing and crying can arise in any contacting phase, but they have something like their home port in the phase of full contact where subject and object merge. The reason for this is that in laughing and crying – as in the timeless emotions – the sense of time gets lost. They express a condition, a timelessness beyond the transient, each moment containing eternity. This is why clear laughter is the brightest expression of **joy**, and deep, dark crying is the most significant expression of **grief.** In *grief* and *joy* time seems to be suspended. And it is just the same in the other emotions of full contact: *awe* and *bliss*, being overcome by beauty, the emotional experience of having an intellectual *insight*, and above all else, *love.* All these emotions are beyond time. "Time is righteous and has no concept of intimacy" as beautifully expressed in a poem written as part of some Gestalt therapy work.[10]

The peculiar timelessness of **love** and other emotions which I consider here consists in having left behind all motivation; in phenomenological terms, they have no intentionality. They are Ego-less emotions because they already have what other emotions seek: a connection, through which contacting subject and contacted object are completely absorbed in each other where the "I" has disappeared into the "Thou".

Perls & Goodman (197) call these emotional experiences transcending our sense of time "concerns", a word which entails having somebody's well-being at heart.

These emotions do not seek to change anything: only to preserve. It is important to recognize that they are not just permanent companions of relationships or latent emotional positions which may manifest in full contact, but psychic experiences of timelessly being in union with another human being. Paradoxically, in mourning it would be being at one with the emptiness left behind by the loss.

It is perhaps easiest to understand this when we experience joy, which can present itself as mood as well as a contact emotion. We can enjoy this and that without it being anything special that we're enjoying; joy is the expression of an existential state, making us laugh and our hearts leap. Indeed, the whole body becomes the medium of expression, as we know from the manner in which children jump and leap in their characteristic expression of joy.

Awakening joy does not require a particular connection to something; indeed, at times the unexpected is more effective. For example, an appreciative affirmation of some habit or character trait or a flattering recognition of some ability are more likely to generate satisfaction than joyous delight.

It is harder to see that the timeless emotions are not connected to relationships, especially where love is concerned. But what I mean by this word is, as we all know, difficult to clarify. The sentence "I love you!" can mean very different things – like "I want to possess you", "I find you sexually irresistible", "I want to share my daily life with you", "I admire you", "I approve of your actions", "I find it easy to picture you as the father/mother of my children" – or simply "my heart overflows right now in your presence". Only the last sentence speaks of a contact emotion of love; all the others are wishes, attitudes and judgements. Love as an emotion is similar to joy but has a slower, gentler motor expression, as if heavier in body and more intense, even while it has less brightness about it than joy.

But language and its images quickly fade; there is good reason why timeless emotions are favoured by poetry, for the art of poetry entails merely hinting at something by omission, preferring metaphor. Love as an emotion spontaneously appears in the contacting process and of course, disappears with it. Indeed, we may be blessed with a special person who is able to evoke these emotions in us again and again. But in that case other people too will benefit from this overflow. Because the essence of this emotion we call love is an over-flowing, being filled with the respective you and if it is easily evoked in one person, it flows towards the just and the unjust alike even as they appear in view. Love is not an emotion of attraction: it does not differentiate between "I love you – but not you". Whoever or whatever stimulated love, as an emotion it is directed towards a "Generalized Other" as George Herbert Mead termed it (Mead, 1934); the general "You" appears before our eyes in a specific manifestation. Love as an emotion therefore is not a strong form of (personal) affection but a letting-go into a state where the "I" is so strongly absorbed in the "Thou" that the "Thou" too can no longer be a specific counterpart, being generalized into the existential orientation of this moment. For this to happen, it is not necessary that the heart of the beloved should also overflow at this exact timeless moment.

If this view of the contact emotion *love* is perhaps difficult to verify in our everyday experience, this does not devalue its phenomenological truth. What is special about love as an affect is that it always points beyond even its timeless moment to an unfathomable indescribable phenomenon potentially available to all of us.

Just how much subject and object are transcended in the timeless emotions of full contact is even more obvious in **awe, reverence** and **bliss**, the religious emotions. I already mentioned that Clynes and a student of his were able to discover an "essentic form" first for "reverence" and later for "bliss". When we say that a person or a symbolic object fills us with reverence or that we are overcome with reverence when we see it, it implies that we sense an aura, a charisma exuded by the object or person, generating something like a "holy shiver" – awe. Reverence denotes the emotion arising from something larger, different, transcendent, which grabs our hearts – it is triggered by a person with a particular aura or by a sacred object, or holy space.

Apparently, it is not so easy to expose yourself to experiences of such religious emotions on your own. Alone they are difficult to express and therefore difficult to intensify, perhaps because they directly connect us with the experience of the small and finite nature of our individual existence. It is natural that people take each other by the hand and jointly go in search of what each of them already has within. It has always been and still is the function of religious rituals to provide social forms for expressing such emotional experiences, safely containing the individual in the group.

Miraculously, the emotion of *being blessed* can also arise outside any religious context and sometimes Gestalt therapeutic work in particular creates the conditions for this emotion to arise. "Blessedness" is too strong a word for what I am exploring here, even though it is the same emotion, if slightly less intense. I am talking about the emotional dimension of the experience of suddenly understanding something, a sudden clarity, a Gestalt being completed, a "mini-Satori". This "aha!" feeling as it is sometimes called – the *eureka*! shout of Archimedes – has an element of relief, because the painful search leading into so many cul-de-sacs has now come to an end; there is also an element of satisfaction – the work is accomplished, a solution for the problem found. And yet, the "aha!" emotion is not about the self: it is again a sense of being filled with something other, something not coming from me; a small enlightenment.

The "aha!" experience is a moment of stillness, of thrilling clarity; one's body image is slightly shivery and above all light, just as it is when filled with joy – as when Archimedes is said to have run naked out into the streets, shouting full of joy with his discovery. When, in the context of Gestalt therapeutic work a patient is overcome by such an "aha!" emotion, it is a sure sign that the shared therapeutic effort has succeeded; that the patient has been able to finish a situation, that a Gestalt has been completed. In the therapeutic situation such peak moments are rare, since it is often much later and outside the therapy setting that the insight gained shows its full impact.

Of the timeless emotions, it is **grief** which concerns psychotherapists most. I do not mean sadness, which is a *mood,* but the experience of loss. The significance of the loss determines how intensely we experience grief; it tends to be strongest at the sudden death of "a significant other" (sociology's neutralising language). But we also know the milder forms of grief when we have to say goodbye to loved ones, when going through a separation, or in wistfulness at the end of a significant period in our lives. Grief is the paradoxical experience of being in full contact with an emptiness, with a loss, and so we can understand – as Paul Goodman says – "how terrible (it is) for if there is neither Ego nor 'Thou,' the emotion is as of an abyss" (Perls & Goodman:198). It is part of our special human emotional condition that we cannot say goodbye, cannot separate from the disappearing Gestalt without falling into this abyss. We need to allow time to heal the wound properly rather than leave it to fester. As with any other emotion, grief too has its point of saturation when appropriately expressed, after which it gradually fades. But here the expression deceives, since grief leaves us not satisfied but exhausted and empty; the organism needs recovery. Gradually then the emptiness will be replenished by a new zest for life and new contacting processes will become possible.

Usually a deep sobbing is the strong, spontaneous expression of grief. It shakes the whole body, knees buckle, back is bent (Plessner, 1970). "Grief work" in psychotherapy though is something quite different from this spontaneous emotion of grief. For it is also part of mourning to express the anger and pain connected with the loss inflicted yet often repressed. Here, too, ritual helps. I did not really understand this until in Greece I experienced the truly bone-shaking cries of lament uttered by a woman who had lost her husband very suddenly through heart failure and was now receiving condolences from her friends and relatives at the entrance to the village church after the service. In these cries, rage, pain and grief were fused into a primeval sound, requiring all her strength to eject it. But nobody tried to calm or soothe this outpouring: quite to the contrary, her two strong young sons held this heavy woman tightly; gripped her by the arms to keep her upright; pressed her against the church wall. Without their help she would have slid down to the ground in exhaustion. The next day this widow followed a custom which to us seems barbaric: she shut herself into her darkened room for forty days; food was brought to her. Total withdrawal – a human being barely existing. And while this ritual prescribes the duration of withdrawal without reference to a concrete situation, it seems that it achieves something similar to that which individualized psychotherapeutic guidance and companionship achieves in our modern social context.

Both strategies attempt to resolve the same problem. It is too easy to turn away from the vanished Gestalt and allow new stimuli to capture us instead of daring to stare into the abyss. Ann Clark in her splendid presentation of grief work in the context of Gestalt therapy says:

> This means, though, that we overlook an integral part of transformational processes. De-structuring and forming are inseparable parts of the cycle of change, growth and development. When we plan ahead and search for beginnings before the end is reached, we live for the future without noticing the present and without completing the past. This results in incomplete situations, unfinished relationships, unfinished endings and distorted new beginnings [...] We cannot really move away from our grief, but retroflect it from a sense of depression at the root of it all. It is all-pervasive to the extent that we get in the way of the cycle of growth [...] Grief is a necessary stage, required for the process of de-structuring in the Gestalt cycle.
>
> (Clark, 1982:50)

Grief therefore is a timeless emotion in which the old contacting figure gradually dissolves. Thus it is a painful emotion, naturally embedded in a process of mourning which also contains emotions of anger and rage. Like Kübler-Ross in her work with people dying (Kübler-Ross, 1974), Ann Clark in her work with people in mourning was able to distinguish several stages of this process. At first there is a stage of withdrawal, where one feels small and reduced, overwhelmed by shock or sometimes relieved from longstanding concerns; in any case debilitated and unable to attend to practical matters, "to do the necessary". Happy are those who have help and support in this situation and can afford to do what the organism requires in this situation – just withdraw. After this follows the phase of anger, and thirdly the phase where we have to accept our fate and work through it ("existential acceptance").

The second phase is of special significance for the work of therapy. Ann Clark distinguished three types of anger here which often remain unexpressed: first, anger, stemming from earlier unresolved situations, especially those where grievances were harboured but remained unspoken. In the present mourning situation all the old and buried complaints re-emerge, strengthening the current grief through an added dimension of anger and rage. Added to this is present anger about the other's absence when we need help, when we need advice, when we want support. And finally, the existential rage about fate in general: why do we have to lose in order to win, die in order to live?

I think there are two symptoms to which a therapist should pay particular attention. On the one hand, anger about the dead person or a person who has disappeared is often repressed because expressing it is not permitted – the principle *"de mortuis nihil nisi bene"* (do not speak ill about the dead) is a de facto social norm initially applicable during the time of mourning. On the other hand, there is an insidious tendency to project existential rage – which if anything should be directed towards God – onto the loved one whom one mourns. This creates a double interruption of contact followed by a secretly smouldering resentment towards the dead person.

Grieving as a process of separation and saying goodbye (Tobin, 1971) entails more than just feeling grief and experiencing the pain of loss. The organism goes through a cycle of paralysis, expression and withdrawal and comes into contact with other emotions as well as grief, especially anger/rage; but also of course, fear. Grieving will turn into *grief work* when other long-hidden emotional issues like helplessness, emotions of guilt, of frustration and resentment play a role; left-over affects clouding pure grief. But in a society supporting individual modes of adjustment rather than collective ritual, a coach for instance or some other untrained advisor accompanying the grieving person may be a problem: in any case Clark warns

> … that it is the therapist who has not had opportunity to work through these experiences on a personal basis who is unable to be helpful in this work; who doesn't even notice the problems or explains them away with answers from established diagnostic, religious or philosophical contexts.
>
> (Clark, 1982:58)

Finally, I would like to mention an emotion which shows the integration of full contact in a particularly beautiful way, an emotion rarely counted as such and in German it doesn't even have a name: the emotion for the beautiful. Does it even exist, an **emotion for the beautiful,** a kind of rapture, when we want to distinguish it from our aesthetic recognition of harmonious proportions? Firstly we have to distinguish between causes and triggers of an emotion (especially when any talk of beauty and the attending emotions is strongly conditioned by culture) and then we need to describe the gift of being able to feel it. "Beauty lies in the eye of the beholder" we say, and that is true in a very specific way: it is not things per se which are beautiful, but through them we have the experience of beauty. And yet this experience consists precisely in being touched by things and being stirred in a way which replenishes to the point where there is no longer any room for an observer. The feeling for beauty, no matter how culturally determined our responsiveness may be, has nothing to do with aesthetic considerations – categories and judgements always require distance. Instead, the experience of beauty overwhelms us, wiping out all distance and for a moment dissolving the beholder who becomes one with this beauty. That is why in the face of overwhelming beauty our eyes fill with tears. In the emotion for beauty we merge with the sensual appearance of the experienced object and even when we say somebody is "lost" in the contemplation of a beautiful object, in fact this timeless moment of fusion only lasts for the shortest time. However, we must not mix up the emotion of erotic attraction with the feeling for beauty, since often in such mixing introjected aesthetic standards are used to channel and block erotic arousal which definitely does not have this quality of timelessness-and-beyond-this-moment. Rather, the emotion for beauty has an aspect of surprise, even of shock, and despite all our preparing and searching we will quite unexpectedly get lost in it. And so the first spontaneous expression, similar to being shocked or startled, is that it takes the breath away, and then finds expression in involuntary sound. The vowel for beauty is "o", while that of disgust is "e" and that of satisfaction "a". (For a fuller account of this see Berendt, 1983:40pp). In beauty as in all emotions, access can be blocked by desensitization, or buried through lack of stimulation. This rarely becomes an issue in psychotherapy – perhaps it is mentioned too rarely. Even while – or perhaps because – all aesthetic judgement is extinguished in the emotion for beauty, we feel secure and at home in this emotion so that the emotional experience of beauty has healing power in itself.

7 Post-contact

Appreciative emotions:

At the end of the contacting process, when saturation and satisfaction have either been achieved or turned out to be unachievable, and the Gestalt which was discovered and created starts to pale, the evaluative function (of lesser importance in the timeless emotions) gradually comes to the fore again. The emotions of the post-contacting phase are spontaneous appreciations regarding the contacting situation coming to an end; they show us the degree and quality of satisfaction reached and orientate us with regard to possible action and relationship consequences arising from this contact. In principle such judgments of course can be positive or negative, indicating "More of the same the next time!" or "Never again!" Moreover, the appreciative emotions apply either to the subject or the object as they separate out during this phase of post-contact, becoming differentiated again as parts of the organism/environment field. From the combination of these alternative judgements we get a fourfold pattern of emotions arising in the post-contact phase (see Table 4.1):

Table 4.1 Patterns of emotions arising in the post-contact

Appreciation	*Regarding the subject*	*Regarding the environment*
Positive	**pride**	**gratitude**
Negative	**despair**	**guilt**

These emotions too arise with many nuances and in varying degrees of intensity, but they tend to have a gravitational centre.

By "**pride**" I mean not the character trait, but a spontaneous feeling of contentment with what has been done and what has been achieved. It is an emotion of strength and self-confidence arising from newly-won certainty regarding one's own energy resources and creative abilities; we can now lean back and relax. The emotion of pride oscillates between a rather passive emotion of satisfaction, such as one feels after a satisfying sexual experience; and a jumpy, sparkly joyous emotion about work accomplished, such as following the completion of a task. In other words, this emotion can arise after work as well as after pleasure. We often experience this emotion, but in a repressed and inhibited way because we so rarely allow its expression.

Here, too, it pays to look at children who have not yet strangled their pride by introjecting norms of false humility: their behaviour allows us to best observe the unashamed expression of this emotion. Their eyes gleam; the face is slightly reddened, often still covered with beads of sweat after effort and excitement. And then follows the action motivation which is part of pride: announcing and exhibiting their accomplishment, not just to evoke attention – which of course serves to validate and thus assumes psychological significance – but more to invite participation in the joy of achievement and the riches of fulfilment. Children return from their big adventures and want to show us what they have found, discovered and built. It is this spontaneous desire to share which removes vanity from the emotion of pride as long as its expression is not repressed. Only in such a case do we find that embarrassed puritanical pseudo-modest self-regard, which has nothing of the desire to express our happiness in being allowed to participate in a part of creation. Therefore, people can express pride in having given birth to a child, or even having fathered one, without anybody taking offence or thinking it egocentric. Pride as an emotion expresses happiness; whereas pride as a character trait just covers up the uncertainty of a person of itself.

Gratitude by comparison is a quiet emotion, and much rarer. Just as there are people who never experience love, so there are people who do not know the emotion of gratitude. I do not here speak about a *moral attitude,* a vague feeling of obligation or about a social convention. Those perceptions exist too and there is nothing neurotic or suspicious about them. I already mentioned the fundamental significance of the universal norm of reciprocity, the ferment of very diverse forms of socialization processes. Individual deficits with respect to assimilating norms of reciprocity are disturbances of personality function and especially part of the psychopathic character. Gratitude, as an emotion rather than an obligation, is one of the deepest and most beautiful experiences of which human beings are capable.

"Gratefulness is heaven itself", according to William Blake, thus moving it close to bliss. Of course, it is quite possible to be grateful without specific reason, as if having received a gift from life itself. Even then the emotion of gratitude looks for a way to express itself through giving; just as one feels enriched, to enrich the environment in turn; a readiness to take care of the other. This isn't just a motivation for action stimulated by gratitude but exactly its expressive quality; it is part of the expression of gratitude to turn towards the other, to give them a glance, perhaps a squeeze of the hand, a kiss, a loving embrace – and above all and strangely, with tears. Tears of gratitude are not those of crying; rather a tender wetness in the eyes, not just veiling them but also making them look warm. The quality of giving in the expression of gratitude is generated by turning towards somebody, by warmth, through opening oneself.

Beyond this, gratitude wants to push towards giving in action but without the quality of exchange or compensation, since gratitude as an emotion, utterly different from gratitude as a convention, knows from the outset about the impossibility of restitution and is not unhappy with it – completely different from emotions of guilt.

Certainly, a desire to look after the other can arise from the experience of gratitude, wanting to maintain in them a small part of one's own world. But that is already a result of contacting processes belonging to the realm of personality functions. In the moment of contact itself the point is to find the right sign, to discover the appropriate symbol to carry the emotion, and express this as a turning-towards. In therapy it is important to offer support in this process of finding expression, but particularly to be able to emotionally accept the client's emotion of gratitude. The grateful person needs a counterpart, since without a response their emotion enters a void and may sometimes even turn into hate. It is however part of quite common narcissistic disturbances in therapists to be quite unable to tolerate such gratitude: it is too close for comfort and the gratitude of the other is warded off instead of being accommodated.

In no way do all contacting processes take a satisfying course. Very frequently – too frequently – barriers become insuperable and our strength and abilities are insufficient, or there is a lack which at present cannot be managed. We are frustrated; still hungry, still longing; we feel disheartened, dejected and empty; our emotional sense of self comes close to a zero point. In short, we feel powerless, despairing even. In this emotion, too, the evaluative function is immediately obvious: "This is too big a bite for me, let it go; admit failure, look for another more easily achieved possibility". The emotion of **despair** is the emotional acknowledgement of our weakness in relation to adverse circumstances, in a specific environment, here and now. Naturally, we do not always feel impotent when a contacting process has not gone as satisfactorily as we thought and hoped. Normally we only sense a certain dissatisfaction, something like an ungratified need, leading in turn to the next attempt; and a slight anger which will mobilize energy for the next effort.

The experience of capitulation is the real emotion of feeling powerless; of failure; we feel that we have reached the limit of our strength. The expression of powerlessness is that of despondency: lowered eyes, defeated inward-turned body posture, flat breathing and paralysed motor expression; a weak voice. This minimization of all expressive contacting functions is indeed quite effective: help is offered quickly by people who are so inclined, but exploitative responses are not uncommon either. From this it follows that the power vacuum of impotence creates an undertow. This doesn't make emotions of helplessness any more pleasant; loss of all power is a terrible emotion since the pervading lack is connected with the certainty that it cannot be assuaged through one's own resources. Perhaps the ultimate experience of being completely ineffectual still lurking in our bones is that of the hungry baby crying in vain.

Therefore, it is not surprising that we prefer to avoid this feeling; either we project our weakness onto the other and fancy ourselves stronger than we are – or, more frequently, we use our remaining strength in repeated furious attempts, even when their futility has long been established. This can become dangerous. When a person, either forced or from neurotic fixation, gets stuck with a situation where they cannot move ahead and do not live out their needs and energies in a different way, impotent rage turns to despair and a failure to see any further possibilities; or the organism devours itself in self-destructive psychosomatic illness. But if the unpleasant feeling is allowed (and we are not in an objective situation of lack, for example in a famine), then we see that retreating and renewed gathering of strength is indicated until re-orientation is possible, leading to more fruitful contacting territory.

Felt powerlessness as a contacting emotion, as opposed to a life attitude, informs us of the limits of our strengths and possibilities, protecting us from dangerously overrating ourselves and from unrealistic fantasies and wasteful stubbornness. Implicitly this means that this emotional experience is typical for a society in which the individual is of greatest importance, as is typically the case in modernity. Norbert Elias, as well as Richard Sennett (Sennett, 2013), have argued that the service classes in feudal society did not experience this kind of impotence because the social order of strict hierarchies with their rituals and rules of respect in which everybody "knew their place" compensated for their lack of power. It makes more sense to me and seems more realistic, however, to assume that sheer dread of draconian punishments generated extreme self-control. This was especially true in areas where the inquisition was particularly strong as well as during the bitter religious wars following the Reformation.

If supporting growth is the object of psychotherapy in modern times its first task here is working on blockages of emotions of impotence, while the second must be to support realistic assessments of the patient's limits as well as their talents and power. Neuroses do not just consist in feelings of inferiority but also in feelings of superiority. In this way the American expression "shrink" (originally "head shrink") for psychotherapists has a core of truth.

Things are the other way round when we talk of **guilt** rather than powerlessness. Guilt feelings signal not a diminution of one's own strength and qualities, but of the environment, specifically through our own immediate agency. Damage has been done or an injury inflicted *unnecessarily* to satisfy a genuine need – that is the most important aspect. A spontaneous feeling of guilt in the just concluding post-contacting phase unmistakeably indicates that the environment has been diminished in ways beyond the necessary exchange processes, serving to balance lack in the organism. Destruction and obliteration in the sense of de-structuring of obstacles on the road to the Gestalt one touches are normal constituents of any contacting process. We don't feel guilty after eating a meal (although some vegetarians would qualify this statement) or having killed a midge on our arm; nor when, with justifiable anger, one shames another into contributing their fair share, or gets a disruptive member of a group to shut up! In such cases we mostly experience satisfaction, relief or sometimes regret; but not guilt.

But when we have unnecessarily hurt somebody, either through careless neglect – for example when causing a car accident – or in anger relating to a different situation; or even perhaps consciously taking such damage to the other into account or intentionally inflicting it, then we feel spontaneously guilty. The immediate expression of emotions of guilt is the body drawing back; we bite our lips or automatically take a step back, as if able to turn back the event, undo what has been done. And that is the action motivation belonging to guilt – to repair the damage, to restore the previous state of affairs, to exercise active repentance.

Before we can allow guilt feelings to come into awareness, we easily imagine that we will never be free of them again, or at least that one's Ego, one's own capacities, will be unbearably curtailed. The only solution is to open oneself to the experience of guilt. True – as opposed to neurotic – feelings of guilt are immediately transformed into those of **remorse,** to which in a way they are identical. Remorse now shows the way out of this limbo of guilt: to do something to bring healing for the guilty person as well as for the environment. The fact that in German the word "guilt" ("Schuld") and "debt" ("Schulden") have the same etymological root makes psychological sense, since this kind of guilt also needs to be repaid. But just as we cannot always give where we have received, we cannot always heal where we have inflicted damage. In all crime against life itself, the most dreadful part is that death is irrevocable. In all guilt we experience our transience, and that is perhaps why our resistance is so strong. Remorse will create a change in our attitude towards *everything* in life; it gives a moral dimension to the organism/environment relationship. Therefore, it is really important to show the repentant person ways and means of restitution. That is sometimes a therapeutic task, often a political one, but always a social pedagogical one. Robert Jay Lifton empirically investigated victims and perpetrators of the mass murders in the Holocaust, in Hiroshima and Vietnam and knows more than anybody else about the psychology of guilt problems. He says: "This kind of guilt is the (arousal) anxiety of responsibility" (Lifton, 1979:139).

In the final analysis, guilt always arises when we take more from the environment than we actually need and change it more than is necessary. No psychological theory can determine how much is too much. It can only name the conditions under which remorse becomes an action-orientating force. Morality is a social code intending to ensure the survival of the individual; whereas ethics can be understood as an individual's code for the survival of the species. Guilty emotions will only arise from having harmed moral norms if simultaneously one has also violated one's own ethical norms. And such norms cannot be socially introjected codes of conduct: they grow from the experience of life's richness and its vulnerability. In the end ethics is, according to Theodore Sturgeon, "a reverence for your source and posterity. It is a study of the main current that created you" (Sturgeon, 1953:237). Ethics arise from reverence for life – first of all for your own.

8 The inhibiting emotions

Being anxious and feeling ashamed

It is easy to confuse emotions of guilt with those of shame, although these two emotions differ significantly from each other. Perls discovered early on that there are emotions which do not promote and advance the contacting process, but rather hinder and inhibit it. In *Ego, Hunger and Aggression* he talks about the emotions of **anxiety** and **shame** as "the quislings of the organism" (Perls, 1992)[11], the traitors to needs, inhibiting and impeding. Guilt feelings are not part of these inhibiting emotions, since they only appear in the post-contacting phase and because through remorse further contacting processes are initiated, giving them a specific direction. Also it is not appropriate to lump the inhibiting emotions together with *emotional attitudes and habits*, which are character attributes of personality. They are reaction formations of the emotions, just as a phobic attitude, for instance, develops from the fore-contact emotion of disgust, or repressed anger is gradually consolidated into resentment. In contrast to these "incomplete emotions", as Perls called them and which I will deal with in the next section, shame and anxiety are emotions complete in themselves and have their own discrete and distinctive forms of expression. They are basic emotions which seem to belong to the anthropological endowment of human beings, found in all cultures and in all people.

How is it possible then that emotions – an unalienable part of human nature – can become "traitors" to the very contacting processes which have such elementary significance for our ways of being in the world? What does it mean that human beings are equipped by nature with emotions inhibiting the contacting process? The significance attributed to the emotions of anxiety and shame in the therapeutic process also depends on the answer to this question. Nevertheless, in the first instance they require a *sociological answer*, since the anthropological function of emotions of anxiety and shame rests on their ability to psychically anchor and direct the expression of social civilizing processes.

From the outset, *homo sapiens* is essentially oriented towards symbolically mediated interaction with other human beings and does not know any natural way of being beyond "culture" – culture which we have in our language and also in our bodies from the outset. There is no such thing as a human being not culturally formed; human nature is nothing but this constraint to embody ourselves in culturally available forms as social beings. The exchange between organism and environment can only be seen as self-directed if one considers specific enculturation as a necessary and essential part of the process itself and not as a neurotic or pathogenic deviation of a primary natural process. If this were not so, the theory of the contacting process would be nothing but a biological relapse away from the insights of philosophy and sociology as applied to the anthropological significance of work, language and expression (Honneth / Joas, 1980). Nor is it the case that in normal emotions of anxiety and shame we find unpleasant introjects of social origin manifesting themselves. In fact, emotions of anxiety and shame are a direct expression of the elementary socialized nature of every individual; of our always being socialized from the beginning. We find them in all types of societies, even if their function in Modern society is closely connected with issues of our ongoing or endangered civilizing processes. In present-day therapeutic work, it is important to distinguish between neurotic introjects and healthy *internalizations* in the service of the preservation of the standards of our civilization (Dreitzel, 2019).

In order to understand the essence of the emotions of anxiety and shame we have to start with understanding what is positive about these inhibiting emotions. I'll start with the emotion of **anxiety**. As already discussed in the context of aversive emotions, I do not mean fear of a concrete threat or danger, but rather the unpleasant experience of excitement anxiety which shows in a feeling of constriction in the chest and throat, sometimes appearing as arousal in a new strange contact and always connected with a disturbance of the free and easy flow of breathing. "The excitement is interrupted; breath is held: this is anxiety", in Goodman's succinct description (Perls & Goodman:188). But excitement is not a state – it is a movement, a flow. Interrupting an arousal is like damming up a river; the energy no longer turns outward but is directed towards "averting the attention, distracting interest in other things, holding the breath, gritting the teeth, tightening the abdominal muscles, retracting the pelvis, tightening the rectum etc." (Perls & Goodman:189). It is as if the threat were arising from one's own organism. And indeed, other than in fear of external dangers (including the fear of illness in one's own body which can, paradoxically, be experienced as an environment outside of oneself, because we not only are our body, but we also have it) it is one's own needs and appetites exuding the threat, whose unfolding in sensorimotor excitement is inhibited by anxiety.

One's own needs, though, can only become a danger when their immediate satisfaction – by these means and to this extent – touches social prohibitions and instructions which have already been internalized. They have become inveterate, second nature, and in Gestalt therapy terminology, they have become *assimilated.* Hence under these conditions the satisfaction of needs would damage the very social nature of the human organism, whereas if we violate un-assimilated introjects, we will experience vague guilt feelings not leading to remorse. This means they do not really motivate us to change our behaviour since introjects inhibit life, our individual pursuit of need satisfaction, without necessarily interfering with basic rules or values of our society.

This can lead to chronic anxiety conditions seriously damaging the organism. The difference between neurotic and healthy anxieties lies in the difference between fully assimilated "display rules" (Ekman / Friesen, 1972) and neurotically introjected ones. Of course, there are social conditions whose rules of expression are so hostile to life that they can never become second nature. Hence they will usually be sabotaged, often subconsciously, and therefore not function perfectly (Dreitzel, 2019). Always, excitement anxiety will be an emotional reason for a dissonance in the organism/environment field, for touching a sore point in the always fragile relationship between individual and society. Only in the shape of social interests can needs be legitimized; *only in the shape of needs can societal interests enter the motivation of social role players* (Dreitzel, 1980). Thus there is always an un-integrated residue of needs and emotions remaining, which are impossible to assimilate and keep setting off arousal anxieties.

Such anxieties have nothing to do with fear of punishment; when one disregards them and allows the action to take place anyway there are no guilt feelings. The quintessential pervasiveness of the civilising process regarding all aspects of the unity of body, soul and mind, which Perls & Goodman call organism, penetrates more deeply than the cultural norms of conscious behaviour; it concerns the general capacity for excitement in the organism, which is somehow suspected of wanting to override with animal immediacy the requirements and necessities of the social intermediation of need satisfaction.

This applies particularly to the context of production and distribution of goods requiring division of labour which entails the social organization of desire. Be there in time, never be sick or tired, do not get pregnant, don't demand vacations and be neither tempted nor victimized by sexual harassment. These workers do not need cafeterias or toilets; they don't smoke; they are not prone to moods, don't need emotion for orientation and motivation. They do not waste time chatting and they don't criticize their superiors. In short, they could be said to be perfect and function like machines. Human labour must compete with robots and artificial intelligence – these machines never go on strike, are always active and more civilized than people – if we define civilization simply as a set of rules restraining the needs and instincts of our bodily nature. This would, of course, be a rather primitive definition of civilization. Actual civilization is much more, it entails cultivation, a refinement of our gifts and talents for understanding this world and creatively adjusting to its challenges. Yet the disciplining pressure of this one-dimensional world of capitalist production, distribution and services is constantly growing – and perhaps this is one of the reasons why outbreaks of uncivilized actions and the appearance of shameless behaviour seem to be on the increase in Western societies today.

With anxiety and even more with shame, society protects itself against the demands of the individual through countermanding arousal and by temporary interruption of the contacting process. Therefore in some ways all anxieties are social anxieties. How do I act in such a way that I do not violate a taboo, ensuring that others continue to consider me one of them? And since it is never completely clear what is taboo, and to what extent, or how I should behave in order to be like others, there are reasons enough for being anxious. But only people who have internalized too few standards of behaviour – whose socialization regarding norms and values has been chaotic – will experience this kind of social anxiety as a pervasive character trait.

Normally, anxiety only appears when the organism is already quite aroused and the expressive functions, arising where the motoric will to express emotions encounters socially determined standards of expression, the "display rules". Excitement anxiety regulates expressive human behaviour so that these "display rules" are normally complied with.

But where these rules are very rigid, there will be a great deal of excitement anxiety and there will be forms of behaviour (reaction formations) with the function of preventing such anxieties from arising. This can easily be observed in therapeutic situations: anxiety kills arousal even before tears can show in a man's eyes, securing the maintenance of a social standard of expression. Or anxiety paralyses a woman's motor expression just at the moment where she senses anger rising up, and through that she guarantees the socially expected passivity of female expressive behaviour, perhaps by smiling or keeping her voice low and soft. If anxiety and shame are traitors to the organism, in the same way they are the *spies of society;* they react like a seismograph to the merest deviation from the current standard of the civilising process preventing malfunction or even its break-down.

Autonomous behaviour, therefore, can never mean behaviour free from anxiety. Indeed, what matters is not to avoid anxiety, not to ban it from experience through the many forms of defence (see Chapter VI, 2) which are part of everyday practice for all of us, but to feel the anxiety and to stay with the breath. Only in that way can anxiety turn into action-motivating emotions like fear or rage or quite simply the desire to create and to express oneself. As we have seen, this can easily be understood when we investigate stage fright (see discussion in chapter IV, 2): The catalyst for transforming anxiety into the ego functions which the respective contacting process needs is the breath. In letting go into the breath when exhaling the individual gathers themself anew and enters into relationship with society again.

In the emotions of **shame** and **embarrassment** we can recognize even more clearly the civilising function. In any case, excitement anxiety and the emotion of shame are two sides of one and the same phenomenon: anxiety appears *before expression,* shame *follows;* both have the same function – to safeguard the social dimension of the organism – and both work according to the same principle: they inhibit and potentially prevent a person's initiative, activity and especially their expressivity in the contacting process. In excitement, arousal becomes paralysis; in shame, desire becomes agony.

The first important point in understanding the emotions of shame and embarrassment is to note that we are dealing with one emotion manifesting itself with very different degrees of intensity. The words confusion, embarrassment and shame mark differing degrees of intensity of the emotion. It expresses a *diminishing capacity to distance ourselves from the experience which provoked it.* For example, a compliment can make us bashful, but usually it is not difficult to overcome the bashfulness through a distancing action. And even when I feel embarrassed about something, at least post hoc there is a subject capable of acting to try to expunge the embarrassment. In shame, though, we are not dealing with something that "happened", an action or an uncontrolled expression in relation to which I can take a position, even while I myself originated this act. I myself am at stake. I feel ashamed of myself, I as the source of all my actions, as a whole, am the origin of the offence. Therefore the wish for the earth to open up and immediately devour me follows – my personal identity must disappear. Such reaction presupposes the existence of a social environment in which the individual as such has a high value – as is typical for modernity. Many sociologists have called individualism the most important mark of modern societies. Georg Simmel, one of the founders of modern sociology, observed this development early on in an essay on shame (Simmel, 1911):

> The deep alternative permeating life in every aspect requires a prior cultural decision – whether the individual is to be considered part of a whole or whether he is himself a whole – before we can understand whether the emotion of shame can actually be experienced. Only the concept of the totally independent individual completely responsible for himself constitutes the context for this tension to even arise, depending on whether individuality is emphasized or played down. This characteristic friction is incompatible with close relations between the individual and the group as a whole. [And importantly he added] Groups that completely absorb the individual are characteristically free of feelings of shame [...] As soon as we feel solidarity with a group, the contrast between what we are and what we should be vanishes.

These last remarks were particularly perceptive at a time when the study of the psychology of the masses had only just began (Le Bon, 1885). Simmel's observations are important in my present context – because they seem to indicate that the civilizing process shows that shame is an important internalized safeguard against the danger of lapsing into inappropriate responses. It is potentially – and quite frequently – weakened through participation in groups or group activities, according to the norms it endorses. There is, indeed, much evidence for this observation which requires further analysis.

Thus, it seems safe to argue that shame is the typical emotional indicator of the second phase of the civilizing process. It requires that we re-evaluate whether the individual should be considered as a personality in their own right. This development began with the urban bourgeoisie during the Renaissance in northern Italy. Of course, this process took centuries to gain enough momentum to become the new basis of the civilizing process in its second stage: it was characterized by previously externalized rules of behaviour becoming internalized, a development spearheaded by the new middle classes especially in Protestant countries and their Puritanical enclaves. In these social environments, deviance from internalized rules and values was at first punished by smear campaigns initiated by religious and secular authorities, just as shown in Nathaniel Hawthorne's famous novel *The Scarlet Letter* (Hawthorne, 1850). Simultaneously, this process also began to generate private feelings of shame.

A significant proof that shame and embarrassment are shades of the same emotion, with different intensities, is that the "sentic form" of their expression is identical: blushing, the wish to cover oneself, to hide. In bashfulness we blush easily and we turn blood red in shame. Whether this reaction appears to the same extent in all people – assuming that the expression of this emotion is not repressed – is difficult to say. Darwin noticed that the phenomenon of facial engorgement also happens in dark skinned races. The wish to cover oneself indicates that the origin of embarrassment is experienced as nakedness, even if we are not dealing with "skin shame".[12] The disguising smile of embarrassment is a gesture of concealment, simultaneously asking for forgiveness. And if we cannot turn away and hide when we are embarrassed about being overcome with emotion, we cover our face.

The more intense the emotion of shame, the more we are inclined to hide anyway, to make ourselves invisible; but even with the lesser feelings of embarrassment we can observe a slight turning away of face and upper body. The function of these different forms of expression is always the same, namely that what is visible of my person – that which, involuntarily and unawares, has become visible from behind my controlled social façade, is to be veiled and hidden so that my nakedness is covered, the embarrassment effaced. The catastrophe experienced when we are overcome by a very strong feeling of shame also implies that it is no longer possible to express it, since if the whole person originates it, the offence can only be removed by removing the whole person. In shame the individual aligns with society and extinguishes itself.

The second important point for understanding the emotions of shame and embarrassment is that they are triggered either by damage to or destruction of one's social identity, through a temporary loss of bodily control or interactional competency. Perhaps this can most easily be understood when we compare emotions of shame once more with emotions of guilt. The latter are responses to norm-violating behaviour, avoidable since the person had all the relevant competencies: they trigger sanctions geared towards a subject which acted consciously and with free will or possibly through negligence. Conversely, emotions of shame and embarrassment are triggered when something "has happened" to the person as a physical body, normally a loss of self-control or containment or of good social form – a "loss of face". It is possible to excuse oneself by falling back on something which in turn triggers shame: reduced mental capacity. But significantly, by observing shame and embarrassment instead of sanctioning it, we overlook the behaviour in question, saying to ourselves that "it is just too embarrassing". The social identity of the person is in question.

Significantly, shame occurs in modern societies when the supposed autonomy of the individual fails and is felt and experienced as helplessness in relation to events and developments beyond our power. Hence our societal culture generates a strange mixture of shame and guilt feelings at any time. It has been suggested (Hermann, 2017) that a general bad conscience can be easily mobilized in the educated middle classes of the West with respect to past crimes of colonialism, racism and wars and is in fact a secularization of the old myth of the fall of man – an idea particularly focused on in Lutheran theology. While Catholicism believes that Original Sin is forgiven through baptism, Martin Luther claimed that the fall of man can only be made well through unconditional belief in God, even though this cannot be achieved as such but only be given as *grace* by God himself. Whether this theology penetrated *all* forms of Protestantism to such an extent that its secular form is now completely pervading our culture seems to me debatable. Yet the conspicuous general morality of the liberal middle classes is an interesting phenomenon which needs explaining. In any case this "Protestant morality" is either cause or symptom of our shame- and guilt-generating culture. This culture is now strongly reinforced by the growing awareness that our moral problems are not confined to the sins of our ancestors but manifest themselves in neglecting the causes of climate change.

Modernity's stake in individualism excludes any concept of *collective* guilt. Thus the descendants of generations of perpetrators of environmental misuse may feel a responsibility for being part of an exploitative nation or the Western world as a whole, or for being part of our present culture of consumerism causing the ongoing destruction of nature, and will tend to develop feelings of shame as the emotional expression of their moral attitudes – sufficiently uncomfortable for many to try to make financial donations to dispel such feelings. Only as individual members of our society can they emotionally shift into guilt feelings which motivate them to get involved in practical work – for instance work in relief organizations. As Robert Jay Lifton has pointed out (Lifton, 1979) such practices – emotionally driven by remorse – are experienced as a relief and may even lead to joy in facing present disasters. My own experiences with helpers in the German refugee crisis of 2015 and with NGO people fighting for human rights or against the destruction of the environment confirm this observation. This is of great importance for any psychotherapy dealing with contemporary perpetrators. Therapists may be confronted with symptoms of generalized cultural shame such as looking away, being resigned, feeling helpless in view of the complexity of the problems, and other forms of reaction formation. Thus it seems that the ambiguities of moral standards in modern society can only be resolved by an emotional shift from collective feelings of shame to individual feelings of guilt.

There is no way of protecting oneself from emotions of shame, except by accepting the social role in which being diminished is the normal state of affairs, as in early childhood, in very old age and in severe illness or disability. To the extent that in these roles the person no longer needs to feel ashamed about their lack of self-control, they also forgo the right of self-determination. And since in addition the threshold of shame is deeply internalized, even with adults in such roles and situations, emotions of shame only very gradually become blunted and only become repressed through severe pain and the hardship of physical suffering.

In shame, society asserts itself against the individual; in guilt the individual affirms itself over society. Guilt presupposes a subject capable of action and of taking responsibility for themself. Emphasizing the individual person's capacity to feel guilt has been one of the great achievements of the emerging bourgeoisie of the Modern Era. In experiencing feelings of shame and embarrassment the individual surrenders claims to individuality in favour of the collective. Shame is always an expression of powerlessness but feelings of guilt assert the individual's capacity to decide. This can be a lonely stand, however. It must be emphasized that the liberating effect of "doing something about it", of personally getting involved in compensatory action works only if the individual is embedded in solidarity with groups of activists! The psychoanalyst Peer Hultberg, a specialist in the study of shame, observed that emotions of shame often are warded off with guilt feelings (Hultberg, 1987:94). As a last claim of individuality against the anonymous collective, this makes a great deal of sense when the same society in general honours individuality. Sometimes, this may reach the point where the ashamed person actually sets out to incur guilt. Erik Erikson warns: "The person who is ashamed wants to force the world to look away, not to notice his nakedness. He wants to destroy the eyes of the world" (quoted by Lifton, 1979:464). Of course there is the opposite strategy too, the avoidance of guilt feelings through projecting one's responsibility onto others. This mostly happens with the small faults and failings of everyday life, when it is more comfortable to admit one's incompetence with regard to adverse circumstances rather than owning up and declaring oneself guilty of sloppiness and inattention.

Shame and embarrassment are deeply social emotions and they are attached to the group rather than to the individual. We don't feel guilty for others, even if they are close associates. But we feel shame for all those with whom we identify, whether partners, parents or children; one's own gender or one's own nation; in certain situations, even for complete strangers whom one witnesses. In Modern societies particularly in embarrassing situations, we are able to observe what community means: instantly everybody pulls together trying to block out the embarrassing event (for a more detailed sociological analysis see Dreitzel, 1983). That can be achieved through ignoring or playing down, through quick assistance or by putting the whole thing in perspective through joking. In any case the individual is not, as in guilt, shown up or denounced and publicly exposed; instead, and quite to the contrary, they are hidden, and taken to the most private part of the backstage. Society's way of dealing with shame is to excuse the actor, to ignore the event. In embarrassing situations everybody contributes to repairing and restoring social normality. Emotions of shame and embarrassment are triggered then by a transient loss of body control or interactive capacity in myself or other people relevant to me in this situation. Shame is the polar opposite to pride; when I feel ashamed, I hide my deficiencies: with pride I show my talents. Pride reveals: shame conceals. And just as I am able to feel shame for others, so I can be proud of others if and when I am identified with them.

It must be kept in mind, though, that these phenomenological descriptions do not apply for pre-Modern societies sometimes called "shame societies" still to be found in Japan or China where they survive in rituals of forcing the perpetrator to publicly admit to their shameful behaviour, thereby offering them a chance to excuse and unburden themselves. These rituals, for better or worse, obviously belong to an earlier, the second stage of the civilizing process.

As I already mentioned, emotions of shame and embarrassment can be triggered by permanent impairment and damage to one's *sense of identity,* as well as through transient *diminution of social competency* or *bodily control.* Though any of these causes can either lead to slight embarrassment or to terrible feelings of shame, the diminishment of one's social identity tends to weigh most. Referring to these three causes of shame and embarrassment, I would like to distinguish between identity-related shame, social shame and body-related shame.

Identity-related shame refers to what I am or what I am not in the context of my reference groups. In the final analysis the question is always – do I or do I not *belong*? In archaic societies exclusion from the tribal community was a punishment always followed by psychic death, often physical death too. In traditional pre-modern societies, social identity is often based on status-specific concepts of honour; violating those standards was experienced as shaming one's membership group, which often could only be repaired through the death of the person shamed or shaming. Today however, most clearly-defined membership groups like large families, guilds, monastic communities or the aristocracy as such have been dissolved. For most people these havens of social identity have changed into widely varying individual fates. For some merely managing their life can be a daily challenge generating identity-related shame. People who are chronically ashamed about their own existence are common in the clientele of psychotherapists, although such embarrassment is often kept secret for a long time. They were unwanted children, whose parents resented their appearance in the world, and those who were always rejected, superfluous, considered "no good for anything," "unworthy to be alive," and all those who from the beginning received the message that "you are not welcome here." But in our age of mass mobility and mass migration this message is often applied to whole groups, which then can have murderous consequences.

Social shame on the other hand arises when social competency is lacking or insufficient. Here we are not dealing with belonging to the wrong group so much as not being allowed to exist in the first place, but with the experience that I am not allowed to be as I am here and now. Perhaps you are poorer than your fellows or you lack education where money is taken for granted and education a matter of course. Perhaps you don't know how to dress, or what to bring when invited to a party; or you lack good table manners, laugh in the wrong place or go over the top in expressing emotion where cool detachment is the norm. There are endless occasions for social shame and they have increased since we have become so mobile that we constantly encounter strangers from social milieus whose codes of behaviour and communication we are not familiar with. Today's society is fragmented into a multitude of identity bubbles with subtle in-group standards of communication, behaviours, and tastes. If one crosses such group boundaries one can quickly land in foreign territories where different rules and behavioural customs apply. This road is plastered with embarrassing situations like stumbling stones.

In **body-related shame** the issue is nakedness. With a plethora of material Hans Peter Duerr[13] has shown that all cultures and every standard of civilization is familiar with original genital shame, a shyness about exposing the genitals; or if nakedness is standard, to look at the other's genitals, especially when in a state of sexual arousal or sexually active. This aspect of body related shame seems to be part of our anthropological endowment and of course a violent infraction of this threshold has devastating psychic consequences, which in people who were sexually abused as children leads to deep identity-related shame. But of course the variability of standards is still very significant, and becomes evident when we look at the varying dress codes in different cultures. Frequently, but not always, women's breasts are supposed to be covered; in India, for instance, the exposure of shoulders and arms is more offensive than exposing the belly in the West; in fundamentalist Islamic countries women's hair or even their faces are to be covered.

In our society, genital shame has perhaps not much diminished but thresholds of shame with regard to defecation, chewing noises and cleanliness in general are significantly higher in Christian cultures than they used to be, while nakedness now triggers far less shame than it did in our grandparents' generation. Norbert Elias argued convincingly that the precondition of this development was and is an internalized restraint of sexual aggression. Yet even with the loosening of standards regarding nudity, what always sets off body-related shame is the temporary loss of standard body control and disarray of one's clothing: an open zip or an incidental belch are harmless examples here. More serious ones are forced disrobement of the body and especially of the genitals, as in the form of "degradation rituals" which regularly take place in closed or – in sociological parlance – "total institutions" (Goffman, 1961) like the military, hospitals, prisons, boarding schools, and the like. Such shamings can easily become a traumatic experience. Shame related to the body only becomes neurotic when it does not occur as a situational signal for having overstepped assimilated cultural standards; only if it chronically hampers need satisfactions – as for instance in anorexia where inhibitions based on having *introjected* body images create significant pathology.

We cannot argue with the fact that thresholds of shame and embarrassment have changed in history even if we follow H. P. Duerr's proposition that public exposure of the genitals has always been offensive in all societies. True, emotions and their sentic forms are the same everywhere. But still they are experienced in very different shades of intensity according to the social settings and cultural contexts in which they appear.

Let us again consider shame that has been caused by shaming. There is no doubt that important factors here are power and rank: in monastic times the King was beyond shaming – his occasional nudity could not disturb his god-like superiority. Even during the 1950s a friend of mine studying at Oxford University and sharing a room with a young English lord told me how astonished he was when, according to agreement, that lord left him alone one evening to offer him privacy for a date with his lover but failed to take his butler along. When my friend complained, the lord answered with surprise "But he is only a butler!" On the other hand, historically masters of all kinds could shame their inferiors by forcing them to undress. And more recently, the taken-for-granted "culture" of sexual assault by film studio bosses and directors in Hollywood and elsewhere is proof that shaming is still a frequent strategy to exert power as "the chance to get one's way against the will and interest of the subjected person" – as Max Weber famously defined power.

Today the *sources* of power seem to have changed. It appears that public shaming has returned as a means to exert power. In struggles over the sources of power the balance is shifting from those who through their position in the professional hierarchies have the power to force their subordinates – especially women – into submission to the power of the New Media to publicly disgrace suspected perpetrators, who often not only "lose face" but also their jobs and their reputation. The culprits of this power to blame and shame – whether or not guilty of the (often anonymous) accusations – may be prominent, powerful or influential actors in all public realms: politicians, actors, media moguls, journalists, sport icons, pop stars etc. This development can be interpreted as a progressive step in the direction of a more equal distribution of power: the #MeToo movement is certainly another move in women's process of emancipation. The problem with this power shift however is that it quite easily sidesteps, negates or surpasses the state's monopoly of power to investigate and punish transgression. This power is guaranteed and reserved to the judiciary as a third and independent pillar of democratic societies. Even though we are aware of serious flaws in its functioning, in reality we must recognize that the principle of lawful states guaranteeing that nobody will be punished without a fair trial – the core idea behind the age-old habeas corpus – is actually becoming obsolete in view of the smear campaigns facilitated by the New Media.

If the speed with which thresholds of shame and embarrassment are changing today has become a pathogenic factor accelerating psychic disturbance, not only psychotherapists but lawyers too have a new client group in those who feel they have been victimized by sexual harassment and in those who feel they have been victimized by smear campaigns – both will feel deep shame. It is important therefore to remember the development of the civilizing process (in modern Western societies), whose focus is indeed this type of change. In the first chapter of this book I described how this process develops in three overlapping phases, cutting across each other. At first we see a multiplication and strengthening of external rules of conduct, followed by internalization of external restraints, so that a strong "Super-Ego" develops. Eventually these external standards of behaviour, guarded by the inhibiting emotions of shame and embarrassment, loosen up through a process of manners becoming more informal. This, though, does not work effectively as far as the expression of emotions is concerned. Instead, this new phase – the informalization of behavioural standards – shows a scissor-like divergence. We see increasingly contradictory processes; more and more informal everyday manners meet with increasingly cooler emotional expressivity in the public sphere, especially in the ever-growing areas where technological processes are involved and questions of security are at stake. At the same time, populist movements as well as separatists fight aggressively against their cultural foes and feel entitled to break the rules of civilized behaviour which they have insufficiently internalized.

In our society all three phases are in operation simultaneously, even while the significance of the first phase is strongly diminished and the significance of the third is only now gradually increasing. The simultaneity of these overlapping phases of the civilizing process also shows in the class-specific differences of behavioural standards.

Regarding the emotions of shame and embarrassment we can say that the first phase is concerned with concepts like "honour" and "insult", both of which always refer to a collective (tribe, class or family) from which the individual derives their identity, and whose representative they feel themself to be. Violations of expected standards are experienced as "dishonouring" the membership group. This phase survives when immigrant families or tribes are not integrated into the new culture, but also in certain subcultures in our own societies, especially in some violence-prone groups at the extreme right like Neo-Nazis or street gangs.

In the second phase – and against the background of the evolving separation of public and private spheres – there is a gradual differentiation of this experience into emotions of guilt and shame. The individual is now seen as a separate, self-responsible subject capable of differentiating taken-for-granted expectations of control and competency on the one hand and rationally accessing norms of behaviour on the other. With the bourgeoisie emerges the idea of a responsible individual, capable of guilty actions. In order for this idea to work in the social world it needed mechanisms for relieving this burden, social "traffic regulations" consisting of assumed competencies and control expectations. Consequently, when they fail, not punishment but help is the result.

It seems likely that long-term social development processes are accompanied by certain moderating surges which increasingly emphasize individual responsibility and liability. In this process new behavioural standards arise which later become internalized. And the process of such gradual internalization perhaps always develops via rediscovering and emphasizing individual culpability and a renewed emphasis on the ability to experience shame. Hultberg apparently has something like this in mind, when he thinks that our society "seems to develop from a culture of guilt towards being a culture of shame, or perhaps it is on the road to a mixture of the two" (Hultberg, 1987:89). "Protean man" at least (Lifton, 1968), a social character seeming to become more and more widespread in our society, seems to have few guilt feelings and is always tumbling into embarrassing situations. Strong, all-consuming feelings of shame have become rarer outside neurotic constellations, while embarrassing situations lurk everywhere.

Let us resume what has been said so far about shame and embarrassment:

1 Phenomenological analysis reveals that expressions like "shame," "embarrassment" and "confusion" referring to an emotion indicate different degrees of intensity of the same emotion. The degree depends on the extent of identification with what is being exposed or lost, and therefore is experienced as embarrassing. Moreover, this emotion has a succinct expressive Gestalt, blushing, covering, hiding, holding up; and is sensed as hot, burning and altogether unpleasant.
2 Shame and embarrassment are social emotions, arising through no fault of one's own and for which one cannot be held responsible. We can feel

shame and embarrassment for anyone with whom we identify. Embarrassing situations, regularly set off collective efforts to restore "normality" in everyone who is part of the situation or the social in-group.

3 Particularly in a therapeutic context it makes sense to distinguish between shame related to identity, social shame, and shame related to the body. Shame related to identity is the emotional reaction to not being allowed to be oneself, not feeling at home where in fact one is at home. Its extreme form is existential shame for being alive at all; getting something wrong in one's relation to others when everybody else naturally seems to know how to get it right. A new mixture of identity shame and body shame can be observed in Western societies in the increasing number of people who do not feel at home with the gender of their body given them by natural birth. This seems to be an extreme expression of the insecurities caused by the high degree of individualization which is commonly and increasingly characteristic for Modern societies. Body-related shame is the sensation of having physically denuded oneself at the wrong time, in the wrong company, and in the wrong place. Genital shame seems to be universally prevalent. But the feeling that one's own biologically-given body identity is somehow "wrong" is something new in Modern society and is probably related to the vision of surgical solutions for this problem in a highly technological culture.

4 The threshold for emotions of shame and embarrassment has been pushed further towards the social environment – at least in our own civilizing process – to the same extent as expectations regarding individual body control, control of affect and interactional competency have increased. In these developments there are disruptions and surges, leading to generational differences regarding internalized shame thresholds. At the same time extremely strong emotions of shame have become pathologized through the individualising process of Modernity. Since social identity today is only marginally constituted by family and status group membership, significant shame related to identity refers to the core of one's being.

5 It must be added that identity differentiation is now sought amongst a multitude of relatively small in-groups or milieus. They are united by specialized work, educated high-brow cultural tastes like scenes for opera fans or art collectors or also low-brow hobbies like collecting militaria or playing collective computer games. There are a plethora of associations for people sharing a passion for sport; or for those interested in pursuing spiritual, religious, ideological or sexual preferences. Hobbies such as gardening, exploring wilderness areas, or hunting, fishing and other outdoor activities, playing with model railways or collecting things bring people together. The problem here is that contact and communication are more and more restricted to isolated circles of insiders, excluding all

> others with whom one shares the larger communities of habitat, traffic, language, political groupings – all of them displaying a tendency to segregate "them" from "us." As Georg Simmel noted, feelings of shame tend to lose their restraining power in the context of in-groups and their relationship with out-groups. This may lead to militancy and even violence toward out-groups, particularly in radicalized political and religious environments. Within one's own group, however, feelings of shame may appear more easily in their function of protecting group cohesion just as the old forms of honour did for tribes and families. I don't need to emphasize that this is a dangerous development undermining peaceful communication within the public sphere at large.

It is according to this fivefold description of the emotions of shame and embarrassment that we must understand their role in psychotherapy. This is where they appear more frequently than in everyday life, since here the reaction formations (defence mechanisms) normally used to control and avoid these feelings gradually become more permeable or even disappear. Indeed, if and when such emotions occur it is a sign that the course of therapy is progressing well. Of course, after a while in any therapy, with growing trust in the therapist, these kinds of embarrassing experiences in the life of the client will become topical.

In a process-oriented therapy, though, something else is even more important; that is, when in the therapeutic contacting process *itself* emotions of shame and feelings of embarrassment arise, attention needs to be paid to the triggers causing them. In the context of Gestalt therapy one can typically observe four such triggers or "reasons":

1 I am ashamed for being embarrassed about something.
2 I am ashamed to be a patient.
3 I am ashamed that I am moved and showing my feelings.
4 I am ashamed for being a burden to you.

The first situation has something to do with historically shifting boundaries between public and private spheres; we all remember earlier times when "certain things" were only allowed to be mentioned or talked about in private, if at all. But which themes belong to this sphere today and which don't differ significantly from generation to generation? Many of today's older people grew up in an environment where marital problems were largely kept hidden even from close friends, or perhaps only talked about with one's pastor, whereas younger people incessantly talk about their "relationship issues." Psychotherapeutic groups contribute to this development: Psychoanalysis has an explicit or implicit rule that the client should talk about everything that goes through their mind or heart. This situation is contained in the intimacy of an individual therapy setting and protected by rules of confidentiality. In group therapy settings, typically for Gestalt approaches what originally mattered was "authenticity," "opening up" and "following one's own process." These values sometimes were pursued under significant group pressure. Without even noticing this, beginners amongst Gestalt therapists sometimes increased this process by pressuring their clients with incessant questions like "How are you feeling right now?" or "What's happening for you?" Even: "How do you feel being with me?" If patients were able to answer such questions with a clarity helpful to the therapist, they would not need therapy. But the main fact we tend to overlook is that one of the major ways in which interactional competency shows is the inability to say "No" i.e. to reject a demand or proposal of the therapist with a clarity and authenticity helpful to one's own therapy. To draw a line demarcation line between self and others and to safeguard one's own space is an essential capacity to be worked towards. There is a certain danger inherent in Gestalt therapy's emphasis on the *contacting* process, that we often do not sufficiently recognize: that *withdrawal,* too, is a core function of the organism/environment field. If this function is interfered with in therapy, rather than being respected, there is a chance that the patient feels embarrassed and will later remember this experience with a (vague) sense of shame. Often the behavior of the patient will be interpreted by a therapist who is not sufficiently at ease with the topic of shame as resistance. Not that Gestalt therapists, who will often in their work encounter such behaviour, usually refer in such a situation to "breaking" through the apparent resistance, but – just from my supervision experience – they will often use seduction methods and charming methods instead.

If Perls described the inhibiting emotions as "emotional resistance" he seems to place them somewhere near Freud's ideas regarding mainly intellectual resistances, whereas actually he strongly emphasizes physiological ones.[14] This draws attention to the fact that we need to deal with emotions of shame and embarrassment in the same way we deal with other kinds of "resistance"; they are to be touched, but also need to be respected; they need support in becoming conscious, and this means they need to be experienced and felt psycho-physiologically, but they are not to be conquered and vanquished. They are also strengths and skills.

This process starts right at the beginning of therapy. Even today many people looking for psychotherapy feel embarrassed about being a patient. After two years of therapy, a theologian consistently called it "our conversations", while I equally consistently chose to speak about "your therapy" or "our therapeutic work". Without doubt it is important that clients sooner or later learn to identify themselves with their patient status, since otherwise there would be disturbances of the personality function of identification. This does not need to be a condition of therapy: it can be a result of it. In classical psychoanalysis this may be different, since it is dependent on developing and later dissolving a "transference neurosis".

The structural reason for emotions of shame arising in this context is the experience of an incapacity, a lack of competence in conducting one's life – the very experience which brought the patient into therapy in the first place. Here the therapist who lacks clarity regarding the social character of shame which involves them, too, can make two kinds of mistake. Some therapists share the patient's emotions of shame to such an extent, empathize so much with them, that they never broach the issue of the client's patient status and tend to treat their clients more like friends. Naturally, then distance and authority are lacking. Other therapists don't feel safe until clients have explicitly and whole-heartedly accepted their patient status. Essentially, they need a gesture of submission from the client, since they do not fully trust their own therapeutic authority. In analytic terms one could safely say that shame can very particularly evoke counter-transference processes. But Gestalt therapy aims to help the patient to see clearly how, within limits, their incapacities, limitations and disabilities truly are riches, too. Gestalt therapy is fuelled by the conviction that people only become whole and complete when they can perceive and experience themselves exactly as they are here and now, no more and no less.

Of even greater therapeutic significance is the third trigger for shame and embarrassment in the therapeutic contacting process, and that is when the client is touched, deeply moved, and wanting to express this, yet fearful of losing self-control at the same time. Though this fear is typical for persons with a strong tendency to engage in narcissistic neurotic processes, beyond all pathology we always experience an emotion of embarrassment exactly when a spontaneous emotional expression runs counter to prevailing manners, i.e. where cultural rules of expression inhibit an emotion from fully unfolding. It is this inhibition which is embodied in shame and embarrassment. In the educated middle classes, from which most clients of psychotherapy originate, these barriers can be so strong that outside the therapeutic situation it is rare that such experiences are encountered. In this social milieu people may already feel embarrassed when they breathe heavily or shout loudly or witness such behaviour coincidentally. At the beginning of the third stage of the civilizing process, when in the 1960s the standards of everyday behaviour became more and more informalized, some members of the educated middle class – at least for a while – loosened up and grew more tolerant of emotional expression by participating in newly fashionable cultural inventions like encounter groups, bio-energetic exercises, "dynamic meditation" and a whole range of other self-awareness groups offered by the cultural market – last not least Gestalt therapy group sessions.

None of this applies to the currently downwardly mobile sections of the middle class and – perhaps with the exception of strict religious milieus – never applied to the lower classes where the cultural barriers of shame were never strongly internalized. Working therapeutically with patients of this social background presents therapists with a different challenge: how to sensitize people to the rich potential of their emotions, a treasure which if owned is their true birth-right. The challenge is how to facilitate their discovery of the many varieties of emotional expression.

But even without employing therapeutic techniques aimed at facilitating emotional discharge, therapy always touches repressed emotions and brings the client into situations where the effort of repressing spontaneous emotional expression becomes fore-ground, becomes the painful figure of experience. Most frequently we notice people attempting to stop the flow of tears and stifling the urge to cry, an effort which creates painful burning sensations in the larynx. More subtle but definitely no less important is the slight hardening of the features and a barely noticeable bodily freezing when people make an effort to interrupt the process of their controlled facial expression slowly melting, as they are expressing positive emotions like love, gratitude or pride. Breathing deeply needs to be encouraged.

Dealing with existential shame in therapy is the most difficult task, since this is the worst form of shame directly relating to identity. These patients perennially experience themselves as a bother to other people and therefore their misery also as a burden for the therapist. Close observation reveals what seems to be a rule in body-related shame: *where there's embarrassment, there's also desire!* In such cases it pays to help the patient to discover what this might be. It seems that in bodily experienced shame the best way forward is to go with the hidden desire without pushing; carefully and lovingly, with joy in new discovery and excitement. In shame related to *identity* we find nothing like this – rather the traces of an introjected negation of one's very existence which may arise from being unwanted from birth. In existential shame the task is to accept and to exude joy in the very existence of one's *incarnation as an embodied person.* Here desire does not exist per se: we are dealing with a bare *élan vital* which has supported this person up to this point in their life. For this reason in therapy with such patients I think that the focus on working with the breath is of central importance, for in breathing and with the pulse beating we are undoubtedly and tangibly *alive.*

In other forms of identity shame, the task is to uncover wishes for *belonging* or *to be recognized*, making people conscious of and working on adequate realistic identifications. The sense of being a burden to others rests on a discrepancy between one's introjected (negative) self-image and experienced reality. This can be strongly pronounced in people who are in some way or other physically disabled: after all, in relation to the standards promoted by the media, we are all disabled! With this form of shame related to identity, the work of therapy is to focus on insight into one's own limitations, the frailty and mortality of the body, identifications with one's own nature instead of societal heteronomy.

Generally speaking, psychotherapy has three tasks in relation to the emotions of shame and embarrassment:

Firstly, we are concerned with restoring sensitivity regarding our own and other people's shame barriers and thresholds of embarrassment by distinguishing assimilated shame barriers from emotions of shame which are nothing but the introjects to which we, as excessively socialized human beings, are all prey, and which we often sabotage – if mostly subconsciously.

Secondly, therapy should achieve an identification with one's own limits and handicaps, helping emotions of shame and embarrassment in this sphere to disappear altogether. That may mean using therapy for learning a bit of "stigma management" (Goffman, 1963). And let us not forget we are all handicapped!

Thirdly, we are concerned with establishing that emotions of shame and embarrassment are the obstacle on the road to freely developing our emotional sensitivity – recognizing through this work that some people's shame barriers are too strongly inhibiting – while others with different social backgrounds lack them, are too unashamed.

Thus, in psychotherapy working with shame always involves a socio-political perspective keeping in mind that the emotion of shame, while it can be extremely suffocating, is also an important protection against relapses into barbarianism.

This last point is true for excitement-raising anxiety also: emotions of anxiety and shame are the keepers of the temple of our desire for emotional expressivity – only those who do not fear them can enter here. As soon as we sense this anxiety consciously, as soon as we stay with the emotion of embarrassment, these emotions wondrously change into what they conceal: arousal and excitement, energy and competence. In existential shame, though, we are concerned with experiencing just being alive. The emotions of anxiety and shame, therefore, are the cardinal point of any therapy. Perls writes:

> The awareness of, and the ability to endure, unwanted emotions are the *conditio sine qua non* for a successful cure; these emotions will be discharged once they have become ego functions. This process and not the process of remembering, forms the via regia to health.
>
> (Perls, 1992:216; my emphasis)

Simply attending to the way excitement anxiety blocks energy is going to restore the blocked flow. And staying with an emotion of embarrassment will liberate the desire already hinted at in the embarrassed smile.

It is important not to imagine that this is a simple process, especially when we think about narcissistic disturbances so much discussed these days. In this situation the therapist may easily repeat what characterized the childhood experience of the patient: to fail in giving them enough space for self-discovery. What Hultberg, alluding to the work of Alice Miller (Miller, 1978), writes about the narcissistically disturbed children of psychologists may also be true for many therapists' clients:

> Without intending to, some psychologists cannot help but communicate to their children the commonly expressed "I know you better than you know yourself" or, as it is called in the terminology of theories of narcissism and the new explorations of empathy, there is a preponderance of active "intrusive" empathy at the cost of passive, nourishing, receptive forms. Without fail the child experiences this as a forceful intrusion into the Self, and tries to defend himself by barring access to the Self through chronic shame. Through this, he also bars his own access to the Self and this shows in depression which is often defended against by bright or manic adaptation, a disturbance which under the name of "the gifted child" has now gained world-wide renown.
>
> (Hultberg, 1987:98).

In any case, there is nothing a patient resents more than being shamed by the therapist. If and when a therapist exposes a patient in front of a group, uses labels, performs voyeuristically or gets caught in therapeutic introjects, the therapist becomes a representative of social norms and socialising institutions instead of being an advocate of the patient's individual creativity, implicitly repeating the parental "Shame on you!" which has already spoilt the life of the child and corrupted their pleasures. Whether it is the ruling norms of the ruling classes or the subcultural norms of a group in the "therapy scene" – what is critical is that this is a renewed attempt at totally socialising the individual. The patient has little chance to resist this therapeutic take-over, since they are just trying to open up, just starting to trust the therapist and engage with a new experience. This therefore may not be discovered until much later and is then experienced in a situation where they cannot defend themself – a humiliation. The pain of such memories is often defended against by idealising the former therapist or through resenting them. Therefore, much time has to be spent in psychotherapy on working through previous therapies.

Notes

1 For a critical appraisal of the academic part of this literature see Benjamin Seyd, a sociologist of Friedrich Schiller University in Jena, Germany, who has specialized in this field (Seyd, 2018). For its popular contribution to this boom the bestselling book by Daniel Goleman, *Emotional Intelligence – Why it can matter more than IQ,* was one of the first and may still be representative (Goleman, 1995).

2 Hunters and hunted, pursuers and pursued seem to constitute a central myth in American culture, in which confrontation with the indigenous peoples lives on in a myriad of ways. Countless books, films and TV shows testify to this fascination, which in specific characters can intensify into an almost archaic passion.

3 See chapter "Action Theory" in Clynes (1976), which I do not further consider here.

4 For a self-inquiry of subtle tension patterns in connection with emotions and moods, the exercises developed for the Tibetan Kum-Nye relaxation are very helpful since they slow down each movement to such an extent that with practice, it is possible to reach an unusual degree of body awareness (Thartang Tulku,

1978). At first glance this book may look like just another collection of relaxation exercises for people stressed by civilization, but it definitely is not!

5 Clynes (1976:26pp). A "sentic form" for bliss was demonstrated by Janice Walker, only after Clynes' book had appeared. Compare "*Sentic Newsletter*", Vol.2, No.1, March 1980, 2.

6 You cannot take your finger off the sentograph with Clynes' investigative method, since then it cannot register what happens.

7 In photographs showing Western politicians visiting Mao Zedong, one could see a large spittoon next to Mao's chair. We might think of the civilizing *history* of spitting: N. Elias analysed the history of spitting in a special chapter of his book (Elias, 1969b).

8 Compare Peter Gleichmann (1984).

9 Clynes' view is that laughter has its own "sentic form" and therefore can be expressed in a medium other than our voice box. For these somewhat surprising ideas, which I will not examine further at this stage, compare chapter 16 in his book: *A New Form of Laughter: A Prediction of Sentic Theory*, undated, pp.207.

10 The workshop was conducted by Erving and Miriam Polster.

11 The expression "Quisling" for traitor is no longer widely known. Quisling was the name of the leader of Norwegian collaborators during the German occupation in the Second World War.

12 According to Agnes Heller, certain tribes in New Guinea have a concept of "skin shame" and "deep shame". Compare Heller (1980:4). This indicates that what I will call body shame and identity shame are universal forms of the emotions of shame and embarrassment.

13 Compare Hans Peter Duerr (2005). This book also contains a fundamental critique of Norbert Elias' theory of the civilising process which was rejected with rigour and in-depth understanding by Michael Schröter. Compare Schroeter (1990).

14 F. Perls (1992) speaks of "emotional" resistances, which he differentiates from physiological and cognitive ones. The advantage of this differentiation at that time consisted in the fact that it was possible to see that the body and the emotions also were parts of the psychic processes. Nowadays we rarely speak of "resistance" in Gestalt therapy. Compare here Breshgold (1989). To interpret a behaviour as "resistance" is problematical because it implies on the one hand that the therapist knows the client better than they themself, and on the other hand, it implies that this behaviour is an impurity in the client's organism which has to be removed for the client to become "well". In fact this behaviour used to be a creative solution in a difficult and threatening life situation, usually in childhood, but still binding a great deal of energy which currently the organism urgently needs elsewhere.

Chapter V

The impact of emotions on personality and society

On the many ways our civilization depends on the refinement of our feelings

1 The problem of violence

The limits of emotional freedom

Emphasising the positive aspects of aggression or assertiveness in Gestalt Therapy does not, of course, mean that we have a predilection for violent solutions! There are many different roots to our human inclination towards violence. Strong *frustrations* and *de-sensitization through dulling habituation* are probably the most important causative factors; simple accumulated affect offers no *sufficient* explanation. In endless discussions about how we might reduce the hostility human beings display towards each other, it often remains unappreciated that by revitalising affective sensibility we should not primarily focus on empathic identification with the pain and suffering of the other – but sharpen our sensitivity for our own aggressive impulses and emotions. In contrast to genuine compassion, moral admonishments do not really help against violent excesses of aggression because they tend to become introjected and therefore prey to internal sabotage (Dreitzel, 2018). In Gestalt therapy groups it is easy to observe that once greater sensitivity has been achieved to one's own hostile emotions and once people re-discover and re-vitalize direct modes of expression for the first stirrings of anger, great bellows and rants and especially violence become superfluous. This is also demonstrated in a new development in meditation exercises: the American Zen master Jun Po Kelly Roshi has developed a new form of kōan practice working with *emotional kōans* rather than with the more intellectually oriented cognitive ones practised by the traditional Japanese Rinzai School.[1] These exercises aim at discovering the emotions which often underlie our aggression, feeding it on an unconscious level with energy – for instance, anxiety, despair, feelings of impotence and dissolution. It is true that genuine compassion is a reliable companion of awareness; how could I possibly hurt another person if I am fully aware of the fact that on a deeper level we are essentially identical beings? But this degree of awareness or mindfulness is difficult to achieve, if we are unaware of the deeper realms of our own aggressiveness. The Buddha pointed to ignorance (of the Dharma), greed (desires going beyond what we physically and emotionally need) and hate (the anxiety of identifying with the other) as the main causes of human suffering. This list could certainly be extended and differentiated. The important point is that we need internal signposts and stop signals for when and where the expression of aggressive emotions might become harmful to another person's physical integrity.

As Norbert Elias pointed out, the eventual internalization of such psychological brakes against violence is a second stage in the historical civilising process, following the successful establishment of external rules of behaviour. But today it seems that this development does not take place with necessity. There is always a danger of regressive setbacks, even catastrophic breakdowns of civilization in a culture. The civilizing process is always a struggle at all levels and must always be carefully protected. This is particularly true in times of anxiety fed by the threat or reality of economic loss and the dangers of climate change against which most people feel powerless. An interesting case of this struggle is the recent charge by two French lawyers of mass murder against a number of prominent European politicians at the International Criminal Court of Justice in The Hague because of their tolerance and indirect support of the drowning of thousands of refugees in the Mediterranean Sea. Not that anybody believes that the court (claimed to be illegitimate by Trump) will actually take action against these people (including the president of the European Commission, the president of France and the chancellor of Germany) – but to direct public attention to the guilty parties in this dramatic break of human rights is a courageous step forward in the endless struggle for a civilized world.

Some Gestalt therapists argue that Perls & Goodman would have been better advised if they had made an effort to distinguish between "good" and "bad" aggressive attitudes and emotions, or at least had drawn a clear line between healthy aggression and violence. But in the middle of the last century sociologists had discovered the "over-socialized" conception of man (Wrong, 1961) as the dominant ideology not only in American sociology but in the Western post-war societies mirrored by it. This ideology is just what Perls & Goodman criticized in their book of 1951. They developed the concept of *"creative adjustment"* in which the assertive elements of aggression have an important role. Today, psychotherapy could not work with depressive processes or with the many kinds of "retroflective" behaviours without these notions. If the emotional life of people becomes repressed by strict and internalized rules of expression, the civilizing process becomes suffocating.

Neither can a distinction between "good" and "bad" kinds of aggression be supported by phenomenological analysis. Of course, we should draw a red line against violence but even this is difficult to do clearly. What about rebellions against oppressive political regimes? Where are the limits of self-defence, so differently interpreted in Europe and in the States? And do we agree with the modern state's claim to have a monopoly on the legitimate use of violence if this includes the development of a society in which electronic surveillance of everybody is the norm? All these questions may be answered in different ways – even within the framework of agreed rules and values defining a democratic society – but they must be openly discussed and therefore made public. It is a failure of democracy if the state feels legitimized to put its citizens under surveillance secretly and then pursues so-called whistle-blowers as criminals.

In fact, the experience in Gestalt therapy is that no amount of repression and self-control will be a sufficient safeguard against violence because repressed emotions tend to re-appear the moment our psychological organism becomes over-strained by experiences of frustration, anxiety and insecurity. But on the other hand, the phenomenology of emotions shows that the more emotions can be expressed with appropriate intensity, the more likely it is that the expression will reach its point of saturation without manifesting itself as an "attack" or "outbreak". For instance, many people have difficulty in simply saying "No!" with conviction or giving enough weight to their voice when expressing justified demands. But the very same people can readily be encouraged to shake their fists, shout loudly, stamp their feet and possibly even kick out when they are in a crowd and encouraged by political "cheer-leaders". In the realm of aggression, too, there are more mature behaviours corresponding neither to regressive ranting nor to repressive silence. Our capacity for emotional sensibility can only develop when we manage to steer between the Scylla of childishness and the Charybdis of repression in our search for means of self-expression connecting subtlety with intensity.

This may sound somewhat naive in a world which appears to be filled with violence, wars and terrorism wherever we look. But this is a wrong impression. In fact, we have less violence in the world in spite of prevalent Islamic terrorism and growing violence emerging from the extreme right. Statistics show that crime rates have declined in all Western societies, even in the United States, and worldwide death rates from wars, epidemics and famine have declined considerably. This is proven by the huge research effort presented by Harvard historian Steven Pinker in his remarkable book *The Better Angels of Our Nature: Why Violence has Declined* (Pinker, 2011). Its findings have been confirmed by many statistics since. But how do we explain the extraordinary brutality of IS fighters and terrorists, or for that matter, of youth gangs and criminals in our own cities? There are no naturally born killers, torturers or suicide bombers – they have all been trained and indoctrinated by fundamentalist religious or fascist ideologies. In other words, systematic violence always has its roots outside the "nature" or the "personality" of human beings.

Of course, there are individual cases of failure of the civilizing process. But a larger re-occurrence of violence is usually caused by repression enforced by a ruling minority abusing state power and religious ideologies, or a whole culture failing to provide satisfying values and meaningful standards of behaviour, especially for the young – as is the case with those IS fighters who come from Western countries. Their passionate hatred is caused by a combination of frustration with the perceived lack of meaningful values in the West and political and ideological indoctrination by Islamists combined with the unleashed greed for sex and power typical in still insufficiently civilized youngsters who respond to being given a legitimizing *ideology* and the *opportunity* to follow their instincts to become violent. The same was true in the case of the extraordinary brutality inspired and legitimized by the Nazi ideology during the Second World War.

2 Unintegrated affects and emotional habits

Emotional attitudes and character

We cannot fully explain the efficacy of cultural rules of expression by referring to the existence of inhibiting emotions alone. Even while we frequently touch on emotions of anxiety and shame in the therapeutic contacting process, they are still relatively rare in everyday situations. Most of the time we live without even noticing these guardians of the temple of our expressive desire. How is this possible? Emotions of anxiety and shame cannot be avoided by an act of will, but only through appropriate emotional attitudes and the stances we take. These emotional attitudes, as I call them, are specific forms of reaction formation which *develop when excess affects connect with introjects.* This process results in affective character structures – rules of expression become independently operative.

This needs an explanation. Of course, we cannot always immediately discharge our anger or immediately express our joy. No special external or internal pressures need conjuring to understand that the fullness of one's emotions cannot always be completely expressed and when not so expressed in one situation, they tend to flow over into another. Joy is a good example: how wonderful to meet somebody who – for reasons unknown – is full of joy and allows me to participate in their laughter and dancing! Feeling like that, a person may give a kiss of joy to an unsuspecting stranger or hand them a flower. Unfortunately, and far more commonly, negative emotions spill over into a new situation: we may encounter unexpected anger, puzzling tears, sometimes without a cause, sometimes apparently quite disproportionate to the occasion. Apart from joy, anger/rage and grief can most easily become excess affects – perhaps because all these feelings are naturally expressed with a ferocity which makes them easy targets for rules of behaviour geared towards reining them in. What is problematic with these excess affects is that they neither have an orientating function nor do they adequately fulfil the normal communicative function of the emotions: cause and object of the emotion in such moments do not belong to the current situation; the person one is angry with has not necessarily given just cause for one's reaction. Furthermore, this person is now wrongly informed about the angry person and vainly looks for a cause in themself. In this way, excess affects easily cause irritating situations instead of preventing them, since they represent instances in which interactional competency is in short supply.

That is why – being subject to the same expressive limitations in the new situation as in the original – the excess affects rarely become visible outside the therapy situation. But when emotions cannot ever be fully expressed, gradually our emotional sensorium becomes blunted and we are less and less able to rely on its orientating function. In the end we are strangers to our own emotions: they have become alien to us and in therapy, when emotions are just beginning to arise, excitement anxiety shows itself. Societies with very restrictive rules for emotional expression become emotionally desensitized. Consequently, people suffer from general motivational weakness and need more and more stimuli in order to warm towards anything or anybody. In fact, the capacity for experiencing excitement can be blunted but it cannot be repressed, and everyday triggers activate rage and hate, grief and joy, impotence and pride, so that over and over again we experience the frustration of emotional expressivity being impossible to assimilate.

In this situation the classic defence mechanism of "identification with the aggressor" offers itself. If we manage to cross over to the side of repressive rules of expression, our own emotional desolation can – as a "cool" life style or an ability "to keep things in perspective" – even add to our sense of self-esteem. But this kind of identification cannot easily be assumed today; our culture is highly inconsistent as far as rules of emotional expression are concerned. After all, what is frowned upon in public is just what is required in intimate relationships: the capacity for intense emotional experience. And even in the public sphere there are not only the enforced routines of the working world and traffic flow, but also media and sporting events entering into ever more experiential realms and requiring varying degrees of sentiment, concern or Dionysian emotional expressiveness as for instance in football.

When emotional expression is connected with early introjects, emphasizing the value of self-restraint as a character attribute, and if such a world of values has been maintained (for example in military or economic organizations) and continues to have currency in the membership groups of this person, then they are still able to achieve a "smooth" "identification with the aggressor", and emotional desiccation is still experienced as a victory over oneself. In fact, such mostly paternal introjects – characteristically rules for living, frequently passed on in the form of family sayings or school slogans – are becoming old-fashioned. Today, the demand "to pull yourself together", "to grit your teeth and just get on with it!" – as well as derogatory descriptions like "you are wet!" and appeasing remarks like "he has thrown in the towel" are mainly identified from their literary uses. In other situations, away from therapy, like sports or the military, this social character still thrives in slightly moderated form. Our current culture of emotional expressiveness shows such enormous fissures that a direct encounter between these antagonisms usually generates violence: we see such escalations in police operations confronting youthful rioters.

In this context I must return to the problem of guilt feelings. For these are an aspect of what the Frankfurt School of Critical Sociology importantly has called the "authoritarian character" (Adorno et al., 1950) that characteristically, constantly develops *neurotic guilt.* The "aggressor", with whom they are identified after all consists of those un-assimilated introjects which as alien bodies have lodged themselves in the organism and are directed against one's own self, against one's very own needs and emotions the moment they stir. They cannot be extinguished; they awaken with every stimulus and unconsciously assert themselves in a multitude of ways. Authentic guilt feelings grow from hurting others; neurotic guilt is generated by one's own compulsions and defences against being attacked. In comparison with authentic guilt feelings, no desire to make amends grows from neurotic emotions of guilt, but merely a gnawing discomfort with one's own fallibility and an unconscious inclination to quickly repeat the process. Neurotic guilt feelings emerge through sabotaging one's own introjects. And – of course – that is connected with secret pleasure, the pleasure fed by repressed needs (H. P. Dreitzel, 2019).

Through attention and experiment in Gestalt therapy, this fact allows us to clearly distinguish authentic from neurotic guilt. Even as the client tells the story which triggered the guilt feelings the first time round, the attentive therapist will notice what in the end – after telling the tale several times as requested by the therapist – the client will also be able to experience: forcibly restrained excitement will be apparent in an animated voice tone, sparkling eyes and frequently in a half strained smile. Through working on authentic guilt, self-accusation gradually turns into the seriousness of a new, more mature responsibility, whereas in working on neurotic guilt feelings the first step is to liberate whatever gleeful pleasure is part of the deed itself, which drives the perpetrator to keep repeating it. Therapy of neurotic guilt moves on from "identification with the aggressor" (introjected rules of behaviour) via identification with the "saboteur within" to a resolution of those introjects through assimilation or evacuation.

Distinguishing between authentic and neurotic emotions of guilt has a tradition. It is now known that some of the neural cells in our brain are actually capable of renewal even in old age, a discovery that has altered our understanding of ageing history. Although Freud never gave up his strange theory – developed in *Totem and Taboo* (Freud, 1912) – of guilt originating from patricide committed by the Ur-horde: he later also developed ideas and theories of the civilising process in *Civilization and its Discontents* (1928), where he differentiated between the general emotion of guilt, the immediate reaction of a strict Super-Ego to sinful thoughts, and the specific emotion of guilt followed by remorse after an actual deed. This distinction however was never taken up properly by psychoanalysis, which perhaps became blinded by too many other constructions about "guilt neuroses". Guilt is simply a terribly painful and damaging emotion which needs to be healed by involving the self in reparative actions (Lifton, 1979). From the perspective taken here, our capacity for responding empathically to any disruption of the organism/environment field is the socio-psychological basis for taking responsibility as an aspect of social competency.

Looked at in this way, neurotic guilt feelings are indeed "incomplete". They keep the capacity for taking responsibility enchained in introjects, so that instead of becoming part of the driving force and a desire for responsible action, repressed needs turn against this capacity and sabotage it. Lifton graphically speaks of "static guilt" – where self-accusation or strategic manoeuvres of avoidance in fact prevent the experience of real responsibility – and "animating guilt" "through which we may gain energy for renewal and free ourselves from self-damnation" (Lifton, 1979:139). After all, liberating the animating power in our capacity for responsibility is the aim of all therapeutic work on guilt – neurotic as well as authentic.

Where smooth identification with such controlling character norms is not successful, since culturally they are gradually fading, we quite often see the emotional habits of a more modern form, the "sullen" *social character* emerging. What is being introjected here are not the norms and value standards of a disappearing patriarchal world, but the experiences of frustration and discouragement of a childhood in a "fatherless society" (Mitscherlich, 1969). If spontaneous expression of elementary contacting emotions is perennially choked off, curbed or disregarded by a dominating, yet weak and irritated mother, and when this experience is again and again fuelled in the course of one's life, then emotional habits may develop where the contradiction between emotional irritability and a curbing of emotional expressivity is fused into one behavioural Gestalt.

Here are some examples: A persistent indicator of this kind of emotional habit is *sullenness*. Such a temper is particularly marked in people whose sense of delight was often spoilt, as if spontaneous expression of *joie* de *vivre* was inhibited by exhortations like "Not so loud!", "Watch where you are going!", "Stop larking around!", "Look how you messed yourself again!" Part of the motor expression of joy is jumping and leaping, and in adults it is singing and laughing. And how many people feel shy and awkward, "self-conscious", as the precise English word will have it, when – with sullen envy – they watch dancers move on the dance floor! And even more importantly, part of joy is wanting to share. That pre-supposes a minimum of attention. For example, a child wants to share a discovery, tell what has just happened. Often, adults react with sullenness to their own inability to share joy when they respond with a blank stare to a child full of the joys of life. It is comforting to see how children in this respect often become educators of the adults; they are able to light up even shrivelled hearts.

Repeated experience of remaining alone with one's joy and having its expression inhibited by perennial nagging, or respectively as an adult being ridiculed as "childish", eventually leads to an inability to experience joy at all. Eventually these limitations are anticipated when emotions want to be expressed, and one limits oneself to so-called "silent" joy. But even this can be spoilt when perhaps a slight smile shows on the face and evokes enquiry and exposure: "What have you got to be happy about, then?". When, having been told, the emotional attachment figure – the "significant other" – decides that the whole thing is ridiculous, the destruction of joy is complete. Eventually, reasons for joy are excluded from perception or at least stubbornly avoided. What we encounter now is a person of slightly grey-weather-sullen character.

In the realm of emotional habits, the best-known phenomenon is the result of perennially repressed anger: *irritability* and *resentment,* and on a physical level stomach problems. Irritability follows most strongly where continuous frustration originates from a beloved person whom one does not wish to irritate. This is often the origin of irritability between marriage partners or in mothers overtaxed and rattled by their offspring. True resentment goes deeper though: it is an emotional habit in people who permanently repress their anger and destructive rage. A person full of resentment wishes for the other person to change – of their own volition. Since change cannot or will not be achieved by direct aggression, one reverts to the indirect route; one projects one's own inhibition for expressing anger and blames the other until they become angry, thereby legitimising one's own anger.

Especially in couple relations this can lead to an escalation where the people concerned are helpless and cannot change except through intervention from outside – as has been shown in systemic family therapy (Watzlawick et al., 1967). What is being avoided in such situations is actual contact with others as people. This can take the form of an angry explosion or an act of generous forgiveness. Often actual contact-making is inhibited by fear of aggravating a conflict which may lead to a separation. But the repression of whatever fuels the conflict is an act of self-conquest. The weakened self then usually projects and constellates a game of guilt and reciprocal reproach, immediately raising neurotic guilt feelings which are forever the accompaniment to each new violation of an introjected inhibition of aggression. Thus the spiral of reproach is endless, since reproach triggers neurotic guilt in the reproaching person instead of triggering authentic guilt in the person towards whom the reproach is directed.

The other kind of anger – that which can escalate into a cold rage, hatred against the obstacles to be removed at all cost – if held back and dammed up is channelled into another kind of emotional habit, *contempt.* Whoever I cannot destroy and remove, in contempt at least I can feel superior to them. In this way projections always become part of contempt. Contempt dismisses in two ways: it refuses appreciation, and also simply disregards the other, not finding something/someone worthy of attention.

But when the object of disdain does not disappear from sight – it could be one's boss whom one encounters daily; a competitor amongst one's colleagues or certain characteristics of one's partner – when even contempt does not succeed, then we see contemptuousness or at least disparagement, a habit of considering everything with a degree of disdain from the start. Disparagement is the product of one's "removing" aggression failing to achieve its object, when neither leaves the field. In any case this constellation has its worst effect when directed towards one's partners or other emotional attachment figures, since

> We can't afford to destroy, to annihilate what we need, even if it frustrates us. Permanent anger results where appetite and removal are interconnected, leading to an inhibition of appetite itself, thus becoming a wide-spread cause of impotence, withdrawal, etc.
>
> (Clynes, 1976:60)

The anonymity of the internet provides new opportunities to express resentment and to experience frustration: it affords safety from the reactions of the objects of one's hate – and frustrates because this object does not react and in effect remains untouchable. Whether this leads finally to violence is an open question.

Emotional habits are as diverse as human character. Most of the time it is not possible to recognize clearly which kinds of excess emotions have combined with which introjects to form specific emotional habits. Possibilities are almost endless – and everyone will have made their own observations. For example, refusing to surrender to grief – teeth clenched and tearful eyes – in conjunction with earlier experiences of renunciation of something to which some value was attributed – can lead to generalized *bitterness* about anything or anybody. Or pride which could not be displayed can – in conjunction with introjects about achievement – become deformed into *conceit* with exhibitionistic tendencies. Probably the emotion which most frequently becomes visible in therapy is sadness, displayed in set facial traits as an emotion which is forever re-stimulated. The real grief hidden in this chronic sadness must be discovered in therapeutic exploration; it may well be a traumatic experience. Often it is a mixture of unexpressed anger and unexpressed grief, connected to resignation and introjects like "There's nothing to be done!" and "That's life, sadly!", i.e. mild depression.

If one gets caught in the fore-contacting emotion of longing, one can gradually turn into a *sentimental character* – as happens with passive people in whom the aggressive functions are inhibited. Conversely, in active people longing may coagulate into hope which then becomes their psychological form and character orientation. I have already mentioned that gratitude can turn into hate when the recipient makes themself physically and/or emotionally unavailable – or if they subtly devalue the emotion of gratitude. An inability to truly surrender to the emotion of love, especially when there are introjected ideals about motherliness, can turn (love) into a caring/worrying *helper's attitude.* I have already mentioned the connection between disgust in conjunction with certain introjects and some *phobic attitudes.* And finally, very secretive people who keep everything to themselves and sometimes have an inclination towards meanness have often experienced too much disappointment and discouragement when they wanted only to spontaneously show pride and joy, to share such emotions.

These are a few observations from my own therapeutic practice: I mention them in this context to stimulate reflection on how to find one's way in the endless complexity of human orientations and characteristics. Every therapist will have different experiences helping them to orientate themself. It is true that we can offer general descriptions about the structure of emotions, but rules of expression introjected socio-culturally and historically vary to such an extent that even in our own society, a therapist's observations and experiences with specific emotional habits depend on the patient groups they are working with. In this respect, too, there is a world of difference between lower-class patients in a psychiatric clinic, formerly drug dependent young people with a petit bourgeois background in a "Release" community, and upper middle-class New Age tourists with a mid-life crisis. On occasion, even successful high-tech entrepreneurs who have never felt a tear in their eyes, appear in a Gestalt therapy workshop. And beyond that, everybody works with and through their life experiences in their own way.

More useful than any system of personality diagnostics is the grand world of literature with its rich and nuanced descriptions of human character. We can learn more from Balzac's novels, his *Comedie Humaine*, or Tolstoy's *War and Peace* than from psychological teachings about character. A theoretical map can only draw attention to what one should be alert to, what one should focus on, which elements enter into typical conjunctions and may have done so in this specific human being – who just now happens to sit in front of me – and on what is going to be catalysed between us in our singular encounter. What we can finally say is that in any therapeutic attempt to dissolve or loosen up specific excess emotions, we have to pay attention to three factors: to the specific excess emotions from a specific unresolved situation; to the partly assimilated, partly introjected rules of expression; and to the character-forming introjects from a person's early socialization milieu.

3 Forms of sympathy

Contagious emotions and shared emotions

Emotions have an orientating function, not just for the person who feels them but also for their co-players, the people with whom they act and share experiences. Motor expression of an emotion, increasing the intensity of an experience for oneself indicates to the exterior world the action intention and relational quality of the subject feeling the emotion. This is exactly the reason why emotional expression is socially regulated and repressed: anyone unable to control their emotions cannot rein them in; whoever immediately shows what is going on with them is immediately considered capricious and transparently obvious – which in our society means childish. It is a functional requirement of modern societies with their long action chains and their profoundly intertwined functions that behaviour should to be predictable.

Relative inscrutability on the other hand is part of the character requirements for specific interactional strategies aimed at gain or conquest. Sociologist Erving Goffman created the concept of *"impression management"* for this situation where people frequently show a "poker face", an impenetrable mask of emotional indifference, i.e. a form of social "mimicry" – Manfred Clynes' fitting name for the art of dissimulation.

> In **mimicry** the "sentic drive" is not connected to its motoric expression. Producing the expression is a purely intellectual act, without the no experience of an emotional state which would correspond to the expressed form. Neither does mimicry lead to a process of empathic attunement. It is an unemotional production of expression. Its funny aspect, wherever it occurs, is based in just this disconnect.
>
> (Clynes, 1976:7)

There are good social reasons for fearing "to show oneself" and "letting go" emotionally. But without the possibility of sharing emotional experience, we can neither begin to think about collective action, nor about work when it is based on division of labour, nor of interacting in personal social roles. These possibilities rely on the fact that we can use the other's emotional expression to orientate ourselves. It is not necessary to intellectually comprehend the forms of emotional expression – we don't need to learn to read them, since we experience the other's emotional state empathically and intuitively. Clynes called this phenomenon "the principle of complementarity"; production and recognition of "sentic forms" are coordinated in our brains in such a way that a precisely expressed form triggers the same form in the person who perceives it – on condition that the capacity for emotional apperception in turn has not been blunted by introjected rules of expression.

In his classical treatise of 1923, still worth studying, the German Philosopher Max Scheler, a leading representative of the phenomenological school, analysed the different forms of sympathy and empathy as the glue that holds society together in the emotional realm (Scheler, 1923). Importantly, he made the distinction between sympathy and empathy which Clynes, too, follows in his studies.

Scheler defines sympathy as the development of a similar or equal emotional state of another person based on the common existential ground of being a human being with the same potential for emotional experience. In his analysis each of these emotional states appears in two forms:

Sympathy as a form of going along with others appears as

- Emotional contagion or as
- Intuitively shared emotion ("unmittelbares Mitfühlen").

Empathy as a form of emotional identification with another exists as

- Compassion ("nachfühlen") or as
- Pure empathy ("einfühlen" or "Einsgefühl").

In the following pages I will explore these fruitful distinctions.

We are most familiar with **emotional contagion** from experiencing the contagious character of laughter. Everybody has had the experience of helplessly joining in with the laughter gripping people around us, even if we have not understood the joke and cannot tell what is so funny about it all anyway. Apparently the gap we experience as human beings incarnated in a body in this world constitutes such a tense existential situation that we are easily seduced to take advantage of a chance to recuperate through laughter whenever possible. Laughter – like crying – is a direct expression of a temporary break-down of this inner distance or gap.

Crying, too, can be contagious, even if less readily than laughter; here, one's own self is not directly involved and only the outer circumstances are relevant. In crying, though, a person has to let go of itself in order to loosen up, which is hard for adults, especially in public. Therefore, we may find emotional contagion in crying under the protective cover of darkness in the cinema, when there is a gradual increase of sniffing and blowing of noses. A teacher told me how during a school excursion and just after everybody had gone to bed, one child started crying – most likely from home sickness – and after the shortest time the whole class was crying. When the teacher asked why they were crying, the children answered "Don't know!"– Having tried in vain to reassure them, the teacher could only think of drastic measures – getting them all out of bed again, and sending them to take another shower.

Emotional contagion is not limited to laughing and crying but also occurs in conjunction with actual emotions – precisely because they can be experienced as pure qualities – that is without psychic or social triggers, without an object. Just seeing an intense emotional expression can touch off a resonance, a similar emotional disposition in the observer. The evolutionary function of this phenomenon most likely consists in the fact that through this kind of readiness, groups can be quickly motivated to action. Emotional contagion is an important element in a group's coherence, its cohesion. In that fact also lies its danger. When emotions like curiosity, longing and destructive rage are perennially frustrated through social, political and economic circumstances, they are ready to be whipped up into enthusiasm by demagogy and diverted towards the most absurd of aims.

Emotional contagion creates a felt experience of collective unity ("Gemeinschaftserlebnis"), a we-emotion, which can drown out any rational consideration of the action's aims and consequences. Unforgettable are the roars of "Yes!" in the Berlin Sportpalast in response to Goebbels' rhetorical question: "Do you want total war?". Violence is always close to breaking out when aggressive moods become contagious – if an enemy is at hand, be it the fan club or the football club "we" don't support. Of course more than one person is necessary for this phenomenon – and so it is not surprising that it happens most easily in mass situations; if animated and agitated in this way the joy of one person turns into a "storm of enthusiasm"; the anxiety of one turns into mass panic reactions; from various personal emotions of anger, anonymous collective violence can be generated. And in the age of mass media, of mass tourism and mass advertising there are many experts who know how to fuel moods to fit the desired purpose (Perhaps this is also the only antidote against totalitarian demagogy!?). Emotional contagion is so dangerous because it usually doesn't stop at objectless emotional experience per se but activates otherwise frustrated and repressed emotions, offering scapegoats and other compensatory objects. Open and hidden persuaders can more successfully build on this in societies which cultivate an overall "cool" image.

It is crucial to note here that possibilities for being manipulated through emotional contagion increase the more a person shows neurotic object avoidance constituting an unrelieved reservoir of emotional dispositions. It is very important to work on this kind of avoidance in psychotherapy. We mustn't be satisfied with the client gaining insight into such behaviour: instead Gestalt therapy must focus on enabling the client to experience through their senses how they block their emotional expression. We can start with the knowledge that inhibiting emotional expression and avoiding objects – including fixations on substitute objects – are two sides of the same process. At the very moment that expressive blockages, introjects carried by the body, start melting, the person discovers and develops new and unfamiliar ways of expressing their emotions, and such expression automatically finds the right objects, since only through that process can the promised satisfaction of unmet needs become possible. Unfortunately, psychotherapy is often limited by cultural boundaries. For instance, one might speculate that the violence of young men who turn into Islamist fanatics is fuelled by the sexual frustrations generated when contact with women is forbidden outside marriage, forced on them by their family culture.

In a more subtle way we perennially succumb to the emotional influences of our environment. Our lives are always embedded in what Clynes calls our "sentic environments". Wherever we share a group environment with other people, we are influenced by their specific emotional atmosphere. In therapy workshops, when small groups are together for a few days and share intense experiences with each other, it is possible to observe this as if under a microscope. Sometimes the whole group is overcome by an atmosphere affecting the theme of all further work on that day. And if the therapist is themself strongly pre-occupied with a subject – as ideally they should not be – this has an even greater effect on the group. But therapeutic groups can cope with and even benefit from a high degree of emotional intensity, since the contract which underlies all interactions allows making the atmosphere itself the theme for exploration.

This is not easily possible in other kinds of situations: indeed, everybody knows that emotional environments can be hostile as well as pleasant, not just cheerful but also depressive, not just loving but also rancorous. In addition, it is a characteristic trait of our civilization that we are exposed to rapidly alternating emotional climates: emotional frostiness in the public realm and emotional shock in the media. In such a climate the individual's sensitivity cannot help but gradually become blunted. People who try to seal themselves off from these influences might pay for doing so by becoming socially isolated and losing the chance to influence what goes on. Clynes describes the consequences:

> We have to create a society where the individual isn't under sentic attack from all sides *and* so that he is liberated from an avalanche of sentic insults which from his own creations and re-creations rushes towards him in such a way that essentic forms can be enjoyed in relation to that specific, human Gestalt from which they emerge: the single/specific individual.
>
> (Clynes, 1976:71 footnote)

This is *one* good reason to protect all victims of "shit storms" and uninhibited hate mails in the social media! One step on the long road towards this goal is the recovery and continuing development of the individual's emotional sensitivity, and one of the vehicles towards this end is Gestalt therapy. But before this goal could ever be achieved it is – in my opinion – necessary to overcome the taboo against abolishing the protection which everybody enjoys by the guaranty of anonymity in the internet. After all this rule undermines the *basic norm of reciprocity* underlying *all* socialization processes.

At first glance, Scheler's second type of sympathetic emotions, the **intuitively shared emotions** ("unmittelbares Mitfühlen"), seems less problematic. In it there is after all an object triggering the emotion which is shared by the interacting partners. Examples may include people sharing the fear of a danger threatening everyone at once (people clinging together in cellars or basements during a bombing raid; refugees trying to cross a river or even a sea); a group of people experiencing shared anger about an authoritarian leader, or gratitude about their boss (perhaps there will be a decision for a shared protest action or a shared present); or people feeling deeply connected after a shared loss (the shared character of the loss has a comforting quality). And of course there is joy associated with projects accomplished together (which may be expressed in a shared party). In all these examples the individually experienced emotion is strengthened by the experience of sharing the same sentic expression with other people, being present. Thus we can say that synchronous expression of the same emotion on the same occasion has a sympathetically strengthening effect.

But here we encounter some problems too. Closer, more detailed observation reveals that a group of people having been affected by the same emotion can also react with a reciprocal strengthening of their affective controls, as is quite frequently observed in a group of mourners. Here we encounter an interesting sociological problem. The way people control affects is always relatively homogenous, and the public nature of the group space in itself creates a shame barrier containing personal emotional expression. But the degree of intensity, and what forms of expression are chosen differs widely, even while they have the same "essentic form". Shared emotions therefore need a medium, so that whatever it is that is shared can be actualized as such – and that is precisely the social function of *ritual*. Depending on people's expectations and needs, such a ritual can consist in particular kinds of music, hymns, threatening or submissive gestures, battle cries, presents, the quotation of holy texts, prayers or acts of devotion like the kissing of feet.

History offer boundless examples of such rituals. They say that in antiquity armies directed volleys of insults and diatribes at each other before actually engaging in battle, doubtless in order to get into an aggressive enough emotional mood to summon up courage for action. In the present – and in a society where many traditional rituals have lost some of their significance – it is interesting to note that we need to invent ever-new rituals able to carry and express a shared emotion, most obvious where a social form is founded in emotion. The fan club and its more widespread minimalist variety, the couple relationship, offer themselves as fields for observation, showing the marvellous creativity which goes into people creating their own rituals. In any case, the emotionality of smaller groups (as long as they are not the theme of reflection, as happens in therapy groups) is under pressure from two directions: they need to find a collective way of expressing shared emotions, which tends towards ritual; and on the other hand there is a danger that emotional experience is hollowed out when emotional expression becomes a repetitive habit.

A more special case of shared emotion with particular significance has still to be mentioned: **reciprocal emotions.** In them, the feeling subject is at the same time the object of the same emotion in the other – and the other way round; we love each other, we hate each other, we are frightened of each other, we are sexually aroused by each other, or we are grateful to each other. This reciprocity of the subject-object relationship in the contacting process generates deepening intensity of emotional experience, based on the fact that here we are not just experiencing our own emotional expression but also that of the other person, creating a feedback effect on what is experienced together. We are particularly familiar with this phenomenon in sexuality; the arousal of one person provides an added stimulus for the other and vice versa. This increase in intensity is the organic expression for the peculiar tension which grows from reciprocal emotions, due to the fact that each partner is also the object of the other's emotionality. Through this the contacting process gains a dialectic which points beyond its normal intention – satisfaction of needs, balancing a lack in the individual. This dialectic also operates in many other contacting processes, and always when the subject of one contacting process also becomes the object of other people's contacting processes. It therefore will pay to continue tracing this dialectic where reciprocal emotions are concerned.

As far as the praxis of our interactions is concerned, they are stamped by attitudes and theoretical positions referring back to a stock of cultural traditions. There are three possible positions we can take with respect to reciprocal subject-object relations in specific interactional contexts: It is possible to emphasize the importance of either the (1) object, the other, or the (2) subject in the contacting process, or (3) one can stress what they have in common and through this go beyond the dyadic relationship. Freud for example focused on the role of the object. While his libido theory remained vague even as psychoanalysis developed, it is his teaching about the psychic positions, about resistance and the content of consciousness and particularly that of objects of drives which has been continually developed, reaching a climax in Kohut's theory of object relations.[2] In consequence, we now find a pseudo-scientific language of "objects" instead of processes, which has affected psychotherapeutic thinking to such an extent that Gestalt therapy and this writer have a hard time freeing themselves from it! But Freud indeed was part of the tradition of enlightenment; we still have to thank this tradition for achieving some freedom from ideological ties and promoting greater precision of thought, as for instance Kant – completely object related – without further ado declared marriage the legitimate mutual possession of sexual organs – and so surely added one of the few clarifying words about this ineradicable social form.

Emphasising the role of the *subject* in the contacting process is always the concern of those who justly or unjustly feel disadvantaged. For in this case, it is the lack in one's own organism, the significance of one's own needs getting a raw deal, which is emphasized. This perspective is characteristic for all emancipatory movements; the first concern is to get to know one's own needs properly, followed by "self-realization" via better need satisfaction. Gestalt therapy, too, as it was developed and represented by Perls & Goodman, understood themselves as advocates of the needs of individuals. They conceptualized the greatest disturbances as arising from people's inability to experience their own needs; normal neurotic disturbance here is a failure of specific ego functions when need satisfaction is attempted in the organism/environment contact. However, this way of accentuating the issue becomes problematical when we fail to acknowledge that where a person is the object of a contacting process, this object is also a subject; that there is a *reciprocal relationship.* Or when (as with some radical feminists) in the heat of the battle for liberation and during such journeys of discovery into the world of one's own needs, the "object" of such needs is simply experienced in an instrumental way and therefore in principle becomes exchangeable – this is a problem since in this case reciprocity is gone. The danger in an interactional perspective of over-emphasizing the subject is that it leads to a narcissistic overvaluation of one's own needs – a danger we have to take seriously, especially in psychotherapy.

The third possibility is seeing the relationship between subject and object *dialectically,* resolving itself either in the partner's similarities ("Your desire is my desire, too") or through a third, arising from an integration – for example, a child comes from the sexual congress of its parents. Initially, this perspective clarifies for us that the reciprocal contacting process between human beings is an *encounter* not completed in mutual need satisfaction, but having a character *sui generis.* Such encounters have their quite specific Gestalt which here, too, is more than the sum of its elements. What develops here cannot be predicted and described in general terms; it is always a new Gestalt, a unique sound created by two people in resonance.

The danger is that a Hollywood (even more so, a Bollywood) type of love ideology suggests an emotional melting of two individuals which in fact leads either to paralyses or to frustration and separation. In our present social reality another concern may be more pertinent – a tendency towards instrumentalizing human encounter for the purposes of mental hygiene, which can be seen in co-operative relationships whose participants understand themselves as sporting comrades and as more or less well-functioning components of the system "couple relationship". Gestalt therapy here speaks of "confluence", neurotically holding on to an Ego-less mutual entanglement, which prevents encounter even as it moves. There is a lot to learn from systemic family therapy; it hasn't only shown that where two or more people continually interact, more things happen than they ever wanted *individually,* but also that what is happening now is not the same as what they had intended and are intending together. In other words, the properties of a dynamic, continually moving system of role relationships asserts itself behind their backs and often against the intentions of the people concerned, determining their actions and behaviour in non-transparent ways.

Understanding these extra-individual systemic forces is core knowledge for therapists today, and should also be part of the social knowledge of clients. However, systemic family therapy is committed to maintaining the system, which is their true client. Whatever new Gestalt arises from the mutual and always conflicted emotional engagement with the other, it too has its time and grace and, short of mummification, cannot be protected from change. What remains is not the shared riches of what one perceives individually, but the individual richness of awareness gained together in the process.

4 Forms of empathy

To be emotionally sensitive to others and to identify with them

This now is a particularly difficult issue, because it reaches into the yet unexplored depths of subconsciousness/consciousness/awareness, and because the capacity of humans to share even dimensions of their consciousness seems unfathomable.

When we feel in *sympathy* with somebody, usually it takes no effort to emotionally be with and alongside the other's emotional expression and resonate to it, since our attention is attracted to the same stimulus and is responsive to the same emotional trigger. We then share a mood or atmosphere. Often we notice this "tuning-in" only in post-contact or even after separation as an afterglow – or else when it is interrupted, perhaps by the unexpected presence of less sensitive (or merely embarrassed) people. This is different in *empathic* emotions, where emotional expression is itself the object of attention. As a stimulus it can be so strong that it is almost impossible to get away from it, or – more normal nowadays – so weak that it requires an effort of attention to even recognize the emotional tone of the over-contained emotion, as for instance in the strange behaviour of gaping spectators at street accidents and other public horrors. Everyone unintentionally turning away from or blunting their attention is emotionally affected by a strong emotional expression. This being touched by the inner experience of another is completely different from just being swept along, as for example by infectious laughter. It is barely possible to remain emotionally cold when we see another person shaken by desperate crying or painful moaning. Even if we do not know the person nor the cause of this pain. When we talk about the "heart-rending" crying of a child, we do not mean the heart of the child, but that of the person who feels with the child. Apparently there is always an aspect of identification which enters into empathic emotions, even if the other person and their circumstances remain anonymous.[3]

There are two forms of **empathic identification**:

1 when we recognize and enter into what the other person is going through – something we have experienced ourselves. What I experience as the same or similar, *entering into someone's experience* does not have to have the same particular trigger; it could be the same general situation (affliction, loss, threat, etc.) or just the *emotional state* which feels familiar. This can easily be demonstrated: A child yelling their pain to the world – bitter pain about a broken toy or the existential anxiety following losing their mother in the crowd. We can easily enter into this emotional expression, not because we are still touched by those triggers, but because we emotionally recognize the situation and can spontaneously relate to it, because for almost everyone these archetypal experiences of unhappiness and being lost are familiar memories – and

also of course, because the uninhibited emotional expression of a small child appeals to our sentic sensibility.

2 when we attune ourselves to such an experience, *even if it is alien* to us, thus truly putting ourselves into the other's position, "taking the role of the other", as George Herbert Mead has called it. We slip into their skin. This astounding capacity of human beings may be easier to understand if compared with the quite different experience of identifying with what is causing the felt emotion because in this case we know it from our own life. What is striking in case of pure empathy is precisely that there is no spontaneous emotional recognition from our own experience but at best it stimulates some part of our cognitive experiential memory bank. That is the case when we cannot really *feel* another person's physical pain. (If the trigger had been the same, we would be dealing with a shared emotion, but that would in many cases be hardly bearable, probably evolutionary impossible as in case of the pain of giving birth; a midwife will *know* how the woman she is helping feels but she will not at this moment experience her pain). We might say "I can really feel for you!" when we are in a general way familiar with the kind of misery displayed but it isn't a problem for us right now. Therefore the emotional intensity of this sharing is of a lesser degree.

It is quite different and we are more emotionally distressed when another person goes through what we are *frightened* of ourselves; experiences which we know will or could happen to us, too: death, accidents, illnesses. Of course there is a touch of projection in this moment of emotional identification with another person (the psychoanalytically-orientated reader might recognize a special case of transference), since identified emotion may become very intense when we recognize ourselves in the other, truly enter into their experience. But it is more important to acknowledge here that in this sympathetic sharing we receive a shocking reminder that both of us, I and the other, are subject to the same *conditio humana*.

In this way entering into somebody's experience always contains some human solidarity. The more I can identify with the situation, the more I'm affected, the more easily **compassion** grows, motivating us to offer comfort, support and help. There is a difference in explaining compassion as solely reflecting the survival interest of the individual or seeing it rooted in the fact that this individual is also a member of our species and only able to survive in a community of others. Perls & Goodman illustrate this inconsistency impressively, and perhaps inadvertently, by offering two contradictory statements about compassion: Completely caught up in the psychoanalytic perspective, they remark "Compassion is avoidance or over-coming of a personal loss by helping another" (Perls & Goodman:187). Yes, avoidance importantly plays a role when the experience of seeing and hearing a fellow human being in pain fends off the *feeling* of sympathy to protect oneself against infection – a necessity in medical helping, when emotional neutrality provides the necessary distance.

Elsewhere, however, Perls & Goodman describe compassion beautifully as *the concern of the therapis*t, differing from other kinds of concerns due to its process character:

> Compassion is the loving recognition-of-the-defective-as-potentially-perfect, and what is processual about him is the realization of the possible in the object. […]. Compassion in action is not based on some interest of the Ego, but in the process of integration of the Thou.
>
> (Perls & Goodman:198)

This means that *true compassion* is neither about being kind to another person, nor is it intellectual understanding. Also it is not about love, whose intentionality it is lacking, nor is it pity, which is the sentimental version of contempt. In compassion I am completely myself with all the ego functions and resources accessible to me since I am not directly affected. Precisely because that is the case, true compassion entails no distancing. At the same time – and that just isn't clear in the psychoanalytic perspective – one's resources are fully utilized in the interest of the Thou, since it is this Thou, feeling this or that, which fills me, which creates a unified Gestalt with me: compassion is a therapist's Eros, completed in moments of full contact with the client. Entering into the experience of another and its special climax in compassion is generated as we perceive the "essentic form" of an authentic emotional expression and identify with the other's experiences, problems and situations. In order to share someone's emotions by sheer identification we must keep our attention focussed on them – and we will be carried along with the other's emotional expression, rather like hearing music. Yet the therapist paradoxically needs to keep a certain amount of distance in their work not to become confluent and hence disable themself from the task of alleviating the patient's misery and facilitating their growth. Thus I was told that Isadore From excused himself for "making a mistake" when, listening to the misery of the childhood experience of his patient during the Nazi occupation in Poland he had begun to weep. Still that was genuine empathy, true compassion. There are occasions when this is more important than to regain the necessary distance for doing therapy – in my own experience especially if the patient suffers from being caught in a narcissistic process disabling them from giving up the emotional self-control for a moment of full contact. The capacity to experience emotions without attachment to objects discovered by Clynes helps to understand this phenomenon.

Compared to this process, empathic **attunement** is an intentional act where the encompassing constructive element of perception in a receptive mode is dominant. For this, the process of attunement does not require the strong stimulus of an intensive emotional expression. Indeed, to be able to take the position of another person is one of the most amazing capacities of all human beings, which does not mean that it is highly developed in everybody. Cognitively this capacity has been conceptualized as "reciprocity of perspectives" and has become a basic element in sociologically understanding human interaction.

On an emotional level we are dealing with the ability to experience in ourselves the emotions which the other person is experiencing in their contacting process with the environment. The necessary pre-condition for both processes is, in Clynes' words "that we must project the condition and the personality of another human being into our own awareness, so that in imagination we are this personality" (Clynes, 1976:71); in other words, *full* identification, a complete experience.

Of course we are building up this identification from the reservoir of cognitive and emotional experiences we have had with this person. But this does not only lead to a static picture but to a personality with a life of its own in our imagination; able to act and decide; with attitudes and opinions not (yet) realized by this person, but consistent with it. In other words, in attuned identification with the other we are potentially capable of perceiving in this person possibilities as yet unrealized. Attunement goes beyond stepping into somebody's shoes in that it does not just makes intelligible what is possible, but it allows us to recognize what might become so.

This doesn't of course lead to giving advice – another kind of fantasy cheaper than the reality of experience. **Empathic attunement** is special in that it also shows the other's limitation. But it makes us *well disposed* towards this person, and strangely, well-disposed also towards people whom we otherwise hate, despise or even just experience as a nuisance. "As we make the decision to allow another being to live in us, we also turn our own survival powers towards this individual which now is alive in us – in short we have good will" (Clynes, op. cit.:72). Empathic attunement is non-judgemental. It is interesting to note that we can no longer judge somebody – or for that matter something – with whom or which we truly identify, neither can we admire them or it any longer. In identification we have left behind our usual standards of judgement and are completely filled with this other person but still keep our own norms and values.

In dealing with a person, how much experience is required in order to attune ourselves "well" to them? This question cannot be answered in this form, since for any empathic attunement, apart from the experience of this particular person, we need to have a great ability to generate effective projections which entails that our mental constructions of reality are focussed. Such ability grows from and is sharpened by cognitive and emotional awareness while experience of life seems to help. In addition, we need the ability to bracket ourselves, stand aside, and be empty and receptive. Each of the human Gestalts living in our imagination is compounded from reasonably realistic elements as well as others which are not – no different (or perhaps a little closer to reality) from our self-image. When somebody has good perceptual abilities, they also know what they haven't (yet) seen, what is simply conjecture, and allow the Gestalt as it lives in their imagination to remain somewhat vague and a little out of focus. Only through this do we remain open to the surprises which the creative self of the other is going to offer. One should never deceive oneself to know everything about any other person, including the most intimate partners.

One might make an assumption however that the ability to identify ourselves to others automatically grows with life experience. This is not the case. It is true, however, for being sensitive to sharing somebody's emotional experience: the more one has experienced, the more emotional states and social occasions generating emotions are part of our portfolio of experience, the more we can feel sympathy with others. In attunement, identification is an emotional process in itself, and therefore it is not dependent on a treasure-chest of experiences gathered in life; rather it requires well-honed emotional sensibility. Old people who have a great deal of life experience but perhaps low emotional flexibility are therefore often well able to enter into the emotional experience of a young person, but quite unable to attune themselves to them. Half critical, half tolerant remarks like "I was young myself once" definitely show an ability to recognize how the young person is feeling, but they remain strangely untouched since their attuning to the whole person is lacking. In order to be able to attune oneself wholly to the current and still unrealized emotional reactions of another person, one has to temporarily separate out from one's own self and its emotions, which is often harder for older people because their bodies so often become foreground.

Conversely, children will never be able to truly attune themselves, and young people only rarely – on the one hand, because their emotional sensorium has not yet developed sufficiently; on the other, because their ego functions are still too weak and they cannot separate from their selves even for a short time. Emotional sophistication is not part of the human endowment with which we are born, but a potential – just like other genetic potentials needing to be developed. If this development remains below a certain standard, the person only has a limited chance of survival; but in reaching the necessary level, the development and refinement of various abilities can continue throughout life. Progress here is often hindered by just those social formations which were particularly helpful in the initial formation of genetic endowments. In this way our emotionality, similar to our capacity to express ourselves in words, is shaped and hindered at once through repressive controls and rules of expression – in the realm of emotionality, too, there is no equality of opportunity. Therefore emotionality is in need of life-long purification and loosening-up, refinement and cultivation. Part of this is the right choice of the "sentic milieu", which we need to take care of. In this way only, an emotional sensitivity capable of attunement not only in extraordinary relational situations is able to grow.

Bracketing our Ego in empathic identification means we put it aside, step emotionally into the role of the other – and immediately we are touched by this other being in a way that is more and different from resonating with the other when I enter into their emotions. It is as if I had touched the subjective centre of the other. The specific "essentic form" of the other in empathic identification is experienced "not just as an expression of a specific emotional state, but as if one was connected to the existential Gestalt of this person", the place we occasionally term "the inner Self" (Clynes, op. cit.:70).

Such an experience pre-supposes some kind of continuity of the conception we have of the person whom we can attune ourselves to. This Gestalt of a person can be so well developed even in our *imagination* that it is alive even in our unconscious, so that we can dream of a person whom we have not seen for a long time and who now – in the dream – is capable of triggering intense emotions. How much such Gestalt-persons lead a life of their own in our imagination can also be seen in our ability to attune ourselves to people who have already passed away. The technique of identification with dream figures or dialoguing with imaginary significant others, whose role one adopts – a technique widely used in Gestalt therapy – are deeply experiential ways to cleanse our capacity for empathic identification of any contaminations arising from neurotic projections.

Attuning is not really an emotional process, but a still, wide awake and focussed way of concentrating on the emotional part of the subjectivity of the other. Yet it also is an emotional process, but it is not a specific emotion, since it is not driven by need which would be its motivating force. Attuning themselves, the person becomes an empty mirror, they attend and observe the other person with emotional openness, but without any judgemental attitude or orientation and without an interest of their own, just with the still openness for the movement activating the other at this moment, in the actual or an imagined situation. When we are fully empathic we are fully compassionate and fully self-contained (bracketed).

Our ability for empathic attunement gains us an immense amount of openness towards the world, as well as humanity, but for the Gestalt therapist it is to some extent simply a pre-condition for their work – it is an extension of the basic relationship human beings have with themselves and of our relationship to the other. Empathic identification is a main source of compassion.

5 Catharsis and therapy

On the relationship between involvement and distance in emotional experience

All societies have standards for regulating the expression of emotions: recently this fact has attracted increased attention from social scientists, but it has so far been mostly overlooked in sociological theorizing (see however Seyd,

2016. In this last section of this chapter on emotional awareness we are concerned with analysing two issues concerning what I have called "rules of expression" (i.e. Manfred Clyne's "mimicry"; Ekman and Friesen's "display rules"; Arlie Hochschild's "emotion work"; Erving Goffman's "impression management"):

1. We will be dealing with the intentional or automatic (neurotic) *repression* of an emotional expression which wants to be embodied; and secondly with the *simulation* of emotions which are not actually felt (for example "crocodile tears") or are shown with pretended intensity (as in laughing rather too loudly at a joke which didn't seem very funny). In the first case, a more intense emotional experience cannot unfold, and the person remains filled with excess emotions at the end of this emotionally unfinished situation.
2. We will analyse what happens psychologically if the orientating function of the emotions becomes blunted through continual misuse of the feedback loop between feeling the emotion and expressing it. The person will increasingly become one with their social roles, becoming a social character mask.

This may sound as if all societies are more or less emotionally inhibiting, emotionally repressive – and also, as if without such modes of social conditioning, emotions could always freely and spontaneously find natural means of expression. This is only partially accurate. In their emotionality, too, human beings are by nature self-cultivating. We are born with certain dispositions towards emotion; universally every emotion has its "essentic form" which also predetermines partly their style of physical expression. Yet only through practice and experience do we learn to find the means and forms of expression which fit their "essentic form" or at least come closer to it. In this regard each human being is an artist of emotional expression, learning to fine-tune the instrument of their emotional sensibility so that eventually they become a suitable sounding board for coming close to an *authentic* emotional expression of the "essentic forms" of emotions, always resonating to specific conjunctions of need and environmental conditions. And such practice and experience in turn is a process of culturally-shaped interactions. In other words, no society just represses or distorts emotions, it develops and cultivates them, too. Each society has its emotional culture, be it rich or poor in expression, whether the culture appears to be tender or somewhat violent; whether it emphasizes spontaneous expression or goes for studied gestures.

Our own culture – thus my initial hypothesis – is currently characterized by two contradictory developmental tendencies: informalization of manners, and impoverishment of emotional sensibility through the norms demanding that we restrain our emotional expression, that we keep our cool. Compared to that of the 18th or 19th centuries, our society is rather primitive with respect to emotional expressivity, although – or indeed because – it favours spontaneity and authenticity. Additionally, it seems to be caught in an atmosphere of latent aggression, although – or again, perhaps because – it inhibits it. Looking more closely, we see that this culture does not actually repress emotions. There are indeed two very important realms where emotion comes close to being over-emphasized: the media world of entertainment, which also affects a culture of political expressivity; and the world of close personal associations and subcultural group milieus. In both realms (each deeply affecting the other) standards of expressivity are cultivated, which constitute a counter weight to emotional impoverishment and emotionally chilled conditions of our organized public sphere – and actually generate much emotional stress.

During the 1960s and '70s, when the informalization process took root, new therapies including Gestalt therapy responded by providing *cathartic* methods to unfreeze emotional blocks. This was the time when Shree Rajneesh, the most popular Guru of the counter-culture at the time, introduced his "cathartic meditations" (among others: *Dynamic Meditation, Kundalini Meditation, Gourishankar Meditation*) which he considered helpful for people raised in the West in order to loosen up before starting with more serious Eastern meditation practices such as the Buddhist *Vipassana* breathing meditation or the Japanese *Za Zen*. Both of which require sitting without moving for long periods of time. Some of the dynamic meditation methods may still be helpful outside or in addition to psychotherapy. In Gestalt therapy however, cathartic methods often served to produce emotional highlights with impressive effects for the group, but they often had little lasting effect on the individual "performer".

Both the sociologist Thomas Scheff and the musicologist Manfred Clynes developed different concepts of catharsis inspired by the classical Greek theatre tradition which are worth a closer look. According to Scheff (2007), the dominant norm of emotional expression in the public realm today is to be "over-distanced," while in the media and in the private relational realm "under-distanced" is the norm. In "over-distancing" we talk and *think about* emotions (Perls called such talks in his Gestalt groups "aboutism") without properly experiencing them on a psycho-physical level. Perhaps we say that we are angry about something, but this anger does not manifest itself in the voice, and therefore it is more thought than felt. *Under-distancing* in turn creates emotional outbursts, where self-control is washed away by rising emotions and we are overwhelmed by their expression. In both cases there is a lack of *optimal distancing,* where psychic and physical involvement in this emotional expressive experience is balanced by an inner distancing through self-observation. It is obvious that in our culture the realms of production and administration are over-distanced, and the realms of reproduction and recreation are under-distanced. Our culture therefore teaches us expressive controls on the one hand, eventually leading us to avoid emotion altogether;

and on the other hand, it validates vague surges and undifferentiated bursts of emotion – depending on the social role in which we are currently embodied. It offers few occasions for learning and practising what Scheff calls *"aesthetic distance"*, optimal distancing for creating a balance between the emotionally engaged subject and the self-aware subject which has been shown to be characteristically capable of empathy.

Although Scheff's own theory of emotion (borrowed from "Co-Counselling Therapy") remains phenomenologically unsatisfactory, his differentiation of these three modalities of emotional expression represents a significant advance. Rightly, Scheff points out that it helps to find more satisfactory answers to some important questions which despite great research investment have remained unresolved, such as the question of whether violence and horror scenes in video and television effectively dispose the viewer towards more violence or whether, conversely, they help the viewer to abreact their latent potential for violent expression: It is probable that a cathartic reaction can only be expected if and when these scenes are presented in an optimally-distanced way, whereas the more common under-distanced scenes of "blood and guts" films seem to lead to a blunting of affect regarding violent behaviour. Our culture therefore seems less to stimulate direct violence than to encourage a habituation to an atmosphere of violence, created by the media's emphasis on occasional outbreaks of violence which stir up anxieties further embedded in a flood of crime stories littering our television programs.

Seen on TV, a passer-by pushing his way towards the scene of a traffic accident, could be heard to say: "I've seen it so often on the television; now I want to see it for real!" Perhaps underlying here is a misunderstood longing for authenticity? With respect to the question of violence, recognising that only *optimal distance* allows catharsis is of great significance, concerning not just the actor's representation but the story, too. Awareness is the issue here, since in that awareness everybody knows intuitively that they hurt themselves as well as hurting the other. Even in its rawest form, rage could never be released through rape, terrorist bombing and random shootings or by sexual abuse of children (to name the four most frequent damaging violent crimes in our societies). Children would be too immature to possess such awareness, which makes it so particularly heinous to misuse them as warriors or terrorists. But the problem of violence is no more than the crudest example in recognising the value of this differentiation between over-distancing, under-distancing and aesthetic distancing. It applies to all forms of emotional expression. This will become clearer when we study how these three expressive modalities manifest themselves in actual behaviour. A Gestalt therapist needs to be a very good observer, especially of different modes of expressing emotions.

Everyone has the disposition for such balancing capacity, because only an emotion expressed with aesthetic distance creates an authentic impression which comes closest to its "essentic form". This allows us to enter into other people's emotions and to show empathy. In other words, apparently it is the very nature of "essentic forms" of emotion that they appear *in their purest form when they are expressed with aesthetic distance.* Unsurprisingly, Manfred Clynes also distinguished three modalities of emotional expression which coincide with Scheff's categories, although he discovered them in a different context and for different purposes.

I have already mentioned that Scheff's concept of "over-distancing" corresponds to Clynes' "mimicry". "Over-distanced experience is purely cognitive" (Scheff, 2007:67) and has no resonance. "In mimicry, the production of expression is purely cognitive" (Clynes, 1976:61). This reflects a frequent observation that human beings can become almost completely alienated from their emotions, that they are capable of pretended emotions – albeit at the price of creating an impression of inauthenticity. However, nowadays the essentially accurate observation that we frequently talk in a pseudo-rational way – which may come across as intellectual but is completely devoid of emotional resonance – is raised to the status of a norm against the rationality of discourse. In this situation, accurate use of language may be sacrificed in *the wake of accusations of apparently pretentious or condescending speech.* "Don't talk rubbish! You are just in your head!" Such remarks reflect intellectual laziness under cover of authenticity. Here the norm of over-distancing is simply replaced by a norm of under-distancing: "Speak from your heart; let it all out!" It is as if two people from different cultures are talking, occupying opposing positions, each despising the other: one celebrating an emotionally impoverished, intellectually-orientated sobriety, while the other celebrates a romanticism of emotionality, often disguised in vulgarity. In times when even business people are trained in silent meditation as well as possibly in "letting it out" as is the norm in therapy groups, it seems as if more and more people secretly help themselves to the resources of both cultures to achieve greater psychological well-being, improving their flexibility by moving between different sub-cultures and so meeting the requirements for managerial jobs.

Under-distancing is just as unhealthy as over-distancing. Clynes, taking up Nietzsche's well-known complementary concepts, speaks of *Dionysian* and *Apollonian* modes of emotional experience, modalities which correspond to Scheff's under-distancing and aesthetic distance. In the Dionysian mode, people physically and psychically surrender to emotional expression; in particular, the whole body is drawn into the expressive act. There is no longer an inner distance to the emotion; the person appears to be "outside themself", "ecstatic". Effectively in this *Dionysian* experience, the person loses themself as a self-governing individual to such an extent that it is clear that there always was and still is a need for a collective setting for such kinds of expression. Today we have a culture of "events" like pop-music concerts or a Pope's visit which serve as such social frames for Dionysian experiences. In the therapeutic situation, people sense the danger that they might lose themselves; they may begin to develop various catastrophic fantasies, not suspecting that emotions can be experienced just as intensely in the Apollonian mode. "If I allowed myself to cry now, I'd never stop", "If I allowed my rage to surface, I'd destroy everything". It is not exactly helpful to see so many under-distanced scenes from the entertainment media, for a person who publicly and outside a collective setting behaves in an under-distanced way is in danger of being considered mad. What would happen, for example, if somebody were to dance as ecstatically in the road and in bright daylight as many do in a disco or at pop concerts around midnight?

In the Apollonian mode emotions are felt and expressed from a different position, meditatively relaxed and slightly removed from any immediately pressing demands arising from one's needs so that such a moderate expression becomes possible. Clearly, this mode corresponds to Scheff's aesthetic distance. "In aesthetic distance", he says, "we are participants and observers of our pain, so that we can freely go in and out of it" (Scheff, 2007:65). And Clynes also calls the Apollonian mode the "spectator-viewing mode" of emotional experience and speaks of "sentic fluidity" as the ability to move on from one emotional experience to another without being attached to a particular emotion. In his words

> ... this mode allows the particular sentic states to be enjoyed in their purity, while retaining control of mental freedom. The exercise of this freedom also allows us to switch sentic states voluntarily and to proceed easily from the empathic viewing of one sentic state to another. The faculty that allows one to switch sentic states in the manner described we call "pre-sentic control". Free exercise of pre-sentic control implies sentic fluidity; one is not stuck rigidly in any one sentic state, but can experience the spectrum of states, freely and readily.
>
> (Clynes, 1976:61)

And he adds significantly: "It becomes apparent that the condition of sentic fluidity is an important aspect of mental health" This indeed corresponds with Gestalt therapeutic experience.

Scheff and Clynes made the same discovery – Scheff employing hermeneutic procedures in his research on cathartic release mechanisms in drama, ritual and therapeutic emotional discharge, while Clynes used experiments, intending to discover the key to musical experience. This means that we all have in us an emotionally expressive actor and also a spectator, who with all their senses comprehends emotionally what is going on. As an actor who merely feels, one gets lost in the psycho-physical actuality of the contacting process; as a spectator who just perceives, one loses the sensory reality of immediate participation and the involvement which comes from it. Only in the balance of aesthetic distance does it seem that one does not stand in one's own way, the way of the contacting process.

> It may appear strange to call an expressive mode spectator mode. This is based on the quality of stillness, which in this modality is required both for the creation and for the perception of its essentic form. Inner silence may correspond to the intentionality of the Zen Master, who demands walking two centimetres off the floor whilst still fully experiencing the floor.
>
> (Clynes, 1976:73)

This mode of experiencing I have called and not just with regard to emotion – embodied awareness (*reflexive Sinnlichkeit*).

It is important to recognize that the silence Clynes talks about is an inner silence; it can definitely accompany strong intense emotional expression. In aesthetic distance this effect is specifically achieved by the sparing use of expressive means. "The dog's bark is worse than its bite", we say; but a certain kind of growl can be a clear warning. The reason for this is that the attention and energy of the actor is gathered precisely at the *contact boundary*, instead of wasting energy in over-distanced "talking-about" or in under-distanced emotional overflow.

Quite apart from the significance of aesthetic distance for a cathartic re-living of unfinished situations and the cathartic resolution of deep seated emotional blockages in therapy, optimal distancing of emotional expression and experience is important for the contacting process in two ways: it ensures the organism's concentration on the tasks and resistances of this particular contacting process, and it protects the relevant environment from exploitation and unnecessary violation, thus facilitating reciprocal empathy. From the perspective of Gestalt therapy, therefore, re-constituting and refining our capacity to be sensually aware in the realm of the emotions is definitely at the forefront of our concern.

The social conditions and constellations framing the encounter between client and therapist in doing this work constitute the background from which this task stands out, demanding solution. Therefore, this background too must be clearly understood. The civilizing process which European societies have gone through in the modern era is a path which leads from an initial dominance of the "Dionysian mode" of emotional experience to the ubiquity of "mimicry" behaviours. The "Dionysian mode" is connected to low behavioural controls and great impulsivity, implying that behaviour is hard to predict and may be accompanied by sudden emotional eruptions. Such behaviour always entails danger to the social order and therefore it is contained as much as possible through *cult* and *ritual*. One could probably write a history of the gradual dissolution and individualization of cults and rituals, already quite advanced during "The Waning of The Middle Ages" (Huizinga, 1972). Through this dissolution, the "Dionysian mode" gradually becomes dysfunctional. When cults and rituals are no longer embedded in feast days and holidays, this mode loses its meaning as a connecting point with the

Beyond. We also have to remember that right into the 19th century, days of pilgrimage to the church or monastery on the next hill were the *only* holidays peasants ever enjoyed. Gradually, the significance of religious as well as of secular rituals has been reduced to being considered personal psycho-hygienic measures, including attending special mass events like pop concerts.

The history of our emotionality therefore is also the history of our rituals. In the past, religious ritual – be it Christian or Pagan – achieved something truly great: it developed ways to collectively contain the expression of emotion in the Dionysian mode, where the whole body is fully involved. In the course of modern processes of secularization, religious rituals in churches and villages were initially displaced by secular rituals of state and co-operatives. Eventually their significance was eroded too, leaving private rituals of persons closely connected to each other, family, friends, colleagues, neighbours, where it is difficult to maintain the fine balance between a phobia of rituals emptied of religious meaning and embarrassing sentimentality.

In the course of this development, contacting emotions like joy, grief and gratitude are expressed less often in ritual today, but *emotional attitudes* are ritually performed instead. National pride and patriotism, xenophobia and class consciousness, but also class solidarity and love for one's homeland are stages of the modern history of emotions which have increasingly devalued contacting emotions in favour of character attitudes. Eventually, repressing all spontaneous affects became the celebrated ideal of self-control, of the authoritarian personality. Therefore, there are increasing amounts of overflow affects from emotionally unfinished, incomplete situations, presenting a latent emotional reservoir for all kinds and forms of political mobilization. Additionally, there are the instruments of affective contagion, masterfully handled by the National Socialists and now the Islamist fascists and the populist movements on the political Right. The informalization process as the most recent stage of the civilizing process must be grounded in the second stage: informalization requires the internalization of civilized manners – maintained by the threat of shame feelings – in order to work adequately. At present, it is not clear whether this connection is still functioning well enough. If not, there is a danger that a process of de-civilization, strengthened by the new media, could gain ground.

Overflow affects and emotional attitudes are the opposite of a finely tuned emotional sensorium of the self; they always result from self-repression. Even as they sometimes manifest themselves in an impressive way in demonstrations and other mass events, they are not to be mixed up with the Dionysian rituals which express contacting emotions. One could call the one kind real emotions; the other false ones. Indeed, there are no essentic forms for jealousy, envy, contempt and national pride. Therefore, they can find expression only in over-distanced, self-controlled verbalizations or under-distanced mass behaviours or individual eruptions. They do not orientate but rather disorientate: they are alienated from need.

The "Apollonian mode" of emotional experience was always socially embedded in religious-meditative situations and in such places where meditative practice was undertaken, mostly in monasteries and particularly in Asia. In Europe it was not until the Renaissance changed its perspective from cosmic to human-centred that a secular interest in individual experience and the possibilities of expressing emotions began to develop. Throughout the Modern period then, we find two contradictory, but nevertheless socially complementary developmental tendencies in conflict with each other: the civilizing pressure to restrain spontaneous affective expression, and the search for authenticity and naturalness in experience and style. On the one hand there are extreme attempts at disciplining the body, and a trend towards stylizing expressive gestures; and on the other, we find passionate observation and exploration of "natural emotional expression" and its mimetic and kinetic expression.

These tendencies are to some extent expressions of class differences. Courtly society was primarily interested in questions of character formation and militaristic body control, whereas the bourgeoisie hoped to find and to legitimize its behavioural norms in the natural sphere. While all forms of "Dionysian" emotional expression gradually came to be seen as pathological (or childish), a need for "Apollonian" modes of expression for secular emotions had to emerge. But while "mimicry" standards were still maintained, *sentimentality* emerged as a pervasive emotional attitude in society – in the public realm, in the pathos of nationalistic and Royalist feelings – and in private life, the middle classes developed a preference for primarily soft, flowing and rather passive forms of emotional expression.

By now pathos and idyll have been thoroughly discredited. Eventually there was established a mixture of "mimicry" standards in public life, and a tentatively ecstatic level of feeling in the private realm: now people are starting to talk about "emotional needs". In fact, to some extent we have been "dispossessed" by the media: we live a second-hand version of emotional life. At the same time, it is mainly the media which protects us from relapsing into sentimentality. In the first place, other people and foreign cultures are now plentifully and graphically brought into our living rooms, so an exclusive identification with one's own group is no longer as easy. Secondly, everything in the media is a play, a possibility, a figure. Emotional attitudes are represented by roles, stars and advertisements which one can partially imitate, partially consume as entertainment; spontaneous contacting emotions are represented as true-to-type. In this way, they both extend and limit the viewer's own repertoire.

The immense flood of stories told in literature, in reports and in films now also offers new opportunities for practising the "Apollonian" mode through empathic experience. Ever since the Romantic period and until the beginning of classical modern art, for some parts of the bourgeoisie art functioned as an independent medium for offering emotional experience with aesthetic distance. Of course, presentation and story-telling in art, film and literature can be over- or under-distanced, and often is. But it is more important to notice the amazing extent to which "Apollonian" modes of experience have become available, especially through film.

Even more important nowadays is to *practise* aesthetic distance not just in the role of spectator/reader with passive empathy, but to do so in our own everyday life and experience. This then is the answer demanded at the current state of our civilization. Its great achievement – the internal pacification of wide areas of the world, achieved less by the state taking over the monopoly of legitimized violence than through people managing their affective lives by restraint – has to be maintained and developed. This is definitely not going to happen without affective controls, although hopefully, not through controls rooted in repression and in blocking emotional experiences but rather in the manner of Clynes' "pre-sentic control"; in our ability to make conscious choices between modes of emotional expression.

Controlling our affects does not necessarily have to be identical with impoverished emotional sensibility. Clynes has shown that we can even increase this sensibility by practising the experience of objectless emotional states – "generalized sentic states", since through this practice greater emotional flexibility is generated in two ways: firstly with regard to the ease with which we can move into an emotional state and then leave it behind; and secondly, we can learn to choose creative new modes of expression, no longer attached to whatever we

Table 5.1 Emotions – a summary of the concepts used in Chapters IV and V

Bodily Sensations	e.g. pain/hunger
Passions	love as passion
Contacting Emotions	**affects/emotions**
1. Fore-contact	Emotions of aversion and attraction: *curiosity, erotic attraction, longing, surprise, fear, disgust*
2. Orientation and manipulation	Aggressive emotions: *rage/hate, sex*
3. (Integration) => full contact	Timeless emotions: *joy, love, grief, surprising beauty, awe, Aha-experiences, bliss*
4. Post-contact	Appreciative emotions: *pride, gratitude, impotence/desperation, guilt feelings*
Inhibiting Emotions	*Excitement anxiety, shame and embarrassment*
Sympathetic Emotions	Sympathy: *emotional contagion, empathic emotions* Empathy: *entering into somebody's emotions, being attuned*
Overflow Affects	Mostly *anger, joy and grief,* but also for instance: neurotic *guilt* feelings, *sadness,* resentment, *contempt, bitterness, sullenness*
Emotional Attitudes = character traits resulting from introjects or unfinished expression of emotions	*envy, meanness, frivolity, helper syndrome, neurotic jealousy, hope, permanent worrying* and many others

have learned in the past. The task is to learn in which situations to choose which kind of mode (Apollonian or Dionysian) and medium (facial expression/mime and/or movement and/or music, dance, singing etc.); what to choose to express my feelings to come as close as possible to the essentic form, to make it most fitting with my own motivation and orientation as well as to that of others.

Therapy groups working with a growth model of psychological experience rather than with a deficit model offer a good milieu for this kind of learning. The reason is that they have already instituted something to replace ritual in the modern world – *meta-communication,* reflecting on how we communicate and enter into relationship with each other. Meta-communication does not have to consist in talking about something any more than does its subject, communication. As we talk, we do not only communicate through our language but at the same time we use our senses and feelings, our posture and facial expression. Sensuous awareness is both medium and aim of the process of cultivating the orientation function of our senses and emotions, experimenting with art as well as with therapeutically guided self-awareness practices, but specifically through everyday practice in our own lives.

6 Aliveness and the joy of life

General goals of Gestalt therapy[4]

Gestalt therapy is concerned with two *general* endeavours for achieving something more encompassing than the complex work of treating individual neuroses. The first is, of course, to increase the patient's level of awareness, especially regarding their own body in the context of its relevant social and natural environments. From the beginning, one of Gestalt therapy's central concerns was *heightening* awareness – long before awareness training, arising from the contemporary trend towards self enhancement, began to be part of the cultural market. The second general goal of Gestalt therapy is to liberate our natural *joy of life* from its culturally generated paralysis, from the dimming of our senses, from the routinization of our contacts, from our creativity – all frequently remaining dormant. Clearly, the second overriding goal of Gestalt therapy is to awaken our joy of life by stimulating our sense of *aliveness* through intensifying our capacity for awareness. Gestalt therapy is well equipped with methods and situationally created exercises and experiments to pursue this second goal with which the reader will be familiar.

But what actually is aliveness, this natural basis for any joy of life we might experience? As with the concept of time, everybody seems to know what we mean when we use the word "aliveness," but hardly anybody can define it.

If asked to think about it – or asked to develop a feeling of the feeling of aliveness – most people will spontaneously produce images of *movement* – perhaps of running children, people dancing or engaged in a passionate embrace or erotic pleasures. Or else one might associate aliveness with inorganic forces like the bubbling waters of a stream or the sparkling drops of a fountain. I assume that most of us will either come up with images of moving bodies or objects being moved by water or air – the only two natural forces which we spontaneously associate with aliveness. We can observe these phenomena within the time frame of our own life – unlike the growth and disappearance of mountains or the movements of geological shifts, or stars.

Moreover, few people would spontaneously think of machines here, though they too can and do move – but they are not alive: they are not *living beings.* Life is at the heart of the notion of aliveness, which is immediately plausible if we approach the word from its opposite. Words like freeze or paralysis come to mind but also fright or shock: experiences that stop the breath, this elixir of life. *Rigor mortis* is the extreme opposite of aliveness. The common denominator of all these opposite associations is the lack of movement or inability to move. So deeply rooted in our consciousness is this connection of life to movement that to be tied up is generally dreaded, while to be buried alive represents the ultimate horror. When freedom-loving Antigone, who had preferred to obey the gods, was punished by King Creon for her disobedience, he pitilessly stuck to the law and walled her in. Bereft of movement, she killed herself. That is the story Sophocles told us in his tragedy.

In addition to our ability to move in space like all other animals, our love of movement is also rooted in the fact that *internally* our bodies are always moving. This we take as a sure sign that we are still alive: without pausing, our hearts beat 70 times each minute for as long as we live; our lungs continuously pump the amount of oxygen we need for survival – just like all living beings on our planet. We take our daily food from the environment and our bodies' juices and bacteria busily help to digest it. Moreover, there are countless streams moving inside our bodies which we hardly notice as long as they function without disturbance: our blood always circulates, our brain communicates with billions of cells within itself and also with the rest of the body; hormones shower through our organism, exciting or calming us; our cells constantly grow, die, and renew themselves. The famous sentence by Heraclitus rings true, particularly about bodies: *Everything moves!*

Another property of the living body is quite familiar from Gestalt therapy theory: that it is involved in constant exchange processes with its environments, not just regarding food and oxygen. Our legs and feet carry us through space from one area to another and our arms are capable of reaching out, so that we can *grasp and touch*. And then we have this incredible gift of our senses! They provide the link between the outer world and our consciousness. In close cooperation with the brain – from the data they collect – they construct the image of a reality usually consistent enough for us to find our way through. This collaboration between brain and senses produces a vague but very powerful image of that Self which psychologically for all of us is the centre of the world. Stabilized by our *sense of balance* we walk and reach out into this world, directed by our eyes which mostly have already grasped the object out there. *Hearing,* too, has its role, often making us aware of what we could or did not see, but may also be an important information for us about the environment. We have sensory equipment for *smelling, tasting,* and last but not least for *touching*, with its most intimate functions of contacting the external world.

Gestalt therapy theory calls our senses the most important of the *"ego functions of the self,"* that strange phenomenon which Perls & Goodman defined as the "contact boundary in movement", i.e. a *process* rather than an area or a *substance.* The self then is the process of the living encounter of the human organism with its ever-changing environments energetically charging us by the constant challenge to generate new *creative adjustments.* This process helps to distinguish digestible aspects of the environment fields from its unhealthy aspects (Perls & Goodman's "alienation" and "identification"). That is where aliveness is to be found – and Gestalt therapy is most eager to re-vitalize this potential.

I have said before that the core of the word *aliveness* is *life.* So it will be necessary to understand what *life* really is to extend our exploration a little beyond the particulars of *human life.* But before we come to the biology of life, a special property must be mentioned which in this particular intensity may be unique to human beings: *our curiosity and urge to gain knowledge and comprehend the world.* This urge can be muted early on and it may fade in old age, but it is a source of aliveness and joy of life which never vanishes completely. This is the reason why one of the most important goals of Gestalt therapy is to reanimate and support *curiosity,* even when it is deeply buried and showing no sign of survival.

The urge to know is a gift, a potential with which all human beings are born. For proof of this assertion, just observe children. If left undisturbed they relentlessly explore their world, starting with their own body and as soon as they begin crawling, they extend their search to the limits of their environment, using all their senses and powers of grasping, biting, tasting, pushing, pressing and tearing to comprehend how things function. Later, when they begin to have some command of language an endless stream of questions follows, many of them unanswerable by adults due to their existential nature. Etymologically, the word curiosity has its roots in the Latin *cura* = care as for instance in *custody* or *curator* or even *cure.* So the original meaning of curiosity is finding something worthy of attention, worthy of careful inspection, worth knowing more about. Indeed, especially in the 17th and 18th centuries during the Enlightenment the adjective *curious* denoted something of special value.

But slowly, at the same time to be curious also became a negative trait, meaning inquisitive, prying, and nosy. In German, the Latin *curiositas* completely disappeared and was replaced by *"Neugier"* which literally means "greed for the new." This was due to the influence of Protestantism, especially in its Lutheran version. Martin Luther is reported to have answered the question: "What was God doing before he created the world?" with "He was sitting behind a bush cutting rods for idiots asking stupid questions!" But today the question of what was happening before the Big Bang is one of the hottest in cosmological research – and not attested to have been "thanks to God"

The American writer Ambrose Bierce, known for his critical comments on his contemporary society in the middle of the nineteenth century, defined curiosity as "an objectionable quality of the female mind". But then he continued surprisingly: "The desire to know whether or not a woman is cursed with curiosity is one of the most active and insatiable passions of the masculine soul." And with this shift in perspective Bierce almost sounded an early feminist note.

For a long time, curiosity was eschewed as a dangerous folly of children and the vice of female addiction to gossip. From a sociological point of view, it should be noted, however, that gossip and the exchange of rumours always have a survival function for the powerless who desperately need information about their oppressors. This is why harems were supposed to be breeding places of gossip and rumours: the women were dependent on the whims of their male owners. Today it is a political issue: Just think for instance of the fate of intellectuals and journalists in Erdogan's Turkey today or indeed in any other non-democratic society.

In essence, *being inquisitive is searching for truth and knowledge.* Or to put it differently as quoted above: in Gestalt therapy, *curiosity* is what in psychoanalysis used to be *libido* – this is the brilliant insight of Michael Vincent Miller (1987;18–32).

Clearly curiosity is the heart of aliveness. There is a joy inherent in searching for truth and gaining knowledge, not least because it empowers us to better deal with the problems of life. After all we are borne into this life without any instructions and with a complete lack of information. And although we will receive instructions from our seniors and will endlessly discover and learn new data about the world surrounding us, these are never ever sufficient. Even in our contemporary scientific culture *trial and error* remains among the main cognitive means of survival. In the end we die – one of the very few things we safely know about our existence – without having learned many of the important secrets of life. And yet there is this urge to know about them, to decipher what we experience and do not understand – and to go on asking questions even while we know that all answers generate new questions.

This passion directly relates to our joy of life. Nothing is sadder than meeting people whose curiosity has got lost in depression or is imprisoned by ignorance, because the passion to know was suffocated early on, like in the story of a father wandering with his little son in the mountains: The child asks: "Dad, what is really behind these mountains?" and the father puts him down by saying: "Shut up and don't ask such metaphysical questions!" – If, however, that passion for knowledge is supported (even when the adults do not know the answer) it may inspire the life to persist right into old age. There does not have to be an end to learning with growing age, even though memory weakness will impede the process. Also, one may experience symptoms of tiredness – a sense of *déja vu* occurs, related to having seen and lived through so many situations. Much seems familiar and too boring to engage with yet again. *The excitement of curiosity will diminish with the weakening power of our senses – that is the tragic fact of getting older.* But always many secrets remain and so there is some consolation in the recent discovery that for a limited period of time some brain cells are capable of recovering even in old age.

There is, though, one new and significant problem with this positive view of curiosity. Now that the smart phone has become a household item, it can no longer be dismissed as a passing craze for the new, though it does indeed have a new plausibility: the pressure to constantly look for new messages, news, "likes" and all kinds of information has made many people dependent on this small but powerful instrument. *This is a neurotic addiction,* not a healthy curiosity in search of relevant knowledge! To heal it most likely the same drastic therapeutic methods we have learned in working with drug addicts will have to be applied.

To avoid getting overloaded by information, we need to distinguish between *data* and *knowledge.* The flood of data we are exposed to via the media or the internet is in itself meaningless, just burdensome to our brains. Real knowledge consists in knowing how data are interconnected in systems and feedback loops, allowing us to decipher *meaning.*

It seems to me that the pleasure of seeking and gaining knowledge can be a companion in life even through the dying process, if one is receiving the gift of a conscious death. In any case, the faces of the dead occasionally show a light of *sheer astonishment.*

There is pleasure in attaining knowledge, in the process of learning, discovering and deciphering, but pleasure is also the gift of having found the solution: Archimedes' *Eureka!* The excitement of knowing, of finding the truth is, like all joy – a very enlivening experience.

The core of the word aliveness is, as I have said, the word *life.* So it will be useful to learn what this actually *is,* if we want to understand the joy of life. This, however, turns out to be not an easy task. There are two unmistakable signs for knowing whether we are alive or not: the sense of physical *pleasure* and the feeling of *pain.* This is due to the *dual tension* which is a property of all life. The Cartesian "I think – therefore I am" no longer rings true in an era of dementia. In fact, we will find that to decipher what life really is demands *phenomenological descriptions* rather than a *scientific definition* in which something always will be missing – just as when we try to define love.

Newton's physics are not applicable to biology, to the study of life,[5] if only because they have different notions of time within which their objects exist. Life does not flow in a uniformly progressing unalterable linear stream, but always has a beginning and an end; it is developing, growing and vanishing; it organizes itself in irregular cycles. "Life is not a succession of cause and effect but a decision" (Weiszäcker, 1997:212). Or rather it is an irregular sequence of bifurcations, as biologists call these intersecting branches where new decisions happen. Life is not structured by *causal connections* but by *functional connections* compressed in dynamic networks of feedback loops in which processes of decay are continuously compensated for by processes of reconstruction.

But each decision at an intersection is irreversible: it cannot be taken back. Even in pre-natal life, cells die. They are just part of an ontogenetic stage of development through which the foetus has to pass. The human body is constantly involved in an incredible, moving process: in the course of 4 to 7 years, all 50 to 70 billion body cells die and are renewed. This, though, is not a *rejuvenating cure,* because the renewed cells, too, are subject to ageing. This means that these processes of renewal become slower over time and eventually fewer and fewer new cells are produced – even if we know today that some of our brain cells, under certain conditions of training, are capable of renewed growth even in older age.

Living systems are highly complex. "Just to build a single germ," says medical researcher Cramer, "the order of one billion pieces of DNA, i.e. genes, has to be reconstructed flawlessly. This high degree of order represents an extremely improbable state." Living systems can only survive by a steadily flowing input of energy from external sources. But even then, they will not escape the law of entropy which entails that all higher order systems will dissolve, or if they are *living* systems they will decay. Death marks a state where the input of external energy breaks down, either because the sources of nourishment have dried up or because the body has become unable to absorb this material (Cramer, 1997:50).

Precisely *when* this state is reached in human beings is a hot topic in medical research at present. Leaving aside transhuman fantasies which blossom mainly in Silicon Valley, expectations are modest because it seems that the weakening of the cell's power to absorb input is part of its genetic program. Reasonable hopes focus on the possibility of somewhat postponing this process of weakening – which, considering the immense time spans of evolution, seems meaningless. A different question is whether this hope for slowing the process of ageing might also hold true at the psychological and cultural levels of human life. A prolonged span of life does not guarantee more wisdom, as we know – but it may improve the chances for those who experience the joys of learning.

What then is life? Let us first keep in mind that living organisms always exist in an eternally ongoing struggle arising from forever changing geological, climatic, and – for humans – cultural environments. Evolutionary life develops through accidental mutations, some of which achieve adjustment to the new conditions and will procreate. Most however will prove to be unable to adapt, condemning their species to extinction. The number of species of animals and plants living today is estimated to be 5 million – but palaeontological research shows that the number of already extinct species is about 500 million!

Nature displays no constancy as far as life processes are concerned. In modern biology, the famous statement of Leibnitz *natura non facit saltus* – nature does not make jumps – is as wrong as Albert Einstein's belief that God does not play at dice. I do not know whether today, after the discovery of quantum leaps and singularities like the big bang, this insight has also arrived in physics. In any case, physicists are busily looking for the universal formula which is to explain "everything." Strangely enough, that formula should conform to the aesthetic criteria of mathematical elegance and beauty. Considering life with its eternal shifts of looking for prey and becoming prey and other fierce procedures, I have my doubts whether God is really an aesthete.

In spite of nature with all her abundance of forms sometimes produces repeating structures – for instance the imitation of plant forms which some animals use to camouflage themselves for protection – she never produces two identical individuals because each body develops according to its genetic instructions, beginning with the first division of cells, and in an endless sequence of decisions, each of which may go in a different direction – that is, if humans do not interfere by attempting to *clone* a living being. So far, nature has punished such attempts with high rates of mortality. Let us recall that genes only determine 50% of a living being, the rest being generated by more or less creative adjustments to the relevant environments. Even identical twins are not completely identical.

Of course, the capacity to *reproduce* is one of the major properties of all living beings. This potential promotes each species' survival, while a successful mutation overtakes the older species in favour of the new. For this astounding capacity, in the past a *vis vitalis* or an *élan vital* was held responsible. But it is more plausible to assume a power inherent in life itself; there are no known living beings not driven by this urge to live, other than human beings who can say NO to life itself. Knowing our mortality, we are capable of suicide – and have now succeeded in gaining this important freedom to destroy our own individual life for our whole species – a very doubtful "achievement" indeed.

"Living organisms multiply as long as the external conditions, mainly its sources of nourishment, suffice for doing it. In favourable circumstances bacteria divide approximately every 10 minutes so that one individual multiplies into several billions within 14 hours" (Cramer, 1997:49). Humans needed a little more time to reach a comparable number – but to make up for it, we – for better or worse – have now become the most powerful of all species. Conditions for life in nature are never the same as life in the laboratory. Life always meets limits; it always tends towards self-destruction or self–transcendence – producing more than it can properly cope with.

An analogue can be found in our culture: people who are compelled to test their limits, push up their hormone levels, thus risking their lives. Over time, I do not think that we can maintain life in a culture of overstimulation. More and more people seem insufficiently alive unless they overstimulate themselves. The normal challenges of life seem no longer to create enough excitement to feel intensely alive, and indeed, special challenges provide ways of stimulating excitement.

But we might do well to heed the biologically imposed advice of older people – to be moderate – which is also age-old philosophical wisdom. Our consumer culture cannot imagine it – but it may indeed be possible to live more moderately without losing any joy of life! The path leading to that possibility is not always another kick but through becoming more intensely aware – the gift of embodied mindfulness.

It appears that the existential simultaneity of order and chaos, of life and death, of an overriding urge to live and self-consuming growth is the hallmark of life and hence the original source of our aliveness, our joy of life. The method for protecting them consists in developing a more sophisticated awareness.

One last remark about *aliveness*: it should not be mixed up with *happiness!* Which has a taste of fullness, of satisfaction, of rest. Happiness belongs to the stage of post-contact: one feels satisfied, a little tired, well taken care of, or even feels loved. One enjoys restfulness or holidays, feels that things have gone well. To achieve happiness was never a promise made by Gestalt therapy; it was to be our patients' endeavour – after therapy. *Aliveness* and the *Joy of Life* in contrast belong to the *vita active* – in Hannah Arendt's word (Arendt, 1989) – of the more energy-mobilizing processes of creative adjustment. It is an active life which produces joy of life, because it strengthens the creative power and competency needed to master life's tasks.

Notes

1 For more information see: Kelly (2014).

2 Compare Kohut (1971), and Kernberg (1986). Regarding the reception of Object Relations theory in Gestalt therapy, compare the debate initiated by S. Tobin (1982) and continued by Yontef (1988). Particularly critical about this incursion of the newer psychoanalytic personality theory into Gestalt therapy is Joel Latner (1983, 1984a). Also compare Sheldon Cashdan (1988).

3 We might ask at this point how it is possible that human beings can systematically torture and plague other human beings, if in identification they hurt themselves. But nobody is born a torturer; instead, torturers have to be trained through methodical desensitization under extremely authoritarian conditions to do what they do. Mika Haritos-Fatouros thoroughly investigated these mechanisms and practices, when she looked at the Greek dictatorship under Papadopoulos (Gibson / Haritos-Fatouros, 1986). It may be, though, that some persons are borne with brain damage blocking their capacity for compassion.

4 This chapter is part of a lecture I gave on the occasion of the New Year celebrations at the Institute for Gestalt Therapy and Gestalt Education (IGG) in Berlin, Germany, on the 11th January 2019.

5 The following text parts regarding biology are mainly based on the German medical biologist Friedrich Cramer (1997).

Chapter VI

Cultural context

Humankind's transformations in the age of environmental destruction

I Looking down from the Moon, or the end and eternity of nature

The cultural context in which our patients' life is embedded in the Western world is extremely complex and multi-faceted. But whatever we might say about it, in my view it is or will be dominated in the next two decades by just one dominant theme: *climate change*. How we respond to this phenomenon will – politically, economically and culturally – determine our future including the fate of the civilising process. In the West survival concerns will be mixed with ethical issues and both will severely affect psychological well-being – our own and that of our patients. In fact, I expect ten years from now this topic will dominate our therapies and create an extraordinary challenge to our craft. Therefore, in this last chapter I will focus exclusively on this theme.

Let me first explain how I came to this conclusion, which will surely surprise many readers. I will begin with a historical observation.

In the 18th century, Europe saw the gradual development of a new kind of aesthetics of nature, matching and complementing the new mode of nature *observation* with its instrumental perspective. Kant's aesthetics conceptualized this development when he distinguished between natural phenomena as either wild and sublime or tamed and beautiful. From that point on, even the rough, the angular, the wild and the crude in nature could be seen as sublime. Romantic painting opened the door for art to develop this mode of seeing, which in turn became the precursor of the wide varieties of nature photography which characterize the Western world's relationship with nature today. At the same historical moment when we escalated our interventions, manipulations and exploitations of nature to the maximum extent, we were able to experience untouched nature as something of particular aesthetic value. This too is part of the dialectics of progress, that we could not discover the beauty of nature in its wildness until we had tamed it and thereby lost our fear of it. This phenomenon is rather important for our topic, since our capacity to see nature from an aesthetic perspective is so far the only counter-balancing position from which to avoid raping nature by using technical means to satisfy our needs, not to mention greed. And we have not yet developed this aesthetic perspective sufficiently.

Today our ways of seeing have been unexpectedly enriched, revealing a host of implications: we can now see the Earth from the Moon; we can consider the view of the whole terrestrial globe from cosmic space. For the first time, Earth sees herself in a mirror – and behold, she is beautiful! (Photographs in: Kelley, 1988). Even before this time telescopes and cameras had allowed us to see early pictures of the cosmos. Through the discovery of a spatial perspective in the Renaissance, human beings discovered themselves in their glorious symmetry, in their divine potentiality.

In the 18th and 19th centuries, when people discovered the beauty of natural wilderness they also discovered the untamed nature of their own desires and needs. As space flight revealed a perspective back from the cosmos onto ourselves, it allowed us a new kind of sensuous experience of our place in the cosmos, forcing us to come up with a new spiritual definition of this position. This is not yet clearly developed. Never before had human beings been able to see our complete habitat in all its beauty, but neither had we seen how small it is and how fragile. They say that nobody seeing this for themselves came back untouched by the experience. For those of us who weren't there, the image has to suffice. But this image alone (if we truly open ourselves to it) will have a profound effect, I believe.

Viewed from the Moon we see the "blue planet", our terrestrial globe, with huge blue seas and slightly smaller brown land masses, pervaded by air currents visible as huge white cloud eddies. In fifty or a hundred years the same view may show yellow-white masses of cloud fumes covering up the face of a greying planet – completely impenetrable and doomed to remain in that state for incalculable time. In photos showing our planet backlit by the sun, we can see the minute habitat available to us humans between the blazing fire of the Earth's interior and the radiant cold of space. If the globe had a circumference of four metres, the human dwelling space with air to breathe on its surface would be no more than four millimetres.

These images matter greatly, because they resonate emotionally and create *emotional clarity,* where cognitively we are increasingly confused. As a research task, the environmental catastrophe is of such complexity, that it cannot be compared to any other problem ever to confront science (Dreitzel / Stenger, 1990). The Gaia hypothesis[1] may well be right when it assumes that the whole globe is a self-contained system of physical, geological, biological and climatic components interacting together. Surely everybody has experienced smog burning the eyes, polluted foam making it impossible to bathe in the seas, rubbish and poison everywhere welling up from the ground. We know enough to realize that rays coming from space itself, cannot be directly experienced through the senses. We know that we are beginning to be less well protected from them.

What is new is that not only astronomical observation but the ever more precise observation of our home planet by satellites travelling in growing numbers around it, have begun to protocol every aspect of how we humans have self-defeatingly wreaked destruction on earth. Satellites notice the fires which extinguish parts of the Amazon rainforest – and recognize the effects caused by oil palm plantations as they grow field by field. Every tree is recorded in Indonesia; they notice the dwindling of the scarce sweet water resources as well as the disappearance of corals in our seas, they register the worldwide melting of mountain glaciers, as well as melting ice caps in polar regions, they protocol the forest fires in Siberia which melt the perma-frost thus releasing huge amounts of methane gas poisoning the atmosphere – as on the micro level our microscopes detect the otherwise invisible Covid-19 virus causing the corona crisis. Here again progress in photographic technology directly helps to increase our awareness of what is happening. The growing quality of nature photography in documentaries contributes to our awareness and speaks directly to our emotions.

What is called *environmental consciousness* is more a function of our emotional sensibility than our cognitive understanding. The emotions have more power of helping us to orient ourselves in our highly complex world than intellectual comprehension.

The situation is quite different when we consider the effect of greenhouse gases on climate change. What the gardener takes as a sunlight-permeable, warming and insulating glass roof of a greenhouse, for the Earth is a layer of gases and dust particles trapping part of the sun's warmth near the earth. Without this layer there would be no life on earth, since the average temperature would be lowered by 35 °C, i.e. it would sink to −20 °C. Humankind has begun to seal in this glasshouse, effectively shutting down the ventilation system by feeding in trace gases, which reflect back to the Earth some part of the emitted warmth, causing temperatures to rise. This greenhouse effect has been known for a hundred years and had been predicted by scientists. But how quickly and how strongly temperatures will rise and what effects should be expected remains unknown – due to their complexity these issues pose very difficult questions to researchers. During the last hundred years our average temperatures worldwide have risen by 1.0 °C, and ocean levels by 20 centimetres. Emissions of carbon dioxide are responsible for at least half of the greenhouse effect. Today it is no longer controversial among serious scientists that warming will happen to an above-average extent near the polar regions, and in consequence the moderate zones will probably have more rain, while the tropical zones will have less. Simultaneously, sea levels will rise by an unknown factor. Researchers are working to find out what consequences this will have and where. But it becomes ever more apparent that the weather anomalies we can observe everywhere – unusually warm summers in Europe; extreme heat and dry periods in the USA; extreme fires and rainfalls in Australia, California and Bangladesh; the fiercest ever tornados and hurricanes – all seem to be immediate consequences of the greenhouse effect. We are sure that sooner or later large areas inhabited today by millions of people, for example the Nile Delta or large parts of Bangladesh, will be flooded and lost. It is also certain that there will be no winners, simply because these intense climate changes, very different from natural variations, happen too quickly for us to have time to gradually adjust – and this is what makes them climate *catastrophes.*

What kinds of changes inexorably hit us can be estimated by considering the role of carbon dioxide.

Carbon dioxide is released each time we burn something: cooking our meals, heating or cooling our houses, melting metals, driving our cars, uprooting our forests, when we burn our dead. In addition animals like cows and the warming of the permafrost by huge fires in Siberia release methane gas, a particularly dangerous pollutant reinforcing the effect of carbon emissions.

Anybody can access the internet and the newest literature regarding climate change and learn everything there is to know about this process, its causes and its burdens (Wallace-Wells, 2019; Rich, 2019; Foer 2019; Scheffler, 2013). It seems as if a part of world society has woken up from its environmental sleep, but largely we become paralysed by exhortations, with appeasements and denials. However even before Donald Trump came to power it was very doubtful whether the Paris agreements of 2016 would be realized. The necessary changes in our lifestyles are too large and too unclear at once for us to develop a truly action-oriented imagination.

The American naturalist Bill McKibben wrote a penetrating and wonderfully poetic book about these concerns, entitled *The End of Nature* (McKibben, 1990). He makes it clear that no longer can we ever or anywhere be certain that nature – wherever we encounter it on this planet – is pure nature, untouched by human beings; as it were "authentic" nature. So a mother's milk may be contaminated; the weather may be entirely taken over by smog; coloured pebbles at the beach may turn out to be bits of plastic. The star turns out to be a satellite; the mushrooms we collect may be radioactively contaminated, and the genetically manipulated animal would never have been produced in this form by evolution. We can never be sure whether and when and to what extent the beneficial and harmful forms and qualities we find "in nature" are the result of human interference or are not. We influence the weather, without knowing quite how we do it. We get into the act but know very little about the effects of our contributions.

While all this is happening, an epoch has come to an end – the time where it was possible, at least theoretically, to adjust to nature, to fit in with it, to entrust ourselves to it. But this is the age of the Anthropocene, the age dominated by our own species and its way of life: Mother Nature is dead, and I grieve for her, even while I know she was just an idea; she was a beautiful invention and discovery of human beings. Still, the life and death of ideas has very real consequences: with "Mother Nature" die many beautiful species of animal and plant which developed on the blue planet. This is the qualitative aspect. The quantitative aspects of these processes are barely imaginable. Up to a hundred species daily disappear from our globe in consequence of climate change. But the expression, the "end of nature", also reminds us a little of the story of somebody painting on a wall: "God is dead – Nietzsche" and a second graffito responds: "Nietzsche is dead – God". Human beings need nature: indeed, we *are* nature – but nature does not need humans. Or perhaps it does?

2 Anxiety and civilization in everyday life on Earth

To look down from the Moon to Earth is not an everyday possibility, but it offers a generalizing perspective. On Earth, we rarely consider this view. The picture of Earth as a lonely space ship in the universe, the one and only known life-sustaining world for human beings, tends to get lost in the foreground business of everyday life – and yet it remains increasingly active in the background, gradually becoming an archetype and affecting us not from the past but from the future. The discrepancy between this background knowledge and the particular everyday contacting processes is huge indeed. How do we live with it? In short, with anxiety – which we ward off. To my knowledge only two authors, F. Franzen (2019) and N. Rich (2019), have had the courage to face the situation openly demanding to stop our illusionary flight: Earlier in this book we have seen that there is a difference between *anxiety* and *fear*. From the perspective of Gestalt theory, fear is a fore-contact emotion: It informs us about the relation between a specific threat and our own strengths; it mobilizes those strengths for flight or fight. Anxiety, on the other hand, is the emotion arising from an interruption of one's natural breathing rhythms: rising excitement is blocked, the natural rhythm of breathing is disturbed, and movement is paralysed. Anxiety paralyses, we say. Actually, it would be more accurate to say that we are *being* paralysed, since it is a passive experience. To be helpless in relation to a threat creates anxiety, and if we feel chronically powerless this anxiety is so depressing that habitually we ward it off. In Gestalt therapy, we get in touch with this anxiety by working on and through our reaction formations, i.e. neurotic defences against this extremely unpleasant feeling. Normally we don't notice it. Excluding the case of anxiety neurosis, clinically a special case, there are two questions:

1 What is it that actually causes us to hold our breath and block excitement so much that we are unable to express ourselves and to act? Why do we "paralyse" ourselves? Or allow ourselves to be paralysed?
2 And how do we frequently manage to avoid sensing the anxiety we create through holding our breath?

The answer to the first question has two aspects. One of them relates to the theory of civilization which has already been discussed. Early on in our socialization we all develop our particular mechanisms of self-restraint, be they healthy internalizations or neurotic introjects constraining the spontaneous expression of pain and desire, rage and love, joy and grief. This is part of the standard equipment of the common personality type in modern society – and part of the reason why we see so much depression and resignation. On the other hand – and concerning the alarming environmental conditions – our motivation to act is paralysed by the impenetrable complexity of what is happening. We are gripped by feeling powerless and helpless; experiences already familiar to us from bureaucratic and technical contexts. These now extend into the crisis of our democracies. When we are dealing with environmental problems, habitual expressive restraint diminishes our capacity for emotional receptivity and adds to disorientation and de-motivation for practical action. Both these factors lead to excitement being inhibited, creating an experience of anxiety so unpleasant that we chronically defend ourselves against it.[2]

I suspect that the most widespread defence mechanisms against anxiety are *selective inattention* and making use of the vast range of *anaesthetics* available to us. In both cases our emotional sensorium has contracted through the affective self–restraint which has become chronic throughout the civilising process. In any case, it is difficult to emotionally touch the dominant depressive-narcissistic social character. We must add to this the blunting effect of the daily horror spectacles of current catastrophes we see on television. They generate a sense that – compared to those worldwide developments – our own scope for action is disproportionately negligible. Ralph K. White spoke of *selective inattention*, and mentioned – more than 20 years ago – our growing environmental problems: White observed this mode of not-noticing, not-sensing, not-responding emotionally, while intellectually knowing what is happening. According to him (White, 1988:73), Selective Inattention applies particularly to four areas:

- we are aware of our own guilt feelings
- of the humanity of our enemies
- of the danger of nuclear war
- of environmental catastrophe.

Selective inattention refers to our capacity for splitting. By way of selective inattention, the Promethean gap which today characterizes our social bodies of knowledge, turns into individual pathology.

The other escape route from our anxiety consists in *anaesthetising* ourselves. It may well be that many people are quite aware of environmental disaster and unknowingly develop unbearably intense feelings of shame which, unawares, they repress. There are innumerable means of giving way to our fear of anxiety and feelings of shame in our Western culture which stop us from becoming aware – and many of these are addictive. This is true for all kinds of anaesthetising drugs, but equally this also applies to certain ways of using old and new media, especially our smart phones, and our cars.

Driving may be a particularly good example demonstrating our lack of environmental awareness, because most of us do it daily. It involves a complex set of behaviours which could bear a close inquiry into the psychological processes involved in loving driving. But driving is not just a personal problem, it is also a political problem. Decades of political neglect of public transportation left many people economically dependent on owning a private car. The car is, literally, deeply rooted into our culture.

It is well known today, that the car despite its catalytic converter is environmentally extremely destructive. It contributes to forest decline as well as to smog development in cities; to the greenhouse effect as well as to the destruction of biological habitats. Yet the worldwide "re-armament" with cars continues with ever increasing speed. The need and legitimate desire for individual freedom of movement – coupled with significant financial interests – seems to kill any satisfactory development of public transportation that could offer a useful alternative. Meanwhile, even the electrification of cars appears to be a doubtful solution considering the environmental costs involved. The amount of energy needed for that change is enormous and perhaps not feasible, in view of the fact that the only unlimited source of energy our planet seems to possess is the sun. Converting sun energy in the necessary amount is not in sight. Meanwhile the damage caused by the speed of climate change increases year on year.

Chronic damage results from regularly repeated short-term need satisfactions, requiring a gradual increase of the dose: a typical feature of addiction, well-known to all of us. In *addictive behaviour*, awareness is reduced; embodied mindfulness may be diminished to such a point that we can no longer perceive or sense the damage we are inflicting – until withdrawal has been achieved.

Just as with most environmental problems, here too the problem concerns the next step in developing our individuality – some people would call this step "conquering our narcissism". We need shared, collective pressure from the bottom up; a readiness to engage with conflicts with the aim of developing an alternative politics of transport; shared cooperative ways of communicating with everybody concerned to discuss better uses of available resources. The same applies to other burning issues – for instance how to reduce home energy use – as well as on a more existential level, how to preserve democracy in our Western societies with reforms to ensure such that everyone's voice is heard.

During the past three years, though, some signs of hope have emerged, obviously due to the growing experience of worldwide observable weather changes – whether correctly seen as related to climate change or not. As Greta Thunberg has emerged as a global star – invited to speak to the assembly of the United Nations in New York or to a meeting of the world's elite economists in Davos – she symbolizes with her movement *Fridays for Future* a growing concern in civil society. This can be seen in many initiatives across the Western World, a development increasingly strengthened by reports and documentaries in the public media. Yet there seems a growing gap between this inspiring development and the prevailing politics of governments caught in out-dated but still surviving ideologies – like neo-liberal economics, real or imagined pressure from the lower classes, as well as very real pressures from the economic power of the super-rich. To this is added a considerable lack of political vision, with a complacency and a determination to hold on to power at all cost.

Without motoric and vocal expression, our emotional sensorium dies, and we find ourselves with a dilemma we urgently need to deal with: Without emotions we are lacking the motivational strength for contacting processes, necessary for examining our relationship with the environment. Therefore, in this respect an "emotional turn" in civil society is desirable. We must work at refining our sensuous and emotional sensorium through increased awareness so that even the smallest forms of emotional expression – by their coherence and authenticity – offer such good orientation to ourselves and others that our needs do not suddenly overwhelm and seduce us into impulsive action. This kind of awareness is not reticence or even asceticism, but what the cultivation of the organism/environment field aims for. Good Gestalt therapy gains strength from its gentle tones, rather than from theatrical peak experiences.

If the civilizing process requires and enforces affect control, then in order to complement and retain some fluidity in this process of cultivating emotions and sensations, we need to develop embodied mindfulness. We need to learn – and this is something Gestalt therapy can achieve very well – that the emotional coherence of an expression, and therefore the intensity as well as authenticity of an emotional experience, is communicated in the melody, the tone of the expression and not through volume or verbal excesses. Introjected affect control may turn into an ability to accurately sense what is going on and to contain oneself, while remaining appropriately involved. Such a sophisticated emotional sensorium the lay person must have and use when encountering experts; or citizens when meeting politicians. In a way, embodied mindfulness is the heart of common sense – the only means we have for reducing the complexity of the available environmental knowledge to proportions which may help us regain standards and guidelines for our actions. Otherwise, the gap between widely available environmental consciousness – in the sense of knowing about environmental destruction – and our hesitancy, even paralysis, regarding hugely necessary action becomes almost unbridgeable.

Discussions of ethics, however necessary, tend towards offering us standards of behaviour which derive from philosophical and theological traditions which people often do not recognize as their own. Only if we have the courage to experience the interaction between human beings and the environment in each concrete case and express this experience in the modality of aesthetic distance will we gain standards which arise from our own experience and therefore have a motivating efficacy.

3 Pressure of time and the fragility of hope

Gestalt therapy values the client's emotional experience over the therapist´s interpretations. It is only by (therapeutically facilitated) working through one's own experience that the client truly realizes what will help them move ahead from other-directedness towards self-responsibility. This is the reason for the "here-and-now" principle at the heart of Gestalt therapeutic work: experience always happens in its particular present; in the place where it happens – any interpretation refers back to something that has already taken place. But it goes without saying that anything that happens occurs within the penumbra of a past which has sharpened or blunted one's senses; helped to unfold emotions or inhibited them; either opened the mind to be receptive for new things or blocked it with prejudices. And the future, too, is always already alive in the present as a horizon of expectation within which in the here-and-now we plan and provide for what is to come or – more commonly – we assume that things will not be significantly different – the next moment, the next day, and the next year.

For an undisturbed contacting process, the shadows of the past are only relevant insofar as they allow us to experience "being different today compared to then", which is constitutive for our sense of biographical identity. Beyond that, psychologically these shadows operate as nothing but a burdensome imprint.

A certain measure of trust that the world we inhabit is not going to be profoundly different in the foreseeable future seems to be an important buttress for our psychic stability. But this trust is being systematically undermined today. We are forever inundated with information and conjectures about all sorts of things that will soon be completely different (mostly of dubious value); changes attributable to practical constraints which supposedly we can barely influence. Since the beginning of the Industrial Revolution, social development has been characterized by the perpetually accelerating speed of technological change which has gradually taken hold of all spheres of everyday life. Those overwhelming fears (for example when railways were introduced) triggered at the time are now forgotten. We remember well, though, the time when all changes marked progress towards a better future. Currently the digital revolution increases the acceleration of change processes even more, though concurrently they seem to worsen our quality of life at least as often as improving it. Hence the world seems ever more complex or frightening for the experiences gained in the past must be part of the present competencies to be effective in the now.

Whatever processes we are thinking about, concern must always be paired with hope: otherwise, such processes would trigger nothing but anxiety. Population growth; urban development; ongoing armament; a worldwide flow of refugees; the chemical and biological industrialization of agriculture; structural unemployment through computerized automation; dissolution of familial bonds; gene technology; the growing percentage of old and very old people; fundamentalist religions spreading worldwide, the rise of populism, etc. This list is arbitrary, and anybody could extend it further. Therefore, the assumption that conditions will be relatively constant, is no longer justified in any sphere of life, although we like to hold on to such notions. Heraclitus' insight that "everything flows" seems to be a post-historical truth. For as far as human conditions and their impact on our planet are concerned, the gently flowing river has turned into a torrent with many cataracts, which does not allow any of us in any way to maintain the illusion of relative continuity.

The speed of time we experience is always relative to our own life span and the time we have already lived or have yet to live. In industrialized countries the average life expectancy beyond infancy has increased by a third. And still, social and economic developments seem to always overtake us biographically. Thus, all social planning increasingly becomes more problematical, as do individual life plans. Everywhere, it is simply the unexpected consequences of planned action which keep us on the run.[3] For example, the population in the developing world does not rise as dramatically due to more children being born, but because Western medicine keeps them alive. But the search for a better life remains active in all of us, and so usually a failed or semi-successful action is followed by a new plan, a further aim.

Paradoxically, the accelerating motor is our deep-rooted longing for satisfaction, the point where having attained everything, no further effort is required. Wherever we are, soon we want to move on, go somewhere else: to another climate; a better job; a more beautiful home; a more satisfying partner; a more authentic experience. The more our lives are speeded up, organized and media-dependent, the more we hasten to find an exit point from this process of acceleration. The higher our expectations, the more we are disappointed; the more frustrated we are, the more we develop higher expectations and the gyroscope of our lives turns faster and faster.

Of course, the one still point is the axis of the gyroscope, the centre of the cyclone. The Archimedean point which allows us to completely revolutionize the situation (and we must use this chance!) does not lie outside of ourselves, but in the centre of the subject. The fulfilment of our longing does not lie beyond the contacting process but in the fullness of its climax, in full contact.

As the pressure of all developmental processes accelerates, society is dominated by "scarcity of time". Modernity's linear sense of time has a tendency to dissolve "time spaces" of experience into the "points in time" of sequential appointments. This gives a sense of breathlessness to the moment, an always-waiting for the next date, the next encounter, the next holiday, the next round of looking at whatever, a permanent rushing from one goal to another. Psychologically it is almost impossible today to gently allow-things-to-arise-and-come-to-me. But there are even more profound connections between the pressure of time and certain social developments. Since the Industrial Revolution, the time perspective through which *families* experience and define themselves has shrunk significantly from an intergenerational continuity, where family extended from the dim past to an undefined future, to the parent-child unit.

This seems to be one of the causes for the carelessness with which we treat the environment. We can no longer understand and intuit the kind of world successive generations will inhabit or would want to inhabit, and thus as a society we are lacking the traditional psychic basis for considering the needs of our children in the future. Of course, since the development of advanced civilizations people have ruthlessly exploited nature – but it was "wild" nature (as the rain forest appears to gold diggers and land seekers as they burn it down) and not their own land, worked on by themselves or undisturbed land offered by God's creation – and they had no idea of the devastating consequences (Weeber, 1990; and Ringhofer, 1988).

In any case, traditional family structures are disintegrating worldwide, and this process of erosion has not stopped with the nuclear family of parents and young children. Sociological research shows again and again that under the pressures of individualization couple relationships are losing their character as an institution intended to last long – even for life – and marked by sharing an *oikos*, a *home* (Beck / Beck-Gernsheim, 1995). Instead, a multitude of different arrangements with very different degrees of stability and commonality seems to prevail, and children can expect less and less to be raised by both their natural parents. And yet most of us secretly believe that it is still possible to achieve an ultimately satisfying relationship and so we keep on seeking it. A kind of serial monogamy is the rule, but psychically we are not geared towards coping with this change, and many people suffer from the threat of separation or from one that is actually taking place.

Similar conditions prevail in the other central component of human life: work. Most biographies show significant breaks in the continuity of their work-life aspect, and this trend will strengthen in the future. Public institutions like schools, career counselling services and pension insurances often still reflect an impression of continuity in working life, something which in fact no longer tallies with the actual conditions of production. Instead, what matters today is professional flexibility, a readiness to be mobile, imaginative and above all ready for life-long learning. In the best-case scenario, a working person can expect to have a career lasting about 45 years, achieving its high point twenty years before reaching pensionable age. As soon as we recognize this situation, a new restlessness is triggered; renewed searching; a midlife crisis. In the worst case, a person loses their job after ten years and is forced to relocate and re-train. But still the hope for achieving a goal, a state of having "accomplished it" lives eternal; hope for a situation where the deepest desires are fulfilled, where one would finally be able to lean back with ease – and here, too, the greater the hope, the greater the disappointment.

On average we now live longer and have more time than ever before in history (Imhof, 1988). And yet subjectively, nobody has any time – apparently for two reasons. Firstly, because most of us want to be somewhere else most of the time, want to do something different, want to be somebody different than where and who we happen to be just now; and secondly, this experience arises from the immense acceleration in the rate of change in our lives. But both these phenomena are interdependent: our endless search for self-fulfilment powers the flow of industrial production as well as our social life to the point where this acceleration of action sequences becomes self-generating and a property of the social sub-systems of which it is part. From that point onward, developments become more and more removed from our needs – to the point that it becomes obvious how vain are our hopes for attaining identity or restfulness. At this moment in time the pervasive goal and growth orientation of our lives and of our society becomes questionable – hollow.

Gestalt therapy therefore rightly insists on an uncompromising concentration on the here-and-now of sensory experience. It is the experience and sensory perception of this specific present alone which liberates us from the pressure of time and opens up the creative treasures of existence. Only through such processes does it seem possible to return to ourselves – not in contemplative seclusion, but – as a self forever waxing and waning in perennial contacting processes – with sensual awareness.

4 The uncertainty of the future and the certainty of death

Planning and provision for the future have gained in importance as economic and social action chains have become longer, and people have become more closely interconnected – while at the same time, the past as a source of legitimacy and a treasure house of experience has become significantly devalued. This shift in emphasis from the past to the future is a marker of the process of modernization. Now, though, we find that a paradoxical situation has arisen: the more important the future is for us, the more confusing is the picture we make of it: the more we plan, the more frequently unexpected things happen.

In fact, we are now dealing not with one future but with many futures. All kinds of developmental processes are being projected into the future by arithmetical or geometrical models. So now there is a future of population growth – soon nobody will be able to be on their own anywhere. Or a future of the car – soon every family in China will have one, yet the promise of more autonomy through individual choice of mobility will be lost in automatic traffic with self-driving cars. Or the future of tourism – soon, ever more hordes of people will be directed to highly organized hot spots of overcrowded cultural highlights or, according to taste, to covered-over tropical paradises with artificial climate regulation. Or a future of water supply – everywhere deserts are growing, and drinking water is becoming scarce. Or a future of medicine – more and more the human body will consist of artificial organs, tissues and fluids. Or the future of flora and fauna – increasingly, we will encounter living beings who owe their existence to human activity in laboratories. Many of our decisions and our behaviour will be governed and controlled by artificial intelligence working with algorithms in anonymous computers.

Everybody can perpetuate this list according to their specific area of information and experience.

Some futures only have local significance. Others seem mutually exclusive. These developmental tendencies are interconnected in a manner so deeply complicated that it is impossible to establish anything with certainty. Even when considered on a fairly long-term basis, some developments have shown a rather absurd continuity as far as their numerical development is concerned. For instance, the fact that the number of scientists working worldwide has for the last two hundred years (!) doubled every fifteen years (Price, 1975), we still don't know when and according to what influences such exponential growth curves enter into a critical phase (i.e. when they grow indefinitely in zero time which is of course impossible and leads into a crisis the nature of which we cannot anticipate) and what happens then. Slowly we begin to understand that it is impossible to predict the evolution of complex systems, because their course is decisively influenced by singular events, often marked by a high degree of improbability, and their feedback loops and interconnections with people are incalculable, because human emotions (i.e. the human brain) seem unfathomable – see the US election of President Trump or the UK's vote for Brexit. Of course, nobody of serious scientific stature predicted the terrorist acts of 9/11 and its enormous consequences. Also, quantitative developments – which we do know – can turn into qualitative ones, generating those differences which alter cases. Many indigenous people considered that the largest part of their tribe always consisted of those who had died and those still unborn; those that were alive were somehow nothing but the tip of the iceberg making up the whole of the tribe – a beautiful concept. Now though, the earth's population is greater than the sum of all those who have died in the course of human history. The future remains uncertain, and hugely alarming.

In contrast, a new kind of certainty is only gradually dawning on us – the certainty that it is not only single human beings but humanity itself that is mortal. This insight is rooted in a qualitative leap in the history of humanity whose witnesses we are. Humanity is about to enter a completely different phase of its development, marked by the following five facts:

1. Humanity as a species has become capable of self-annihilation since it is now possible for the entire planet to sink into a nuclear winter.
2. Through this realization, humanity has irreversibly become a whole. The development of our media of communication and of the means of transportation are necessary but not sufficient conditions for this development.
3. Human civilization can be extinguished simply by an accident of the nuclear war machine or through a series of civil nuclear accidents.
4. Simply by our way of life, we can destroy our own conditions for living and those of many other species. We are capable of making ourselves ill through the way we live and of perishing as a civilization in consequence of our human-made catastrophic changes to our climate.

5 Computer technology and gene technology are taking the first steps on a road at whose end – in the relatively near future – human beings may have found the capability of transcending themselves through biological and engineering technologies.

Nothing can better bring home to us the relationship between power and powerlessness than the possibility of taking our own lives. The power to inflict death on ourselves equals our powerlessness to revoke this deed. This fact may help us to sense that we are mortal, even without making a specific contribution to expedite this outcome.

Here I would like to pick up two connected threads. The first again originates with Robert Jay Lifton (1979). He drew attention to the fact that our human ability to destroy ourselves and our natural resources also affects what he calls our available resources of *immortality experiences* – the inner standards of meaning we attribute to our lives and our relationships which constantly form the background to our actions, even while normally they remain outside awareness. Lifton distinguished between five modes of historical experience people use to create a connection between themselves as individuals and the species:

1 Religious ideas of immortality, whether belief in resurrection or re-incarnation.
2 The thought of living on in one's own offspring as part of an endless chain of biological concatenations.
3 The thought of surviving in one's works; the idea that one's contribution to human culture, whilst not eternal, may constitute a slightly more enduring participation in the history of the species than one's own quickly passing life – *ars longa, vita brevis.*
4 The idea of living on in nature as a part of its elements and thus being part of the breeding ground of future generations.
5 The authentic mystical experience of time and death simultaneously disappearing, which Lifton calls "experiential transcendence".

The fact that humanity is now capable of collective suicide affects these experiential possibilities. How might we picture some kind of spiritual continuity on a planet whose conditions no longer allow any life except perhaps in some sort of microscopic form? If Lifton is right, then all our ideas of a hereafter – apart from the mystical one – are based on the physical continuity of our species and of our biosphere. In any case it is clear that in a culture where humanity is aware of its mortality, we cannot defer anything to the next generation – neither our own survival, nor unlived life chances nor unfulfilled desires. It is more than likely that our children will not have a better life. Instead, our children will pay for everything we are doing – and for what we fail to do – unless we and they succeed in developing a new quality of embodied mindfulness.

The other thought again is concerned with death's certainty. The capacity to commit suicide, in itself is not quite on a par with mortality; it just makes us think – for example, about time horizons. A highly sophisticated audience gathered in the Berlin *Wissenschafts-Kolleg* to hear Stanislaw Lem, the Polish philosopher and science fiction author, report with great seriousness and commitment on a problem concerning the whole solar system in the near future, including the earth – about which he was worried. It involved the fact that our solar system is located at the outer edge of one of the widely spreading spiral arms of our galaxy and – he presumed – we will soon be catapulted like the spark of a Catherine wheel into intergalactic space with dire consequences. After a while a lady interrupted him anxiously, asking when this event was likely to occur. "Oh, soon, very soon", he answered, "it is likely to happen in less than half a billion years!"

The Earth is 4.6 billion years old. That is 4600 million years. We cannot imagine such a number. Perhaps a comparison from an eco-fiction novel by Trevor Hoyle can help us here. Literally taking our breath away, he clarifies just how quickly our planet could run out of oxygen by imagining as an experiment the age of the earth in terms of *our* experience of time (Hoyle, 1983): Let's imagine that the earth just turned 46 years old. We know little about the first ten years; it must have been the time of God separating heaven and earth. The next twenty years were required for the earth's surface to calm down. Only in her forty-second year did the earth manifest primitive life forms, first as plants. The last year is well remembered. It is the year of the dinosaurs, even though they did not last for the whole year. How many species of animals and plants the earth has known during these last two years! Most of them have already disappeared. In her forty-sixth year, events occurred thick and fast: eight months ago, the first mammals appeared. In the middle of last week humans evolved from primates. But they soon had a hard time, since only last weekend, there was another ice age. Historical humans have been populating the earth for just the last four hours; only an hour ago they invented agriculture. The Industrial Revolution started a minute ago. During this one minute we have changed the earth to a massive extent, and perhaps in this very moment we have been as destructive as the impact of large meteors would be.

Measured on a cosmic scale, humanity is a tiny experiment as short as God blinking an eye. Nothing suggests that our species will last even as long as the dinosaurs – a few hundred million years, or just a few months in the course of our planet's forty-six years. Of course, here, too, we must differentiate between quantity and quality: the length of time is not the only differentiating factor. Here, too, nature may squander inconceivable amounts of time to hit the bull's eye once it had created consciousness. But the law of entropy applies to us, too: as a species, humans are unavoidably condemned to die out and we cannot exclude the fact that death may happen very soon due to our own carelessness. It is interesting that as I write of all people two *American* writers pleaded to give up our illusions to stop climate change, i.e. intellectuals living in the country whose last president denied the existence of anthropogenic climate change and whose culture, always generally noted for its optimism, produced "Silicon Valley" with its fantasies of technological solutions for all problems of humankind. Right or wrong, they are the first Western intellectuals (others have followed by now) with the courage to break through the fog of anxiety to confront our illusions: These are Nathaniel Rich with his book *Losing Earth* (Rich, 2019) and Jonathan Franzen, with his essay: *What if We Stopped Pretending?* (Franzen, 2019).

People who are deeply narcissistic, as adolescents naturally are, think of themselves as immortal or rather feel immortal right in the face of the obvious. Of course, they know about death, but this knowledge does not impact on them; it does not make a difference to them. But perhaps humanity is reaching the end of its own adolescence and slowly beginning to allow itself to be touched by its mortality. That is the *biographical* analogy. The analogy with the *contacting process* leads us to a different image; in its relationship with the environment, humanity perhaps stands at the beginning of the full contacting phase and that would really be the qualitative point of change. Interrupting the contacting process at this point we would be holding on to neurotic control needs called narcissism, which is based on the retroflection of melting, opening-up, surrendering to a healthy confluence with high degrees of energy and high measures of awareness. Can we learn something from this picture? Perhaps this is the place where the repressed *anima* is hidden; perhaps here is the place where – as we let go of all intentional, planned action sequences – we could begin to search for the female energy we are lacking in our relationship with nature and repressing in our society.

5 Flight into the trans-human realm and the misery of power

But *homo faber* has not yet reached the end. It is not just the environment we can change, but the human organism can be changed, too. When improvement of the environment hits its limits – even triggering developments which run counter to our intentions – then the question arises of why human beings do not simply adjust to their environment instead of subjecting the environment to their human needs and greeds. Should someone invent a new body for us, less demanding, tougher, more long-lasting? Or is it not true, that the difficulties in the relationship between humans and the environment are actually rooted in us human beings? Are we a flawed product of nature?

The human body in this view is characterized by deficits; we need to use our intellectual strengths to compensate for what we are lacking in instinctual security and adaptation to nature. This is an old anthropological idea – except that there is no natural niche in the environment for human beings to adapt to. It is also an age-old dream that our intelligence may not just help us to cope with our biological deficits by manipulating our environment – that is by working on nature – but that we may become able to undo these deficits themselves. It is the dream of the fountain of youth, of life everlasting, of human beings becoming creators of themselves.

Today humanity pursues the traces of this dream in two scientific-technical ways; a biological one and a mechanical one. At the biological frontier researchers are currently busy working on the most serious biological flaws through embryo-medical and stem cell biological technologies, hoping to eventually improve the physical substratum of our species as a whole. Medical research, of course, also includes pharmacology on which rests no small hope of human *enhancement*, as it is called today. At present, the peak of this development is the attempt to manipulate our emotions, and especially the feeling of love in the form of erotic attraction and even aversion (Young / Alexander, 2014). Here we are finally promised medical cures for love-sickness, vain longing, dying feelings between people married for a long time, fears of being unattractive – the whole enterprise geared not to relieving us from the emotional causes of impotence and frigidity, but to dealing with the symptoms. What a promised land we are entering! The connection of love with suffering and tragedy would finally become obsolete. But would the loss of all spontaneity be acceptable in the light of this paradise? I don't think so: it would be the denial of the end of an age-old pillar of human civilization (maybe even of the universe) – love as an emotion. Already sexuality in its function as the most intimate and very effective bond between two individuals is becoming undermined by the misuse of pharmaceuticals. The possibility and availability of means to manipulate the hormonal dimension of our *feelings* would be a disaster, even for sexuality.

The other frontier of "enhancement" research and development is concerned with constructing materials, machines and control instruments with which to actually replace or at least strengthen deficient organs. "In the light of the far-reaching progress we are expecting in synthetic chemistry, information theory and general systems theory", Stanislaw Lem already wrote in 1964 in his *Summa Technologia*:

> … the human body is going to be shown up as the most imperfect element of the world of the future. Human knowledge will outstrip the biological knowledge that has been accumulated in living organisms. Then plans, which now we consider ridiculous in the light of evolution's achievements, will be realized.
>
> (Lem, 1964:521)

Without doubt, such developmental orientations belong to the inventory of Western civilization, part of the essential nature of the European mind. Who would like to do without dental prostheses, contact lenses or pacemakers? Only when it comes to artificial intelligence do we feel a little queasy, but at the current stage of its development no problems have yet arisen which are essentially different from those that come up with other forms of extensive technology.

In the realm of biological interventions, we more quickly reach a limit where, on a moral level, problems cannot be resolved. Without doubt the huge growth in world population creates inconceivable suffering, directly in the form of hunger and persistent illness, indirectly by creating an ecological disaster. At the same time, our growing knowledge of the prenatal life of human beings makes any thought about abortion difficult to contemplate, even without considering religious dogma. Is it not just an impertinence to have to decide whether a child with a genetic disease should perhaps not be born in view of the amount of suffering for child and parents brought about by such a birth? But such dilemmas are coming up more and more frequently, and they are rooted in our own demiurgic essence. Here emotions run high and aggression abounds. It is "interesting," to use a "cool" expression, that pro-lifers have turned to violence, even murder in the States.

For in trying to improve our physical basis, using the means of instrumental reason, in the final analysis we humans do nothing but follow our instinct for self-preservation. The problem does not really lie in the attempt itself, but in the one-sided mechanistic understanding of nature with which this agenda is promoted. In the research practice of the natural sciences too, increasingly sinister questions arise with urgency. As we gradually learn more about the body's capacity to remember as far back as the pre-natal state – what kinds of psychological consequences may arise from in-vitro inseminations and other techniques of embryological interventions? At present, excessive belief in progress based on a mechanistically delimited understanding of nature is pitted against a somehow religiously inspired sanctification of nature – and there is no common language between these positions.

From a Gestalt therapeutic perspective however, we are mainly concerned with developing a mode of perception which is attentive, concentrated and entails all senses; a perception able to notice all aspects of the presenting situation in their interdependent entanglement. The point is to sense what we touch and to allow it to speak to our senses, before the touch becomes an intrusion. Of course, this does not disregard the fact that some interventions are necessary, but with sharpened perception they might be carried out with embodied mindfulness and empathy deriving from it and therefore also perhaps with other ways and means of establishing limits. From this perspective we are always concerned with a calm, relaxed concentration on our sensuous experience of the world as it is given to our bodies and particularly to our senses. This perspective assumes that only through contact with the senses do hidden interconnections become accessible to awareness, which we have to respect. For the history of the sciences teaches us that the more interconnections we decode, the more mysterious the overall interdependence which is revealed – so that it pays to accept the unknown more deeply and widely than we are currently doing.

The flight into the trans-human realm, into a fantasy of a biologically or technically essentially different form of physicality, thoughtlessly passes by the barely known and as yet unfathomed richness of our senses. For it isn't those prostheses for our senses – microscopes and telescopes and hearing aids – which truly improve our perceptual capacity. Our senses, however expanded and refined by prostheses, are always components of our cerebral being-in-the-world-in-just-this-way. It pays to pursue an understanding of our physical condition, of our evolved bodies, more deeply and widely than we do at present. We should pursue our sensory experience with embodied awareness before we should even begin to think about changing our physical nature, possibly changing it in its very essence. What makes some modern science limited as it spreads everywhere in a technically biased and foreshortened way, is the fact that it seems to always give priority to what is practicable as opposed to allowing space for nature's wonderful complexity, its mysterious constitution to rise into awareness The foremost place in this mysterious realm is occupied by our brain, this "Three-pound Universe" (Hooper / Teresi, 1986), of which our senses and emotions make up an essential part. And exactly here Lem commits a major anthropological error when implicitly he thinks about the brain without a body, an un-embodied brain. The brain thinks and feels with the body; an un-embodied brain is the product of bad science-fiction fantasy, anthropologically unthinkable due to the holistic nature of our organism and the process character of its being-in-environment. We are far removed from comprehending our one and only irreplaceable organ of understanding, but even where it has deficits we recognize its wonders.[4] This is true for all the particular senses: what hearing and seeing, touching and tasting actually mean for our reality construction we may best learn from those intrepid researchers who investigated their own loss of sensory input, who – even in the silence of their deafness, the darkness of their blindness – turned to these phenomena with a great deal of embodied awareness. In principle there is no objection against the undertaking of further developing the "auto-evaluative potency" of human beings (Lem). But even with all our demiurgic capabilities, we humans must always perceive ourselves as embedded in environments on which we existentially depend – indeed, they co-define us. We still know far too little about this interdependent relationship and cannot therefore afford to take action other than with the greatest caution and awareness – very slowly in any case – whenever we think we can improve something in the evolutionary process. It is far less important today to transform the world than to experience it with all our senses – in leisure and with love.

Finally, there is the question of why we have so intransigently declared war on our mortality, even as we know that death will conquer all anyway. It is almost as if we had begun to hate whatever is organic because it is transient. But even in that hate we are still tied to our senses, since it is only through our capacity for sensory perception in human time-span parameters that the transience of organic matter has a special status compared to the transience of inorganic life forms. We just might eventually learn to experience even weakness, decay, dying and disappearing with embodied mindfulness – with appreciation.

The German philosopher and theologian Christopher Quarch summarized in a wonderful way what we are concerned with here,

> Profound humanity – as we can learn from the (old) Greeks – is fed by knowledge about our mortality. To acknowledge this, embrace it with love and to celebrate life – in the knowledge of its unavoidable end – in all its facets as a play – that still has to be the appropriate program for a conscious humanity. Simply to be a human being, this also means not to have to be God, not immortal, not limitless. The expansion of the limits set to human beings as promoted by contemporary trans-humanists and apostles of Human Enhancement like Ray Kurzweil, from a Greek perspective is nothing but hubris, an assault on humanity. Considered in the light of day, trans-humanism is the end of humanity. Deeper humanity will not unfold through technical optimization but will emerge from celebrating our mortality.
>
> (Quarch, 2014)

Those life-denying efforts that go into not wanting to die – so characteristic for our culture – are a consequence of our society demanding autonomy from its individual members even while it increasingly denies autonomy to its collective membership. In consequence, the modern character experiences a deep fear of letting go, of surrender, letting itself fall into full contact – as if when the other acknowledges and touches me I was losing myself; as if I was delivered into the other's power. The *desire for power* is only the other side of fearing powerlessness; loss of individual autonomy. At this point we should ask a question we usually avoid: What is the relationship of power and identity? For it seems as if a stable and secure sense of Ego-identity depended on an oppressive relationship with one's own self and one's environment, apparently dependent on self-control and world domination. The price for this false security is life itself: the feeling of aliveness, and the experience of being enriched. The more we cultivate our ability for embodied mindfulness the less the ever-new processes of self-unfolding-in-contact need to use the crutches of power and identity.

Notes

1 For James Lovelock's Gaia hypothesis, see Lovelock (2000; 2006); also compare Durrell (1986). The best recent summary of the climate catastrophe I know of was for some time: Jorgen Randers' *2052 – A Global Forecast for the next Forty Years*

(2012). But since then the new IPCC (International Panel of Climate Change) report by the UN was published in October 2019 showing that climate change progresses much faster than scientists had been able to forecast in the decades before (www.ipcc.ch).

2 I am not speaking here of the German "Angst", which is a more existential feeling related to melancholia. Compare: Anna Wierzbicka's fascinating book *Emotions across Languages and Cultures* (1999), with a special case study on "German Angst".

3 The unexpected consequences of planned action have been a well-known topic for a long time in the social sciences. Compare Robert K. Merton's classic text *Manifest and latent functions* (Merton, 1957); also compare Dreitzel / Stenger, 1990.

4 Compare the amazing case histories which the neurologist Oliver Sacks reports in his books. See for instance Sacks (1985; 1984). In these books he clearly shows – as Freud said – that even in adults the Ego is first and foremost a bodily Ego.

Chapter VII

Epilogue

Gestalt therapy of environmental destruction

Let us face it: there is no denying any more that climate change is not a future scenario but is a reality here and now; it is worldwide, it is at once measurable and unpredictable in its details, it will bring unimaginable misery to a large number of human beings living now and to be born in future – and it is human-made!

How much of the environmental catastrophe enters our daily working life? What role does the threat to our world play in our therapies? I suspect very little. Silently, the threat remains in the background, but the concerns of one's life take up the foreground, that has been conquered by the sudden advent of the Covid-19 pandemic, as well as the fear of its terrible economic consequences, giving many politicians an excuse to deny it. Yet the dragon is dormant at best. And everybody knows it. Just before the coronavirus hit us, there was a brief moment, when climate issues seemed to come more to the foreground of public and political attention. But the newly elected Donald Trump lost little time in taking the United States out of the Paris Agreement and adjusting his policies accordingly. Only in the very last years as unusual weather patterns worldwide have drawn increasingly the attention of a larger public does climate change seem to be coming slowly into the foreground of media reports and worries of politicians. Now the debate follows simultaneously two paths: one is a growing debate about how each of us could contribute to minimize the so called individual "ecological footprint" we leave by producing the CO_2 that causes climate change simply by our lifestyle – currently 20 tons in the United States and 10 tons in Germany according to J. S. Foer, whose new book, full of valuable and well researched facts, also describes how very difficult he discovered to be his own attempts in this direction (Foer, 2019).

The other path is focused on the question of how we could survive what is already going on, mostly by looking for technological solutions. But one of the principles of Gestalt therapy is that the shackles limiting our clients' ability to form appropriate Gestalts should always be looked for in the *background*, and it is the therapist's task to bring this disturbed background into the foreground! The question is how? For we may safely assume that for most of our clients climate change still rests in the background of their awareness where it is blocked by feelings of helplessness, resignation and anxiety. Thus these feelings have to be brought into the foreground there to be changed into fear of concrete dangers, rage against the passivity of most industrials and politicians, and as a result motivation for action.

For only on rare occasions – and mostly in unexpected ways – does this background anxiety become topical. In Europe, for two or three months after an explosion in a nuclear processing plant at Chernobyl in Russia the situation was – briefly – different; everybody tended to react by amplifying their most familiar neurotic patterns. Depressives became even more downcast, hysterics even more hectic and schizoids even more absent. And everybody felt vindicated. I will never forget the undisguised pleasure of a client, who as a pastor had been active in the peace movement for some twenty years: now, finally his colleagues in the church would wake up – catastrophe as a learning experience (Chu, 1991). In contrast, the more recent destruction of the nuclear plant at Fukushima in Japan did not shock as deeply, probably because it was geographically too far away. The German Chancellor was exceptional in that, to everybody's surprise, she was motivated to make a complete about-turn in her energy policy by deciding to shut off all German nuclear power. But by now even she has come back to "business as usual". For the moment only the children of the movement "Fridays for Future" in their astonishing alliance with thousands of scientists worldwide seem to be seriously concerned – a fabulous coalition of motivating fear with concerned rational thought! How serious the reality of climate change and other forms of pollution today is might be learned from some recent literature (United Nations, 2019 / Wallace-Wells, 2019 / Rich, 2019 / Foer 2019; Scheffler, 2013).

From the range of Gestalt therapeutic ideas of growth, and those of similar approaches, I will distil five tenets which might help to orient our therapeutic actions in the context of ongoing environmental destruction and politically endangered democracy:

First tenet: Anxiety must turn into fear – Getting ready for action

I have been making it clear that the concatenation of introjected affect controls and – in conjunction with a sense of how enormous the threat to our situation has become – the lack of transparency in our living conditions is leading to a paralysis of our ability to act, which in turn generates massive anxiety. We defend ourselves against this kind of anxiety by using various methods of anaesthetising ourselves and also through selective inattention. Our first task is to allow this anxiety to surface. The pathway towards that goal is to interrupt – again and again – our chronic and most favourite forms of self-anaesthetising, and at the same time look at what happens with full attention and awareness. The resultant anxiety will have to be borne for a while since, when no longer defended against, it turns very quickly into fear which motivates action against any actual threat. Soon we don't hold our breath any longer; soon we give vent to our emotions; sometimes we shout. It helps to have company: for a time, we will have to become a self-help group of anxiety-ridden human beings. As soon as we are free again and able to breathe in agitation, paralysis dissolves all by itself, except that now *there is no refuge anywhere;* menace is everywhere. And then all energies flow into wanting to act.

Gestalt therapy teaches that the resulting liberation of our aggressive potential, possibly by reactivating our capacity for de-structuring the presenting Gestalts and for removing the obstacles we encounter, is of crucial importance for ensuring that the contacting process succeeds. Courage under threat requires the liberation of rage from the prisons of our self-control. But not the blind rage of wildly hitting the nearest pillow (or person) or of hectic activity: rather the clear-sighted rage of initiative arising from the connection between our readiness to face conflicts and our awareness. Exactly where each person finds their field of action at this point is not necessarily the concern of therapy, although feedback and dialogue about these matters are important. The core task of therapy is to liberate energy and to increase awareness. Both together transform that vague anxiety of being lost in the dark into a specific fear of a concrete threat. Once the danger has been identified and flight made impossible, only struggle remains. By necessity, readiness to act on environmental concerns entails willingness to engage in conflict. Energy flows into the argument and the argument in turn energizes.

Second tenet: Emotional sensibility instead of environmental morality – motivating resistance

As well as a lot which does need doing, it is equally important to desist from doing certain things. Yet from where do we draw the necessary kind of readiness? Readiness to stop throwing things away while living in a throw-away society; to reduce driving in an automobile society; to use less water and cleaning materials in a society which suffers from delusional addiction to cleanliness; to insulate our roofs and windows while oil is still plentiful. Why choose cross-country skiing when down-hill skiing is affordable for almost everybody? Why always bring your own shopping bag when plastic bags are so convenient? We find renunciation difficult because it demands that we give up so much hard-won freedom, so much only recently achieved pleasure – and also: renunciation costs time, planning and care which in turn increase stress. And to crown it all there is the persistent sense that a single person cannot do much about these problems anyway.

An unfathomable chasm seems to exist between one's own actions and the impending world-wide catastrophe. We are morally over-taxed.

> In order to incarnate the new imperatives of the ecological Mega-Super-ego, we need the emergence of moral mutants, paranoid people of the third order who can say: "I am one with Terra, and the ozone hole hurts me personally"
>
> (Sloterdijk, 1990:722)

There is indeed no lack of exhortation. By now it is publicly and legally sanctioned that fingers are raised about the environmental catastrophe in the media, and philosophers have begun to talk about an ethics of responsibility. Everybody demands a new environmental morality.

Now we have to remember that it was one of Perls & Goodman's most important insights that the Super-ego is not a necessary psychic element of the mature personality, but a conglomeration of unassimilated introjects. Introjected rules of behaviour are perennially violated, because they restrict and interfere with needs which cannot be suppressed. However strong the "top dog", its efforts are always going to be sabotaged by the "underdog". Unassimilated behavioural norms do nothing but guide our creative energies towards developing innovative strategies for reaching the forbidden fruit. Gestalt therapy has taught that there is another way: morality is a question of awareness, and within this realm we need to particularly focus on the issue of emotional sensitivity. From the sociology of the relationship between friend and foe we are familiar with the phenomenon that enmity between people presupposes a significant degree of ignorance of one another. The more we know about the other, experience the other, the more we discover interesting things about each other, enmity lessens; in order to maintain enmity, we must keep each other at a distance. And how salutary that the wonderful experience we create in therapeutic work reveals many loveable aspects in clients who seem to be nothing but boring or even repellent at first. Such experience is created when people come close to each other in therapy and self-help groups.

It could be like that in our relations with our environment. People who eat with awareness taste more and need less. People who really love trees have a sense that a part of their own soul burns when a forest is burned down. And who is beyond reach of that kind of love who ever took the time to look closely at a tree, smell it, touch it, climb into its branches, rest in its shade, experience its seasonal changes? I realize this does not help re-settlers and landless farmers who are pushing ahead with their slash-and-burn practice in tropical forests, since for them the law of Berthold Brecht's Mackie Messer rules: "First, we must eat; morality comes after!" A hungry person cannot yet practice these levels of awareness. There are also environmental problems about which Gestalt therapy has nothing useful to say at this stage.

It isn't hungry people whose emotions are blunted to the wider implications of their survival actions who can make a difference: those who are sated have the real power to affect environmental issues. Therefore, we need to continue to develop new techniques of emotional sensitization and Sensory Awareness and spread it beyond the narrow therapeutic context. Of course, in no way are techniques of Sensory Awareness sufficient for what we seek – just as exercises in meditation are not yet the meditative position – but both are helpful. Unnecessary destruction and wasting of things towards which we have opened ourselves in meditative stillness is as impossible as doing harm to somebody we perceive in their actuality. And we are able to guide people towards such experiences; we can create such opportunities. We do not have to thank Aldous Huxley just for the horror vision of *Brave New World* but also for the most beautiful positive utopia of modern literature known to me. In his novel *Island* (Huxley, 1962), he describes a society where Sensory Awareness and emotional attentiveness have become standard in schools and the wider society. Here, it is important to note that such an attitude is not limited to reserves of quiet contemplation of nature in one's backyard. In fact, the point is that we must show the same kind of sensibility when we are in active relationship with nature, when we work on it, when we build on it, when we travel in it. And then we have yet to discover the Buddha of machines, an attitude towards the technical world marked by loving care rather than by wastefulness and resistance, which Albert Pirsig described in his novel *Zen and the Art of Motorcycle Maintenance* (Pirsig, 1974).

A last word concerning the issue of emotional sensitivity towards the environment: here we are not just concerned with liking but also with disliking. In view of the damage we cause with our lifestyle to the ecology of our planet part of the process of cultivating emotions is that we must also cultivate the *inhibiting emotions,* of *shame* and *disgust*. As I am writing this a new word is establishing itself in the German language: "Flugscham", meaning shame of flying, i.e. using airplanes for vacations and such pleasures. At first it was used ironically to mock the moral sensitivities of the prosperous part of the middle classes but now it has gained a serious moral undertone in the debates on climate change. Disgust would be a more serious reaction. Humans naturally experience two kinds of this extreme feeling of adversity: disgust for their own excrement and disgust for decay, especially rotting meat. This strong feeling has an obvious evolutionary function. Beyond that, disgust is culturally specific: some people are disgusted by the idea of eating dog meat, others by pork, and others again by any kind of meat. We need to work towards a culture where we find our refuse just as disgusting as our excrement, and where we are as embarrassed to be discovered with the one as with the other. Increasing levels of shame and embarrassment are at the heart of our civilizing process. But so far, they only relate to our bodies and our affects. Perhaps we actually do have to verbally express and hence to direct our attention to where the next levels of embarrassment should be focused – for example on our violence, or on how we pollute our world. But in the end our embarrassment and disgust must become our second nature to function automatically as civilizatory restraints. They must become a function of our senses, part of our awareness, not new external norms of moral behaviour.

Third tenet: A principle of assertive non-violence should be the rule for any form of resistance, since that is the only trustworthy expression of our concerns

Niklas Luhmann, founder of the systems theory school in sociology, offers a formulation which says that from the perspective of society both nature and human beings are environment (Luhmann, 1989). A lot can be learned from examining this perspective for a moment. First what we must clarify is that in recent times society has solved the environmental problem of "nature" through the market mechanism; it decides what and how much is taken from nature; what we work on and change, and how we deal with the residue – with slag and cinders – and with our rubbish. There is no other kind of mechanism of similar power and influence in sight – religious or aesthetic ones for example. And other market-limiting norms to contain it through alternative controls – for example, the demand to permit only reversible interventions in nature and only biodegradable products – offer important standards for the political discussion of threshold values but are not powerful enough to tame capitalism's self-serving inventiveness. Perhaps it is necessary to understand society as nature's environmental problem rather than the other way round!

And the other side of Luhmann's paradigm – people as an environmental problem of society? Here we can sense a hint of the merciless untouchability of system-theoretical abstractions, which does not mean they are wrong. And yet, it matters what we declare as our core interest, and what in consequence becomes peripheral – "environment". No sociological or psychological theory, however formal, is politically innocent. There is an increasing number of suggestions and experiments focused on adjusting human beings to climate change and not the other way round, aiming to revoke those climate changes which do not truly serve us and which we ourselves have brought about. In this instance, the formality of sociological systems theory unintentionally aids and abets crude capitalist interests.

Gestalt therapy is marked by its emphasis on the "I–Thou" relationship which originated with Martin Buber. In this perspective the other is no longer the object of desire and planning; of domination and management or, for that matter, psychotherapy, but a subject in its own right, a human being in its uniqueness, which may create surprising inspiration, whose advice and help I may need at some point in my life. I encounter a human being, to whose compassion I owe the halving of my burdens, and with whom I can share and thus increase my joy. We need this "Thou", this other, this companion on the road through anxiety to fear and through courage to action. Only through this detour via the other can we be sure of ourselves; this is why the principles of non-violence must be observed under all circumstances. After all, we pay for each oppression of others with self-oppression; each hurt inflicted on others becomes self-mutilation; each insincerity and deception of others we pay for with increased blindness about ourselves – the other is me in a different garment. It is important to mention this, not because the discrepancy between this insight and its realization in everyday life is so great, but rather because such an attitude is actually being realized from time to time – and the fact is that Gestalt therapy is a useful practice ground for this development. The core method of Gestalt therapy is doing experiments in self-awareness supported by empathy and accompanied by compassion, and its focus is on working through issues as they arise, in the dialogue between "I" and "Thou".

This method has proved its worth in therapy and can show its usefulness in other kinds of situations – as long as it specifically allows the other room for self-realization in valiant contention for the common cause, and as long as it is not misinterpreted as a suffocating exhortation to be nice to each other. In Buber's language, the "I–It" relationship must as often as possible become an "I–Thou" relationship.[1] We should remember that materially we are the main perpetrators of our environmental catastrophe, while the millions of poor people in the developing world – and at home – are the principal sufferers. Even with the best will in the world we cannot change this fact. And in this case too, morality does not help but rather damages; externally, it often leads to misguided aid programs, doing nothing but increasing dependency in the poor; internally it leads to (repressed) guilt feelings. Instead, we need the courage to enter into an exploration of what awareness of those others in their misery and in their otherness does to us. After all, how much can we bear? The answer depends on our political and psychological capacity to act, because only action relieves our sense of impotence. But beware that the emotions raised by populist rallies are not only under-distanced but provide an illusionary feeling of power if and when we delegate the real power of action to the leader they are cheering.

Fourth tenet: Paying attention not just to needs but also to satisfaction – never neglecting zest for life

In the reflections on the subject-object relationship we have seen how we can emphasize the object as well as the subject in the relationship between them. If we emphasize the object, we quickly get to the reality principle: resources are scarce and human beings are greedy – for this reason, we have to pay attention to economics and the law: a Mosaic perspective – Freud's perspective. Or we emphasize the position of the subject. Then we are dealing with drives, which are never quite satisfied: recognition we are still waiting for; hunger still unsatisfied. Wilhelm Reich, Alfred Adler, Fredrick Perls, the rebels of the psychoanalytic movement, shifted emphasis to the subject. And all other emancipatory movements position themselves in a similar way. Yet this is one-sided, unbalanced. We easily give in to such a one-sided search for our need satisfaction while overlooking the fact that learning to sense satisfaction is an equally important part of the id functions of the Self. There are always two sides to the contacting process: beginning and ending; approach and withdrawal; need and satisfaction; growing and passing; breathing in and breathing out. It seems to me that humanistic psychologists too have one-sidedly over-emphasized the growth aspect of this equation.

Yet we know only too well from our therapeutic work that disturbances can also arise at the stage of full contact, or rather at its beginning or even when it "threatens" to happen: the inability to let go; those half-satisfactions with hunger quickly returning; this excess, yet still wanting more. Of all illnesses, bulimia symbolizes most clearly our sick relationship with the environment, with its rapidly alternating gorging and throwing up; greed and aversion in endless repetition. What about other needs? Is there perhaps something similar to compulsive eating and its relation to hunger in other processes? Is there perhaps a television-bulimia, a travel-bulimia or even a relationship-bulimia? The problem of "too-much" does not just consist in the fact that through being sated we also become dulled, hunger subsequently returning even more quickly; but also in the amount of rubbish that is generated. Whoever eats more also produces more refuse. Humans are rubbish-producing beings – this should gradually become clear to everybody: refuse consists increasingly of stuff which cannot be reduced to its constituent materials. We are sending into the atmosphere by-products alien to that environment and, not easily bio-degradable, they create damaging reactions. Micro-plastic particles have now been detected even in the air we breathe. Nuclear waste retains its radioactivity longer than the whole of the known history of humanity. And there are not only material kinds of rubbish. For example, we live in an unbelievably noise-polluted world. If it is true that the ear is the entry gate of the soul, just as the eye is its mirror, then our souls have been in hell for a long time. And that the psyche is polluted too is known to many therapists from their daily work. All introjects are psychic rubbish, and perhaps it is part of our work to name the perpetrators.

People swallow something because they are lacking something. From where does this endless hunger and longing come in a society which has so much? This question is of paramount importance if we want to come to terms with our relationship to our environment; it is worth the effort to follow it alone and with others in careful self-inquiry. My guess is that it will turn out to be devoid of meaning. I think it is possible that in the final analysis we are ruining our world through a vain search for meaning. This search has to remain futile as long as it is directed towards aims, circumstances, results, truths – towards something final. Let's remember the teaching of the Tao – *the path is the aim*. But this sentence has to be experienced *sensuously,* as self-evident: otherwise it remains a meaningless aphorism. And this entails a very great deal: it might entail relinquishing what by now is the world-dominating European spirit; renouncing aims; renouncing what we assume to be the meaning of history. It means that we must invent and discover and spread possibilities of sensuously experiencing the riches and depth of the way, of the movement. Novelist Sven Nadolny points towards one means: he recommends the *Discovery of Slowness* (Nadolny, 2003). Anybody who ever practiced Tai Chi or Kum Nye would agree with him.

Fifth Tenet: It is not nature which heals but awareness – developing embodied mindfulness is the path

Since we replaced God with nature, the idea has spread that nature is good; even that healing is achieved through it. This is a thought from the Age of Enlightenment, further developed in the Romantic Movement, and one cannot help noticing that nature has since been equipped with the classical attributes of God: omnipotence, wisdom, goodness, beauty. Before this point, things were different; nature was alien and dangerous; mountains unfathomable; the sea treacherous and the darkness of night definitely anxiety-provoking. Of course, this change in how we experience nature is owed not to God's tiredness but to our own busy restlessness; only cultivated nature is "good" nature; only countless new safety mechanisms allow us to look calmly at the sublime. In fact, nature is not healing; it is not true that as the title (not his own!) of the essays by Paul Goodman promises "Nature Heals".[2] Instead, having a respectful attitude towards nature could, perhaps, have a healing effect. It is a naïve and sometimes dangerous illusion to confuse untouched nature with the Garden of Eden. People irredeemably exist in a complex and broken relationship with nature. We are never quite at home; must always build a shelter first. Always we must work on nature, reshape, and change things in order to have a chance of survival. The relationship between our organism and its environment is never an innocent one. It is true, there have been indigenous peoples who for a long time in certain ecological niches managed to live in relative balance with their natural environment. But they also paid a price for this, which we should examine closely: less than half of our life expectancy for example, and certainly not living in peace with their neighbours. The method to keep their population constant was mostly so-called female infanticide, killing many female children. Supernumerary men could still hunt, as well as going without a sexual life if required.

It is not nature that heals, but *awareness*: this is our uniquely human potential. There is no such thing as original harmony with nature and we will continue to work on her, to reshape her in future. I also do not believe that this is a question of securing ethical boundaries or even the preservation of

God's creation, and I say that knowing that we are about to make hugely significant steps with gene technology and the new embryology as well as with the development of artificial intelligence. But there is no way in which we can randomly establish *quantitative* limits to growth and to our hunger for increasing knowledge. What counts is the *quality* of our conditions, our products, our relationships; it is the "when" and "where" and above all the "how" of our actions that matters. A beautifully esoteric insight formulates it thus: "God sleeps in the stones, breathes in the plants, dreams in the animals, and tries to wake up in human beings." Perhaps human beings, a movement of God's eyelid, are His/Her eye opening. If so, then it is up to us to keep our still-sleepy eyes open. When we start thinking less in material terms than in terms of consciousness and awareness perhaps we will see that human beings are a transitional phase where waking either succeeds or fails. In any case, everything is moving now very fast indeed, and there is no longer time for being asleep.

Notes

1 Buber (1958). Compare: Judith Brown (1980) and Richard Hycner (1985).
2 Paul Goodman, *Nature Heals, The Psychological Essays of Paul Goodman*, ed. Taylor Stoehr (who created the title), (1977)

Illustrations

Figure

Tables

Bibliography

Adams, M. (2016). *In Praise of Profanity.* Oxford: Oxford University Press.

Adorno, T. W. (1964 / 1973). *The Jargon of Authenticity.* London: Routledge & Kegan Paul.

Adorno, T. W. (1966 / 2008). *Lectures on Negative Dialectics. Fragments of a Lecture Course 1965/1966*. Cambridge: Polity Press.

Adorno, T. W. / Frenkel-Brunswik, E. / Levinson, D. J. / Sanford, R. N. (1950). *The Authoritarian Personality.* New York: Harper and Brothers.

Albright, M. (2018). *Fascism – A Warning*. New York: HarperCollins.

Anders, G. (2002). *Die Antiquiertheit des Menschen. Bd. I: Über die Seele im Zeitalter der zweiten industriellen Revolution*. München: C. H. Beck.

Arendt, H. (1958 / 1998). *The Human Condition*. Chicago, IL: University of Chicago Press.

Bandler, R. / Grinder, J. (1979). *Frogs into Princes – Neuro-Linguistic Programming*. Boulder, CO: Real People Press.

Baten, J. (2016). *A History of Global Economy: 1500 to the Present*. Cambridge: Cambridge University Press.

Baudrillard, J.*et al.* (1989). *Philosophien der neuen Technologien*. Berlin: Merve Verlag.

Bauriedl, T. (1988). *Das Leben riskieren – Psychoanalytische Perspektiven des politischen Widerstands.* München: Piper.

Beck, U. / Beck-Gernsheim, E. (1995). *The Normal Chaos of Love.* Cambridge: Polity Press.

Bell, D. (1976). *The Coming of Post-Industrial Society: A Venture in Social Forecasting*. New York: Basic Books.

Benedict, R. (1946 / 1977). *The Chrysanthemum and the Sword: Patterns of Japanese culture.* London: Houghton Mifflin.

Berendt, J. E. (1983 / 1991). *The World is Sound*. Merrimac, MA: Destiny Books.

Bergen, B. K. (2016). *What the F: What Swearing Reveals About Our Language.* New York: Basic Books.

Berger, P. L. (1963). *Invitation to Sociology: A Humanistic Perspective.* New York: Doubleday.

Berger, P. L. (1969). Zur Soziologie kognitiver Minderheiten (The Sociology of Cognitive Minorities). In: *Dialog*, Jg. 2.

Berger, P. L. / Luckmann, T. (1966). *The Social Construction of Reality: A Treatise in the Sociology of Knowledge.* Garden City, NY: Anchor Books.

Bergmann, L. (1989). Auf Teufel komm raus. Zur Austreibung des Geburtsschmerzes. In: *Niemandsland, Zeitschrift zwischen den Kulturen* 4, 10/11.

Berkenbusch, G. (1985). *Zum Heulen: Kulturgeschichte unserer Tränen. (Crying – A Cultural History of our Tears)*. Berlin: Transit.

Berne, E. (1964). *Games People Play – The Basic Handbook of Transactional Analysis.* New York: Ballantine Books.

Bernstein, B. (1971). *Class, Codes and Control: Theoretical Studies Towards a Sociology of Language.* London: Routledge & Kegan Paul.

Blankertz, S. (1988). *Der kritische Pragmatismus Paul Goodmans. (The Critical Pragmatism of Paul Goodman): Zur politischen Bedeutung der Gestalttherapie.* Köln: EHP.

Blankertz, S. (1990). *Gestaltkritik: Paul Goodmans Sozialpathologie in Therapie und Schule.* Köln: EHP.

Bloch, E. (1954 / 1986). *The Principle of Hope.* Cambridge, MA: MIT Press.

Bloch, E. (1961). Naturrecht und menschliche Würde (Natural Law and Human Dignity). Frankfurt: Suhrkamp.

Boadella, D. (1973). *Wilhelm Reich – The Evolution of his Work.* Plymouth: Vision Press.

Breshgold, E. (1989). Resistance in Gestalt Therapy: An Historical Theoretical Perspective. In: *Gestalt Journal*, 12.

Brown, J. (1980). Buber & Gestalt. In: *Gestalt Journal*, 3.

Buber, M. (1958 / 1985). *I and Thou* (1939). 2nd edition. New York: Scribners.

Buytendijk, F. J. J. (1948). *Über den Schmerz.* Köln: Medizin Verlag Huber.

Buytendijk, F. J. J. (1962). *Pain: Its Modes and Functions.* Chicago, IL: Chicago University Press.

Cashdan, S. (1988). *Object Relations Therapy: Using the Relationship.* New York: W.W. Norton and Co.

Chance, M. R. A. (1980). An Ethological Assessment of Emotion. In: R. Plutchik / H. Kellerman (Eds.) *Theories of Emotion.* New York: Academic Press.

Chaney, A. (2017). *Runaway: Gregory Bateson, The Double Bind, and the Rise of Ecological Consciousness.* Chapel Hill, NC: University of North Carolina Press.

Chu, V. (1991). *Krisenzeit: Nach Tschernobyl: Meditationen eines Psychotherapeuten.* Köln: EHP.

Clark, A. (1982). Grief and Gestalt Therapy. In: *Gestalt Journal*, 5.

Clynes, M. (1976). *Sentics: The Touch of Emotions.* New York: Doubleday Press.

Clynes, M. (1980a). The Communication of Emotion: Theory of Sentics. In: R. Plutchik / H. Kellerman (Eds.) *Theories of Emotion.* New York: Academic Press.

Clynes, M. (1980b). *Sentic Newsletter.* Vol.2, No.1, March.

Corbin, A. (1988). *The Foul and the Fragrant: Odor and the French Social Imagination.* London: Harvard University Press.

Cramer, F. (1997). Leben. In: C. Wulf (Ed.) *Vom Menschen: Handbuch Historische Anthropologie.* Hamburg: Beltz

Crombag, H. / Merkelbach, H. (1996). *Missbrauch vergisst man nicht. (Abuse cannot be forgotten)*. München: Verlag Gesundheit.

Csikszentmihalyi, M. (1990). *Flow: The Psychology of Optimal Experience.* New York: Harper and Row.

Damasio, A. (1994 / 2005). *Descartes' Error: Emotion, Reason and the Human Brain.* London: Penguin Books.

Darwin, C. (1852 / 2008). *On the Origin of Species.* Oxford: Oxford University Press.

Darwin, C. (1872 / 2009). *The Expression of the Emotions in Man and Animals.* London: Penguin Books.

DelVecchio, M. / Brodwin, P. E. / Good, B. J. / Kleinman, A. (Eds.). (1992). *Pain as human experience.* Berkeley, CA: University of California Press.

Döbert, R. / Habermas, J. / Nunner-Winkler, G. (Eds.). (1977). *Entwicklung des Ichs.* Köln: Neue Wissenschaftliche Bibliothek.

Doster, J. A. / Nesbitt, J. G. (1979). Psychotherapy and Self-disclosure. In: G. J. Chelune. *Self-Disclosure: Origin, Patterns, and Implications of Openness in Interpersonal Relationships.* New York: American Psychological Association.

Dreitzel, P. (1963). Selbstbild und Gesellschaft (The Image of Self and Society). In: *Europäisches Archiv für Soziologie*, Vol.3.

Dreitzel, P. (Ed.) (1972). *Sozialer Wandel: Zivilisation und Fortschritt als Kategorien der Soziologischen Literatur (Social Change: Civilization and Progress as a Notion in Sociological Literature).* München: Luchterhand – Random House

Dreitzel, P. (1973). Arbeit und Sinnlichkeit: Zum Elend des Leistungsbegriffs. In: *Sinn und Unsinn des Leistungsprinzips.* Köln, München: Deutscher Taschenbuch-Verlag.

Dreitzel, P. (1980). *Die gesellschaftlichen Leiden und die Leiden an der Gesellschaft: Eine Pathologie des Alltagslebens (Social Roles - A Pathology of Everyday Life).* 3rd edition. Stuttgart: Ferdinand Enke Verlag.

Dreitzel, P. (1981). Körperkontrolle und Affektverdrängung. In: *Integrative Therapie*, Jg. 7.

Dreitzel, P. (1983a). Peinliche Situationen (Embarassing Situations). In: W. Eßbach / M. Baethge (Eds.): *Soziologie: Entdeckungen im Alltäglichen: Hans Paul Bahrdt: Festschrift zu seinem 65.* Frankfurt: Campus Verlag.

Dreitzel, P. (1983b). Der Körper als Medium der Kommunikation (The Body as a Medium of Communication). In: A. E. Imhoff (Ed.) *Der Mensch und sein Körper.* München: Springer.

Dreitzel, P. / Jaeggi, E. (1987). Psychotherapie: Plädoyer für kreative Vielfalt. In: *Psychologie Heute*, Jg. 14, H. 2.

Dreitzel, P. (1988). Zur Theorie und Genese narzisstischer Persönlichkeitsfunktionsstörungen. in: *Gestalttherapie*, Jg. 2, H. 2.

Dreitzel, P. (1991a). Sympathie und Empathie. In: G. Althaus / H. Berking / R. Thiessen (Eds.): *Avanti Dilettanti. Festschrift für Urs Jaeggi.* Berlin: Metropol.

Dreitzel, P. (1991b). Umweltgewahrsein. In: *Gestalttherapie*, Jg. 5, H. 1.

Dreitzel, P. (1992), *Reflexive Sinnlichekit.* Bergisch-Gladbach: EHP-Verlag.

Dreitzel, P. (2003). Soziologie der Angst (Sociological Aspects of Anxiety). In: F.-M. Staemmler / R. Merten (Eds.). *Angst als Ressource und Störung.* Paderborn: Junfermannsche Verlagsbuchhandlung.

Dreitzel, P. (2004 / 2010). *Gestalt and Process: Clinical Diagnosis in Gestalt Therapy: A Field Guide.* (Translation, from the German original). Bergisch Gladbach: EHP.

Dreitzel, P. (2018). *The Art of Living and the Joy of Life: Developing and Maturity in a Changing World.* Siracusa: Instituto Gestalt.

Dreitzel, P. (2019). The Sabotaging of Introjects: Thoughts about Processing Introjects in Gestalt Therapy in a Changing Culture. In: *Gestalt Today, Malta*. Vol. 3.

Dreitzel, P. / Stenger, H. (Eds.). (1990). *Ungewollte Selbstzerstörung: Reflexionen über den Umgang mit katastrophalen Entwicklungen, (Unintended Self Destruction: On the Management of Catastrophic Developments)*, Frankfurt: Campus Verlag.

Dreitzel, P. / Wilhelm, J. (1966). Über das Problem der Kreativität bei Wissenschaftlern. In: *Kölner Zeitschrift für Soziologie*, Bd. 18.

Duerr, H. P. (1987). *Dreamtime: Concerning the Boundary Between Wilderness and Civilization*. London: Blackwell.

Duerr, H. P. (2005). *Der Mythos vom Zivilisationsprozess*. Frankfurt: Suhrkamp.

Durrell, L. (1986) *State of the Ark: An Atlas of World Conservation in Action*. New York: Doubleday.

Ehlich, K. (1980). *Erzählen im Alltag: Herausgegeben von Konrad Ehlich*. Frankfurt: Suhrkamp.

Ekman, P. (1980). *The Face of Man: Expressions of Universal Emotions in a New Guinea Village*. New York / London: Garland STPM.

Ekman, P. / Friesen W. V. / Ellsworth, P. (1972). *Emotion in the Human Face: Guidelines for Research and a Review of Findings*. New York: American Psychological Association.

Elias, N. (1969a / 2000 / 2006]). *The Collected Works of Norbert Elias: The Court Society*. Dublin: University College Dublin Press.

Elias, N. (1969b /1994 / 2000). *The Civilizing Process, Sociogenetic and Psychogenetic Investigations*. Oxford: Basil Blackwell Ltd.

Elias, N. (1969c / 2013). *Studies on the Germans*. Dublin: University College Dublin Press.

Emrich, H. (1983). *Psychophysiologische Grundlagen der Psychiatrie und Psychosomatik: Bewusste und nicht bewusste Wahrnehmungen emotionaler Reize*. Stuttgart: Hogrefe.

Enzensberger, H. M. (1990). Vermutungen über die Turbulenz. In: P. Sloterdijk: *Von der Jahrtausendwende. Berichte zur Lage der Zukunft*. Bd. 1. Frankfurt: Suhrkamp.

Ernst, H. (1991). Leben statt Lifestyle. In: *Psychologie Heute*, Jg. 18, H. 6.

Flannery, T. (2005). *The Weather Makers: Our Changing Climate and what it means for Life on Earth*. London: Penguin Books.

Foer, J. S. (2019). *We Are the Weather: Saving the Planet Begins at Breakfast*. New York: Macmillan

Foucault, M. (1977). *Discipline and Punish: The Birth of the Prison*. New York: Random House.

Foucault, M. (1979). *The History of Sexuality*. Vol. 1–3. London: Vintage Books.

Francesetti, G. / Gecele, M. / Roubal, J. (Eds.) (2013). *Gestalt Therapy in Clinical Practice – From Psychopathology to the Aesthetics of Contact*. Milano: Istituto di Gestalt HCC.

Franzen, J. (2019). *What if we stopped pretending?* In: *The New Yorker*, 8th September 2019.

Freud, S. (1912 / 1999). *Totem and Taboo*. Hove: Psychology Press.

Freud, S. (1928 / 2002). *Civilization and its Discontents*. London: Penguin Books.

Friedman, M. (1977). *The Healing Dialogue in Psychotherapy*. New York: Jason Aronson Inc.

From, I. (1984). Reflections on Gestalt Therapy After Thirty-Two Years of Practice: A Requiem for Gestalt. In: *Gestalt Journal*, Vol. 7 (1).

Fuhr, R. / Gremmler-Fuhr, M. (1991) *Dialogische Beratung: Person, Beziehung, Ganzheit*. Köln: EHP.

Gebhardt, E. (1975). Identity is a Total Institution. In: *International Journal of Sociology* Vol. 5.

Geertz, C. (1973). *The Interpretation of Cultures: Selected Essays.* New York: Basic Books.

Gehlen, A. (1958 / 1988). *Man: His Nature and Place in the World.* New York: Columbia University Press.

Gerhards, J. (1988). *Soziologie der Emotionen: Fragestellungen, Systematik und Perspektiven.* Weinheim, München: Juventa.

Geyer, C. (2004). *Hirnforschung und Willensfreiheit: Zur Deutung der neuesten Experimente.* Frankfurt: Suhrkamp.

Gibson, J. T. / Haritos-Fatouros, M. (1986). Education of a Torturer. In: *Psychology Today.* Vol. 20.

Gleichmann, P. (1984). Die Verhäuslichung körperlicher Verrichtungen. In: P. Gleichmann / J. Goudsblom / H. Korte (Eds.), *Materialien zu Norbert Elias Theory of the Civilising Process.* Amsterdam: Sociologisch Tidschrift.

Gleichmann, P. / Goudsblom, J. / Korte, H. (Eds.) (1984) *Human Figurations: Essays for Norbert Elias.* Amsterdam: Sociologisch Tidschrift.

Gleichmann, P. / Goudsblom, J. / Korte, H. (Eds.) (1979) *Materialien zu Norbert Elias' Zivilisationstheorie.* Frankfurt: Gesellschaftliche Prozesse und induviduelle Praxis.

Goffman, E. (1961 / 1986). *Asylums: Essays on the Social Situation of Mental Patients and Other Inmates.* New York: Anchor Books.

Goffman, E. (1963) *Stigma Management: Notes on the Management of Spoiled Identity.* San Francisco: Touchstone.

Goffman, E. (1967). *Interaction Ritual: Essays on Face-to-Face Behaviour.* New York: Anchor Books.

Goffman, E. (1974 / 1986). *Frame Analysis.* Boston: Massachusetts Northeastern University Press.

Goleman, D. (1995). *Emotional Intelligence: Why It Can Matter More Than IQ.* New York: Bantam Books.

Goodman, P. (1977). *Nature Heals. The Psychological Essays of Paul Goodman.* (Ed. T. Stoehr). New York: Gestalt Journal Press.

Gouldner, A. (1960). The Norm of Reciprocity. In: *American Sociological Review,* Vol. 25.

Graumann, C.-F. (1966). Bewusstsein und Bewusstheit: Probleme und Befunde der psychologischen Bewusstseinsforschung. In W. Metzger / H. Erke (Eds.) *Handbuch der Psychologie,* Bd. 1, 1. Halbband. Göttingen: Hogrefe.

Gross, E. / Stone, G. P. (1964). Embarrassment and the Analysis of Role Requirements. In: *American Journal of Sociology,* Vol. 7.

Gross, S. J. (1985). *Of Foxes and Hen Houses – Licensing and the Health Professions.* London: Quorum Books.

Grunwald, M. (2017). *Homo Hapticus, Warum wir ohne Tastsinn nicht leben können.* München: Droemer HC.

Gurwitsch, A. (1957). Théorie du champ de la conscience. In: *Revue de Métaphysique et de Morale.* Vol. 63.

Gutiérrez, G. (1987). *On Job: God-Talk and the Suffering of the Innocent.* New York: Orbis Books.

Habermas, J. (1971). *Knowledge and Human Interest.* Boston: Beacon Press.

Hager, F. / Haberland, H. / Paris, R. (1973). *Soziologie und Linguistik.* Stuttgart: Metzler.

Hawthorne, N. (1850 / 1962). *The Scarlet Letter.* Durham, NC: Duke University Press.

Heinsohn, G. (1995). *Warum Auschwitz? (Why Auschwitz?)*. Hamburg: Rowohlt Tb.

Heller, A. (1980a / 2009). *A Theory of Feelings.* Plymouth: Lexington Books.

Heller, A. (1980b). *The Power of Shame: A Rational Perspective.* London: Routledge & Kegan Paul.

Hermann, H. G. (2017). *Im Moralapostulat: Die Geburt der westlichen Moral aus dem Geist der Reformation*. Lüdinghausen: Manuscriptum Publ.

Hess, E. (1975). *The Tell-Tale Eye: How Your Eyes Reveal Hidden Thoughts and Emotions.* New York: Wiley & Sons.

Hochschild, A. (1983 / 2003 / 2012). *Managed Heart: Commercialization of Human Feeling*. Berkeley, CA: The University of California Press.

Hoell, K. (2020). (Forthcoming) Friedlander's "Polarity-Principle", "Creative Indifference" and the "Revolution of Egoism": Their Impact on the Theory of Gestalt Therapy. In: *Gestalt Review.*

Hondrich, K. O. (1975). *Menschliche Bedürfnisse und soziale Steuerung*. Reinbek: VS Verlag für Sozialwissenschaften.

Honneth, A. / Joas, H. (1980). *Soziales Handeln und menschliche Natur (Social Action and Human Nature)*. Frankfurt: Campus Verlag.

Hooper, J. / Teresi, D. (1986). *The 3-Pound Universe.* Basingstoke: Macmillan.

Hörmann, H. (1964). Die Bedingungen für das Behalten, Vergessen und Erinnern. In W. Metzger / H. Erke (Eds.) *Handbuch der Psychologie*, Bd. 1 & 2. Göttingen: Hogrefe.

Hoyle, T. (1983). *The Last Gasp.* London: Sphere.

Huizinga, J. (1972). *The Autumn of the Middle Ages.* London: Pelican.

Hull, J. M. (1990). *Touching the Rock: An Experience of Blindness.* New York: SPCK.

Hultberg, P. (1987). Scham: Eine überschattete Emotion (Shame: A shadowed Emotion). In: *Analytische Psychologie*, Jg. 18.

Huxley, A. (1945a / 1976 / 1990). *The Perennial Philosophy.* New York: Harper Perennial.

Huxley, A. (1945b / 2013) *The Doors of Perception & Heaven and Hell.* Important Books.

Huxley, A. (1962). *Island.* New York: Harper & Brothers.

Hycner, R. (1985) Dialogical Gestalt therapy: An Initial Proposal. In: *Gestalt Journal*, Vol. 8.

Hycner, R. (1990) The I-Thou-Relationship and Gestalt Therapy. In: *Gestalt Journal*, Vol. 13.

Hycner, R. (1991) *Between Person & Person: Toward a Dialogical Psychotherapy.* Gouldsboro, ME: The Gestalt Journal Press.

lmhof, A. (1981) *Die gewonnenen Jahre: Von der Zunahme unserer Lebensspanne seit dreihundert Jahren, oder, von der Notwendigkeit einer neuen Einstellung zu Leben und Sterben*. München: Archiv für Sozialgeschichte.

lmhof, A. (1988) *Die Lebenszeit:Vom aufgeschobenen Tod und von der Kunst des Lebens.* München: C.H. Beck Verlag.

Izard, C. E. (1977). *Human Emotions.* New York: Springer.

Jacob, F. (1976 / 1993). *The Logic of Life.* Princeton, NJ: Princeton University Press.

Jacobs, L. (1989). Dialogue in Gestalt Theory and Therapy. In: *Gestalt Journal*, Vol. 12.

Jantsch, E. (1975). *Design for Evolution: Self-Organization and Planning in the Life of Human Systems.* New York: George Braziller.

Joas, H. (1980). *Praktische Intersubjektivität: Die Entwicklung des Werks von George Herbert Mead*. Frankfurt: Suhrkamp.

Jütte, R. (2004). *A History of the Senses: From Antiquity to Cyberspace*. New York, London: Polity Press.

Kamper, D. (1989) "Nature Morte": Mimesis des Schreckens. Über Körpertexte in Schriftbildern. In: D. Kamper / C. Wulf (Eds) *Transfigurationen des Körpers*. Berlin: Reimer.

Kahle, G. (1981). *Logik des Herzens: Die soziale Dimension der Gefühle*. Frankfurt: Suhrkamp.

Kandel, E. R. (2007). *In Search of Memory: The Emergence of a New Science of Mind*. New York: W. W. Norton & Company.

Kant, I. (1907 / 2006). *Anthropology from a Pragmatic Point of View*. Cambridge: Cambridge University Press.

Kelley, K. W. (Ed.), (1988). *The Home Planet*. New York: Da Capo Press.

Kelly, Jun Po D. (2014). *The Heart of Zen: Enlightenment, Emotional Maturity, and What It Really Takes for Spiritual Liberation*. Berkeley, CA: North Atlantic Books.

Kernberg, O. F. (1986). *Severe Personality Disorders: Psychotherapeutic Strategies*. London: Yale University Press.

Kierkegaard, S. (1983). *The Sickness unto Death*. Princeton, NJ: Princeton University Press.

Klaus, C. (1991). *Problemzonen: Eine empirische Studie über die "individuellen Körperpraktiken" in den Fitness-Studios*. Berlin: Soziologische Diplomarbeit, Freie Universität.

Kohut, H. (1971). *The Analysis of the Self: A Systematic Approach to the Psychoanalytic Treatment of Narcissistic Personality Disorders*. New York: International Universities Press.

Korte, H. (Ed.) (1990). *Gesellschaftliche Prozesse und individuelle Praxis: Bochumer Vorlesungen zu Norbert Elias' Zivilisationstheorie. (The Bochum Lectures on Norbert Elias' Theory of Civilization)*. Frankfurt: Suhrkamp.

Kübler-Ross, E. (1974). *Death: The Final Stage of Growth*. New York: Simon & Schuster/Touchstone.

Kuhn, M. H. (1973). Die Bezugsgruppe – neu überdacht. In: H. Steinert (Ed.) *Symbolische Interaktion*. Stuttgart: Klett-Cotta.

Lake, F. (1986 / 1997) *Clinical Theology - A Theological and Psychiatric Basis for Clinical Pastoral Care*. Lexington: Emeth Press

Latner, J. (1983). This is the Speed of Light: Field and Systems Theories in Gestalt Therapy. In: *Gestalt Journal*, Vol. 6.

Latner, J. (1984a). The Kingdoms of Experience. In: *Gestalt Journal*, Vol. 7.

Latner, J. (1984b). The Thresher of Time: On Love and Freedom in Gestalt Therapy. In: *Gestalt Journal*, Vol. 5.

Le Bon, G. (1885). *Psychology of the Masses*. Independently published.

Leidig, H. (Ed.) (2001). *Leidenschaften (Passions) – Symposion zum 65. Geburtstag von Hans Peter Dreitzel*. Berlin: Dissertation.de. Verlag im Internet.

Lem, S. (1964 / 2014). *Summa Technologiae*. Minneapolis, MN: University of Minnesota Press.

Lessing, G. E. (1901 / 1956). *Laocoon*. Oxford: Clarendon Press, English online: https://archive.org/details/jstor-20646767.

Lifton, R. J. (1968). Protean Man. In: *Partisan Review*, Vol. 35.

Lifton, R. J. (1979). *The Broken Connection: On Death and the Continuity of Life*. New York: Simon and Schuster,

Lifton, R. J. (1993). *The Protean Self: Human Resilience in an Age of Fragmentation*. New York: Basic Books.

Lorenz, K. (1980). *The Foundations of Ethology*. New York, Wien: Springer-Verlag.

Lovelock, J. (2000). *Gaia: A New Look at Life on Earth*. Oxford: Oxford University Press.

Lovelock, J. (2006). *Gaia: The Practical Science of Planetary Medicine*. London: Allan Lane / Penguin.

Luhmann, N. (1982 / 1998). *Love as Passion, The Codification of Intimacy*. Redwood City, CA: Stanford University Press.

Luhmann, N. (1989). *Ecological Communication*. Chicago, IL: University of Chicago Press.

Lumley, M. A.*et al.* (2012). Pain and Emotion – A Biopsychological Review of Recent Research. In: *Journal of Clinical Psychology*, Vol. 67.

Maaz, H.-J. (1990). *Der Gefühlsstau (Emotional Jam): Ein Psychogramm der DDR*. Berlin: Argon.

Macho, T. (1993). Die Umwertung der Schmerzen. In: P. Sloterdijk / T. H. Macho (Eds.) *Weltrevolution der Seele; Ein Lese- und Arbeitsbuch der Gnosis*. Zürich: Artemis & Winkler.

Maelicke, A. (Ed.) (1990). *Vom Reiz der Sinne*. Weinheim: Wiley-VCH.

Marcuse, H. (1955 / 1974). *Eros and Civilization*. Boston / Chicago: Beacon Press.

Marcuse, H. (1965). *One-Dimensional Man*. London: Routledge & Kegan Paul.

Marcuse, H. / Wolff, R. P. / Moore, B. (1965). *A Critique of Pure Tolerance*. Boston / Chicago: Beacon Press.

Margraf, J. / Schneider, S. (1990). *Panik: Angstanfälle und ihre Behandlung*. Berlin: Springer.

Markowitsch, H. J. / Welzer, H. (2009). *The Development of Autobiographical Memory*. New York: Psychology Press.

Maslow, A. (1954a / 1981). *Toward a Psychology of Being*. 3rd edition. New York: Wiley.

Maslow, A. (1954b / 1987). *Motivation and Personality*. 3rd edition. New York: Harper.

Mauss, M. (1966). *The Gift: Forms and Functions of Exchange in Archaic Societies*. London: Cohen and West.

McKibben, B. (1989). *The End of Nature*. New York: Random House.

Mead, G. H. (1934). *Mind, Self, and Society: From the Standpoint of a Social Behaviorist*. Chicago, IL: University of Chicago Press.

Merleau-Ponty, M. (1962 / 2012). *Phenomenology of Perception*. London, New York: Routledge.

Merton, R. K. (1957 / 1968). Manifest and latent functions. In: R. K. Merton, *Social theory and social structure*. revised edition. New York: The Free Press.

Metzinger, T. (2010). *The Ego-Tunnel: The Science of the Mind and the Myth of the Self*. New York: Basic Books.

Miller, A. (1978). *The Drama of the Gifted Child*. London: Virago Press.

Miller, M. V. (1980). Notes on art and symptoms. In: *Gestalt Journal*, Vol. 3.

Miller, M. V. (1987). Curiosity and its Vicissitudes. In: *Gestalt Journal*, Vol. 10.

Miller, M. V. (2019). From F. Perls *Psychopathology of Awareness*, an unfinished and unpublished manuscript with commentaries by contemporary gestalt-therapists. St Romain la Virvée: Exprimerie, Institut Francais de Gestalt-therapie.

Milz, H. (1991). *Ganzheitliche Medizin*. 2nd edition. Frankfurt: Athenäum Verlag.
Mitscherlich, A. (1969). *Society without a Father: A Contribution to Social Psychology.* New York: Harcourt, Brace and World.
Mitscherlich, A. & Mitscherlich, M. (1975). *The Inability to Mourn: Principles of Collective Behaviour.* New York: Grove Press.
Montagu, A. (1978). *Touching: The Human Significance of the Skin*. 2nd edition. New York / London: William Morrow.
Morris, D. (1977 / 2002). *Manwatching: A Field Guide to Human Behaviour.* Reprinted, as *Peoplewatching*. London: Vintage.
Morris, D. (1978). *Der Mensch mit dem wir leben*. München: Droemer-Knaur.
Morris, D. B. (1991). *The Culture of Pain*. Berkeley, CA: University of California Press.
Müller, B. (1988). Zur Theorie der Diagnostik narzisstischer Erlebens- und Verhaltensstrukturen. In: *Gestalttherapie*, Jg. 2, H. 2.
Müller, B. (1996) Isadore From's Contribution to the Therapy and Practice of Gestalt Therapy. In: *The Gestalt Journal* Vol. 4.
Müller-Lyer, F. C. (1914 / 2012). *Soziologie der Leiden*. München: Nabu Press.
Musil, R. (2017). *The Man without Qualities.* New York: Picador
Myers, N. (1984). *The Gaia Atlas of Planet Management*. London: Octopus Publishing Group.
Nadolny, S. (2003). *The Discovery of Slowness.* Edinburgh: Canongate Books.
Nietzsche, F. (1882 / 2010). *The Gay Science.* New York: Knopf Doubleday.
Nietzsche, F. (1883 / 1976). *Thus Spoke Zarathustra.* translated by W. Kaufmann, New York: Random House; Harmondsworth, Penguin Books.
Ornstein, R. / Thompson, R. F. (1984). *The Amazing Brain*. New York: Houghton Mifflin.
Peele, S. / Brodsky, A. (1975). *Love and Addiction*. New York: Taplinger Publications.
Perls, F. (1992). *Ego, Hunger and Aggression: A Revision of Freud's Theory and Method.* Gouldsboro, ME: The Gestalt Journal Press.
Perls, F. / Hefferline, R. F. / Goodman, P. (1951). *Gestalt Therapy, Excitement and Growth in the Human Personality.* Book One: *Mobilizing the Self*; Book Two: *Novelty, Excitement and Growth*. New edition. New York: Julian Press.
Perls *et al.* = Perls, F. / Hefferline, R. / Goodman, P. (1952). *Gestalt Therapy.* The latest edition came out in 1994, edited by Isadore From and Michael Vincent Miller, who also wrote a helpful new foreword. Gouldsboro, ME: The Gestalt Journal Press.
Perls, L. (1989). *Leben an der Grenze (Life at the border): Essays und Anmerkungen zur Gestalttherapie.* M. Sreckovic (Ed.). Köln: EHP.
Petzold, H. (1981). Das Hier-und-Jetzt-Prinzip und die Dimension der Zeit in der psychologischen Gruppenarbeit. In: C. H. Bachmann (Ed.) *Kritik der Gruppendynamik*. Frankfurt: Fischer TB.
Petzold, H. (1984). Vorüberlegungen und Konzepte zu einer integrative Persönlichkeitstheorie. In: *Integrative Therapie* 1–2, Jg. 10.
Piketty, T. (2014). *Capital in the Twenty-First Century.* Cambridge, MA: Harvard University Press.
Pinker, S. (2011). *The Better Angels of Our Nature: Why Violence has Declined.* New York: Viking Press.
Pinker, S. (2019). *Enlightenment Now: The Case for Reason, Science, Humanism and Progress.* New York: Penguin Books.

Pirsig, R. M. (1974). *Zen and the Art of Motorcycle Maintenance.* New York: Harper Torch.

Plessner, H. (1953). *Die Deutung des Mimischen Ausdrucks.* Bern: Zwischen Philosophie und Gesellschaft.

Plessner, H. (1956). Unmenschlichkeit. In: *Diesseits der Utopie.* Frankfurt: Suhrkamp.

Plessner, H. (1964). *Conditio Humana.* Frankfurt: Suhrkamp.

Plessner, H. (1970a) Anthropologie der Sinne. In: *Philosophische Anthropologie.* Frankfurt: Suhrkamp.

Plessner, H. (1970b). *Laughing and Crying: A Study of the Limits of Human Behavior.* Evanstone, IL: Northwestern University Press.

Plessner, H. (1979). *Philosophische Anthropologie.* Frankfurt: Suhrkamp.

Plutchik, R. / Kellerman, H. (Eds.) (1980). *Theories of Emotion.* New York: Academic Press.

Portele, G. (1989a). Gestalttherapie und Selbstorganisation. In: *Gestalttherapie,* Jg. 3, H. 1.

Portele, G. (1989b). *Autonomie, Macht, Liebe: Konsequenzen der Selbstreferentialitaet.* Frankfurt: Suhrkamp Verlag.

Pradines, M. (1934). *Philosophie de la sensation.* Paris: Editions Belin.

Price, D. de S. (1975). *Science since Babylon.* New Haven, CT: Yale University Press.

Quarch, C. (2014). *Der kleine Alltagsphilosoph.* Garmisch: Graefe und Unzer.

Randers, J. (2012). *2052: A Global Forecast for the Next Forty Years.* London: Chelsea Green Publishing / PGUK.

Rank, O. (1924 / 1999). *The Trauma of Birth.* London: Psychology Press.

Rank, O. (1929). *Wahrheit und Wirklichkeit.* Leipzig / Wien: Franz Deuticke.

Reckwitz, A. (2017). *The Society of Singularities: On the Structural Change of Modernity.* Frankfurt: Surkamp.

Reich, W. (1927 / 2009). *Die Funktion des Orgasmus.* Köln: Kiwi

Reich, W. (1933 / 2013), *The Mass Psychology of Fascism.* New York: Ferrar, Straus and Giroux.

Reich, W. (1945 / 1980). *Character Analysis.* Basingstoke: Macmillan.

Reinarz, J. (2014). *Past Scents: Historical Perspectives on Smell.* Champaign, IL: University of Illinois Press.

Rich, N. (2019) *Losing Earth: The Decade We Could Have Stopped Climate Change.* New York: Macmillan

Riesman, D. (1960 / 2001). *The Lonely Crowd: A Study of the Changing American Character.* London: Yale University Press.

Ringhofer, L. (1988). *Fishing, Foraging and Farming in the Bolivian Amazon.* Hamburg: C.H. Beck.

Robert, J. (2004). *A History of the Senses: From Antiquity to Cyberspace.* New York / London: Polity Press.

Robine, J.-M. (2016). *Self: A Polyphony of Contemporary Gestalt Therapists.* St. Romain de Vivrée: L'expremerie.

Rosenblatt, D. (1986 / 1999). *Türen öffnen: Was geschieht in der Gestalttherapie?*Köln: EHP.

Rosenfield, I. (1985). *The Brain for Beginners.* London / New York: Allan and Unwin.

Rosling, H. (2018). *Factfulness: Ten Reasons We're Wrong About the World – and Why Things Are Better Than You Think.* Flatiron, NY: Macmillan.

Sachsse, U. (1994). *Selbstverletzendes Verhalten.* Göttingen: Huber.

Sacks, O. (1985). *The Man Who Mistook His Wife for a Hat*. New York: Touchstone Books.

Sacks, O. (1984). *A Leg to Stand On*. Cambridge: Touchstone Books, Cambridge University Press.

Scarry, E. (1987 / 1992). *The Body in Pain: The Making and Unmaking of the World*. Oxford: Oxford University Press.

Scheff, T. (1997). *Emotions, the Social Bond, and Human Reality*. Cambridge: Cambridge University Press.

Scheff, T. (2007). Catharsis and other Heresies: A Theory of Emotion. In: *Journal of Social*. Vol. 1.

Scheffler, S. (2013). *Death and the Afterlife (The Berkeley Tanner Lectures)* (English edition). Oxford: Oxford University Press.

Scheler, M. (1923 / 1992). The Meaning of Suffering. In: *On Feeling, Knowing, and Valuing: Selected Writings*. Chicago, IL: University of Chicago Press.

Scheler, M. (1933). Über Scham und Schamgefühle. In: *Schriften aus dem Nachlass*, Bd. 1, Berlin.

Scheler, M. (1954 / 1970). *The Nature of Sympathy*. Hamden, CT: Archon Books.

Schröter, M. (1990). Scham im Zivilisationsprozess. In: H. Korte (Ed.) *Gesellschaftliche Prozesse und individuelle Praxis*. Frankfurt: Suhrkamp.

Schudson, M. (1984). Embarrassment and Erving Goffman's Idea of Human Nature. In: *Theory and Society*, Vol. 13, No. 5.

Schumann, R. / Stimmer, F. (1987). *Soziologie der Gefühle: Zur Rationalität und Emotionalität sozialen Handelns*. München: Sozialforschungsinstitute.

Searle, J. R. (2004). *Mind, A Brief Introduction* (Fundamentals of Philosophy). Oxford: Oxford University Press.

Seneca (1928). *Moral Essays* I. London: Harvard University Press (Loeb Classical Library).

Sennett, R. (2013). Respect: The Formation of Character in an Age of Inequality, In: *Berliner Debatte* Vol. 3.

Seyd, B. (2013) "How Does It Feel?": Zur sozial- und gefühlstheoretischen Problematik einer Frage. In: *Berliner Debatte* Vol. 3.

Seyd, B. (2016): "It's the End of the World as We Know It (and I feel fine)". Überlegungen zum Verhältnis von Affekt und Utopie. (Thoughts about the Relationship between Affect and Utopia). In: N. Eibisch*et al.* (Eds.) *Endspiele interdisziplinär: Zukunftsentwürfe zwischen Weltuntergang und Utopia*. Göttingen: Edition Ruprecht.

Sichtermann, B. (1986). *Femininity: The Politics of the Personal*. Minneapolis, MN: University of Minnesota Press.

Siglitz, J. E. (2010). *The Price of Inequality: How Today's Divided Society Endangers Our Future*. New York: W. W. Norton.

Simmel, G. (1911 / 2001). *Aufsätze und Abhandlungen 1909–1918*. Band I, *Die Ästhetik der Alpen*. in Gesamtausgabe, Band 12. Frankfurt: Suhrkamp.

Spagnuolo Lobb, M. (2015). The Body as a "Vehicle" of Our Being in the World. Somatic Experience in Gestalt Therapy. In: *British Gestalt Journal*, Vol. 24.

Sloterdijk, P. (1990). Nachwort: Etwas vor sich haben. In: *Von der Jahrtausendwende: Berichte zur Lage der Zukunft*. Bd. 2, Frankfurt: Suhrkamp.

Sloterdijk, P. (2009). *Du musst dein Leben ändern*. Frankfurt: Suhrkamp.

Strauss, E. (1980). *Phenomenological Psychology (Phenomenology, Background, Foreground & Influences)*. New York: Garland.

Strittmatter, K. (2018). *Die Neuerfindung der Diktatur (The New Invention of Dictatorship)*. München: Pieper.
Sturgeon, T. (1953 / 1986 / 2003). *More Than Human*. London: Gollancz.
Tobin, S. (1971). Saying goodbye in Gestalt Therapy. In: *Psychotherapy: Theory, Research and Practice*. Vol. 8.
Tobin, S. (1982). Self Disorders, Gestalt Therapy and Self Psychology. In: *Gestalt Journal*, Vol. 5.
Tomatis, A. A. (2005). *The Ear and the Voice*. Lanham, MD: Scarecrow Press.
Tulku, T. (1987). *Kum Nye Relaxation*. Berkeley, CA: Dharma Publications.
Tull, J. (2016). *Positive Thinking in a Dark Age: Essays on the Global Transition*. New Orleans, LA: Pums Negra.
United Nations (2019), *Global Climate Report 2019*, Internet.
Vincent, J.-D. (1990). *Biologie des Begehrens: Wie Gefühle entstehen. (The Biology of Instincts: How Emotions Function)*. Reinbek: Rowohlt.
Vollstedt, T. (2002). *The work of Alfred Lorenzer, An Introduction*. MSc theoretical psychoanalytic studies, online University Innsbruck. http://bidok.uibk.ac.at/library/schaffrik-lorenzer-work-e.html
von Matt, P. (1995). "Ai mir": Der Schrei und die Dichtung. In: *Merkur* Vol. 2.
von Thadden E. (2019). *Die berührungslose Gesellschaft*. München: C. H. Beck.
Wall, P. D. (1977). The Problem of Pain. In: R. Duncan / M. Weston-Smith (Eds.) *The Encyclopaedia of Ignorance*. Vol. 2, London: Pocket Books.
Wallace-Wells, D. (2019). *The Uninhabitable Earth: A Story of the Future*. New York: Penguin Books.
Watzlawick, P. / Bavelas, J. B. / Jackson, D. (1967 / 2011). *Pragmatics of Human Communication: A Study of Interactional Patterns, Pathologies and Paradoxes*. New York / London: W. W. Norton & Co.
Weber, M. (1968 / 2013). *Economy and Society*. Berkeley, CA: University of California Press.
Weeber, K.-W. (1990). *Smog über Attika: Umweltverhalten im Altertum*. Zürich / München: Artemis Verlag.
Weil, S. (1952 / 2002). *Gravity and Grace*. London: Routledge.
Weiszäcker, W. (1997). In: C. Wulf (Ed.) *Vom Menschen: Handbuch Historische Anthropologie*. Hamburg: Beltz.
White, R. K. (1988). The Stream of Thought, the Lifespace, Selective Inattention, and War. In: *Journal of Humanistic Psychology*, Vol. 8, No. 2.
Wierzbicka, A. (1999). *Emotions across Languages and Cultures: Diversity and Universals*. Cambridge: Cambridge University Press.
Wilkinson, R. G. (1996). *Unhealthy Societies: The Inflictions of Inequality*. London / New York: Routledge.
Wood, R. (Ed.) (1990). *Klima-Aktionsbuch: Was tun gegen Ozonloch und Treibhauseffekt?* Göttingen: Verlag Die Werkstatt.
Wouters, C. (2007). *Informalization: Manners and Emotions Since 1890*. London: Sage Publications.
Wright, D. (1991). *Deafness: An Autobiography*. London: Faber and Faber.
Wrong, D. H. (1961). The Oversocialized Conception of Man in Modern Sociology. In: *American Sociological Review*. Vol. 26.
Wulf, C. (Ed.) (1997). *Vom Menschen: Handbuch Historische Anthropologie (About Human Beings: Handbook of Historical Anthropology)*. Hamburg: Beltz.

Wulf, F. (1922). Über die Veränderung von Vorstellungen (Gedächtnis und Gestalt). In: K. Koffka (Ed.) *Beiträge zur Psychologie der Gestalt*. Psychologische Forschung1. Leipzig: Barth.

Yarbus, A. L. (1967). *Eye Movements and Vision*. New York: Plenum Press.

Yontef, G. (1979). Gestalt Therapy: Clinical Phenomenology. In: *Gestalt Journal*, Vol. 2.

Yontef, G. (1988). Assimilating Diagnostic and Psychoanalytic Perspectives into Gestalt Therapy. In: *Gestalt Journal*, Vol. 11.

Young, L. / Alexander, B. (2014). *The Chemistry between Us: Love, Sex and the Science of Attraction*. London: Penguin Books.

Young, M. / Willmott, P. (1975). *The Symmetrical Family*. London: Pelican Books.

Zuboff, S. (2018). *The Age of Surveillance Capitalism: The Fight for a Human Future at the New Frontier of Power*. London: Profile Books.

Index